Peptic Ulcer Disease

Guest Editor

FRANCIS K.L. CHAN, MD

GASTROENTEROLOGY
CLINICS OF NORTH AMERICA

www.gastro.theclinics.com

June 2009 • Volume 38 • Number 2

SAUNDERS an imprint of ELSEVIER, Inc.

W.B. SAUNDERS COMPANY

A Division of Elsevier Inc.

Elsevier Inc. • 1600 John F. Kennedy Blvd., Suite 1800 • Philadelphia, Pennsylvania 19103-2899
http://www.theclinics.com

GASTROENTEROLOGY CLINICS OF NORTH AMERICA Volume 38, Number 2
June 2009 ISSN 0889-8553, ISBN-13: 978-1-4377-0680-2, ISBN-10: 1-4377-0680-0

Editor: Kerry Holland
Developmental Editor: Donald Mumford

Gastroenterology Clinics of North America (ISSN 0889-8553) is published quarterly by Elsevier Inc., 360 Park Avenue South, New York, NY 10010-1710. Months of issue are March, June, September, and December. Business and Editorial Offices: 1600 John F. Kennedy Blvd., Suite 1800, Philadelphia, PA 19103-2899. Customer Service Office: 6277 Sea Harbor Drive, Orlando, FL 32887-4800. Periodicals postage paid at New York, NY and additional mailing offices. Subscription prices are $256.00 per year (US individuals), $131.00 per year (US students), $385.00 per year (US institutions), $282.00 per year (Canadian individuals), $469.00 per year (Canadian institutions), $355.00 per year (international individuals), $181.00 per year (international students), and $469.00 per year (international institutions). Foreign air speed delivery is included in all *Clinics* subscription prices. All prices are subject to change without notice. **POSTMASTER**: Send address changes to *Gastroenterology Clinics of North America*, Elsevier Periodicals Customer Service 11830 Westline Industrial Drive, St. Louis, MO 63146. **Customer Service: 1-800-654-2452 (US). From outside the United States, call 1-314-453-7041. Fax: 1-314-453-5170. E-mail: journalscustomerservice-usa@elsevier.com (for print support) or journalsonline support-usa@elsevier.com (for online support).**

Reprints. For copies of 100 or more, of articles in this publication, please contact the Commercial Reprints Department, Elsevier Inc., 360 Part Avenue South, New York, New York 10010-1710. Tel. (212) 633-3813, Fax: (212) 462-1935, e-mail: reprints@elsevier.com.

Gastroenterology Clinics of North America is also published in Italian by Il Pensiero Scientifico Editore, Rome, Italy; and in Portuguese by Interlivros Edicoes Ltda., Rua Commandante Coelho 1085, 21250 Cordovil, Rio de Janeiro, Brazil.

Gastroenterology Clinics of North America is covered in *MEDLINE/PubMed (Index Medicus), Excerpta Medica, Current Contents/Clinical Medicine, Science Citation Index, ISI/BIOMED,* and *BIOSIS.*

Printed and bound by CPI Group (UK) Ltd, Croydon, CR0 4YY

Transferred to Digital Print 2011

Contributors

GUEST EDITOR

FRANCIS K.L. CHAN, MD
Chief of Gastroenterology & Hepatology, Department of Medicine & Therapeutics, Prince of Wales Hospital, Chinese University of Hong Kong, Hong Kong, China

AUTHORS

TAUSEEF ALI, MD
Gastroenterology Fellow, Section of Digestive Diseases and Nutrition, University of Oklahoma Health Sciences Center, Oklahoma City, Oklahoma

FRANCES K.Y. CHEUNG, FRCS
Department of Surgery, Prince of Wales Hospital, Hong Kong, China

PHILIP W.Y. CHIU, MD
Associate Professor, Department of Surgery, Institute of Digestive Disease, Prince of Wales Hospital, The Chinese University of Hong Kong, Hong Kong, China

BYRON CRYER, MD
Department of Veterans Affairs Medical Center, Medical Service, Digestive Diseases, North Texas VA Medical Center; John C. Vanatta III Professor of Medicine, Department of Internal Medicine, University of Texas Southwestern Medical School, University of Texas Southwestern Medical School, Dallas, Texas

STEFANO FIORUCCI, MD
Dipartimento di Medicina Clinica e Sperimentale, Universitá; di Perugia, Via E. dal Pozzo, Perugia, Italy

RICHARD F. HARTY, MD
Professor Emeritus of Medicine, Section of Digestive Diseases and Nutrition, University of Oklahoma Health Sciences Center, Oklahoma City, Oklahoma

COLIN W. HOWDEN, MD
Professor of Medicine, Division of Gastroenterology, Department of Medicine, Northwestern University Feinberg School of Medicine, Chicago, Illinois

ANGEL LANAS, MD, DSc
Service of Digestive Diseases, University Hospital, University of Zaragoza, Instituto Aragonés de Ciencias de la Salud, CIBERehd, Zaragoza, Spain

JAMES Y.W. LAU, MD
Department of Surgery, Chinese University of Hong Kong, Hong Kong, China

RUPERT W. LEONG, MBBS, MD, FRACP
Director of Endoscopy, Gastroenterology and Liver Services, Sydney South West Area
Health Service, Concord and Bankstown-Lidcombe Hospitals; and Conjoint Associate
Professor of Medicine, The University of New South Wales, Bankstown-Lidcombe
Hospital, Sydney, Australia

GRIGORIOS I. LEONTIADIS, MD, PhD
Assistant Professor of Medicine, Division of Gastroenterology, Department of Medicine,
McMaster University Medical Centre, Hamilton, Ontario, Canada

KENNETH E.L. MCCOLL, MD, FMedSci, FRSE
Medical Sciences, Gardiner Institute, Western Infirmary, Glasgow, Scotland, United
Kingdom

LENA NAPOLITANO, MD, FACS, FCCP, FCCM
Professor of Surgery, Division Chief, Acute Care Surgery, [Trauma, Burn, Critical Care,
Emergency Surgery], Associate Chair, Department of Surgery, University of Michigan
Health System, University of Michigan School of Medicine, University Hospital, Ann Arbor,
Michigan

ENDERS K.W. NG, MD
Department of Surgery, Institute of Digestive Disease, Prince of Wales Hospital,
The Chinese University of Hong Kong, Honk Kong, China

JAMES M. SCHEIMAN, MD
Professor, Department of Internal Medicine, Division of Gastroenterology, University
of Michigan School of Medicine, University of Michigan Medical Center, Ann Arbor,
Michigan

FEDERICO SOPEÑA, MD, DSc
Service of Digestive Diseases, University Hospital, University of Zaragoza, Instituto
Aragonés de Ciencias de la Salud, CIBERehd, Zaragoza, Spain

Contents

> This article summarizes and appraises the evidence from randomized controlled trials (RCT) and meta-analyses of RCTs on the role of proton pump inhibitors (PPIs) in non-variceal upper gastrointestinal bleeding, with a specific emphasis on peptic ulcer bleeding. PPIs have an established role in the management of endoscopically documented peptic ulcer bleeding. PPIs, compared with H_2-receptor antagonists or placebo, consistently reduce re-bleeding rates. All-cause mortality is reduced in patients with high risk endoscopic signs and in Asian populations. The optimal dose and route of PPI administration in peptic ulcer bleeding has not yet been defined. The role of PPIs prior to endoscopy in patients presenting with non-variceal upper gastrointestinal bleeding is still somewhat controversial; PPIs reduce the proportion of patients with high risk endoscopic signs and may reduce the requirement for endoscopic hemostatic therapy at index endoscopy, but there is no demonstrable effect on mortality, re-bleeding or surgical interventions.

> Acute upper gastrointestinal (GI) hemorrhage is one of the commonest causes for hospitalization worldwide. Endoscopic therapy is effective in achieving primary hemostasis. The shift of management from the operating theater to the endoscopy suite has not changed the rate of mortality over the past 20 years. Several hypotheses are discussed that may account for the lack of improvement in the mortality resulting from bleeding peptic ulcer. One potential way to improve management is to identify those at risk for adverse outcomes, which may improve the initial triage, timing of primary endoscopic hemostasis, and postendoscopic management. Two adverse outcomes generally considered as significant for acute upper GI hemorrhage are rebleeding and mortality. Numerous clinical risk models have been developed to predict these outcomes, and this article reviews them.

> Managing massive bleeding from a peptic ulcer remains a challenge, and it should involve a multidisciplinary team. Endoscopy is the first-line treatment. Even with larger ulcers, endoscopic hemostasis can be achieved in the majority of cases. Surgery is clearly indicated in patients in whom arterial bleeding cannot be controlled at endoscopy. Angiographic embolization is an alternate option, particularly in those unfit for surgery. In selected

patients judged to belong to the high-risk group, a more aggressive post-endoscopy management is warranted. The role of early elective surgery or angiographic embolization in selected high-risk patients to forestall recurrent bleeding remains controversial.

Stress-ulcer bleeding in critically ill patients develops as a result of various risk factors, notably prolonged mechanical ventilation and coagulopathy. The incidence of clinically significant bleeding is decreasing secondary to widespread use of potent antisecretory medications and improved intensive care. This article describes the epidemiology, pathogenesis, risk factors, and management of stressrelated bleeding. The various prophylactic agents should be used judiciously to prevent unwanted drug side effects. Standard algorithms for critically ill patients are needed to identify those at high risk and to delineate criteria for the use of prophylactic therapeutic options in these patients.

Refractory peptic ulcer disease (PUD) manifests as either *hemorrhagic complications* (persistent or recurrent bleeding) or *gastrointestinal (GI) complications* (perforation, stricture, obstruction). Treatment strategies for hemorrhagic complications include Endoscopic therapy, surgery, and transcatheter angiographic embolization. Treatment strategies for GI complications include endoscopic dilation for stricture and surgery for perforation and obstruction. Potential etiologies of persistent or worsening PUD must be considered in these cases and include the following: patient risk factors and noncompliance, persistent *Helicobacter pylori* infection, and non–*H pylori*–related infection, related to underlying idiopathic gastric hypersecretion or Zollinger-Ellison syndrome and gastrinoma. An appropriate and meticulous diagnostic work-up for refractory PUD is mandatory.

Increasing use of antiplatelet therapies is associated with increasing GI complications, such as ulceration and GI bleeding. Identification of high-risk patients and, in such patients, incorporation of strategies to reduce their GI risk would be clinically prudent. After assessment and treatment of *H pylori* in patients with prior ulcer or GI bleeding histories, further reduction in GI risk in other high-risk patients who require antiplatelet agents is primarily accomplished by prescribing drugs that when coadministered with antiplatelet agents protect against mucosal ulceration, primarily proton pump inhibitors (PPIs). However, observational studies indicate a higher cardiovascular event rate in patients taking PPIs along with clopidogrel and aspirin compared with that of patients undergoing dual antiplatelet therapy without PPIs. Whether concurrent use of a PPI with clopidogrel represents a safety concern or not is currently being evaluated by the US Food and Drug Administration. Until more specific regulatory guidance is available, current recommendations are that patients taking both PPIs and clopidogrel concurrently should probably continue to do so until more data become available.

Balancing Risks and Benefits of COX-2 Selective Nonsteroidal Anti-Inflammatory Drugs

James M. Scheiman

The recognition that nonsteroidal anti-inflammatory drugs (NSAIDs) increase not only gastrointestinal (GI) but cardiovascular (CV) adverse events as well has created a dilemma for practicing physicians. Clinicians selecting appropriate NSAID therapy must estimate each patient's baseline risk for both (GI) and (CV) adverse events, and then estimate the impact of each medication (and its dose) for the individual patient. To synthesize a rational current treatment approach, we have developed a 2×2 table to guide NSAID medication choice, considering the use of concomitant aspirin as well as gastroprotective therapy. COX-2 inhibitors were an important scientific advance in pain therapy, and using them in a safe and cost-effective manner is possible when all the competing risks are carefully weighed.

Prevention of Nonsteroidal Anti-Inflammatory Drug-Induced Ulcer: Looking to the Future

Stefano Fiorucci

Nonsteroidal anti-inflammatory drugs (NSAIDs) are widely prescribed for treatment of pain and inflammation, despite their association with gastrointestinal complications, including bleeding and perforation. Inhibition of cyclooxygenases (COXs), is the main mechanism of action of aspirin and NSAIDs. Inhibition of COX-1 derived prostanoids in the stomach represent the underlying mechanism involved in development of gastric and duodenal ulcers in patients taking NSAIDs. Selective COX-2 inhibitors (coxibs) spare the gastrointestinal tract, but their use increases the risk of heart attack and stroke. In addition to prostanoids, two gaseous mediators, nitric oxide (NO) and hydrogen sulfide (H2S) exert protective effects in the gastric mucosa. In rodent model administration of NO donors attenuates gastric injury caused by NSAIDs. This property has been exploited in the development of NO-releasing NSAIDs, also indicated as COX-inhibiting NO-donating drugs (CINODs). NaproCINOD, an NO releasing derivative of naproxen, is a non-selective COX inhibitor. Clinical studies have shown that this agent reduces systemic blood pressure and has better cardiovascular tolerability than coxibs, while causing less gastrointestinal damage than its parent drug. H2S-releasing NSAID derivatives have been recently developed, based on the observed ability of this gaseous mediator to cause vasodilation and to prevent leukocyte adherence. In preclinical settings, H2S-releasing NSAIDs produce less gastric damage as compared to the parent drugs. CINODs represent examples of new anti-inflammatory drugs created through the exploitation of the beneficial effects of endogenous gaseous mediators in the gastrointestinal and cardiovascular systems.

Nonsteroidal anti-inflammatory drug (NSAID)-associated intestinal damage to the small and/or large bowel is frequent and may be present in up to 60% to 70% of patients taking these drugs long term. Intestinal damage is subclinical in most cases (eg, increased mucosal permeability, inflammation, erosions, ulceration), but more serious clinical outcomes, such as anemia and overall bleeding, perforation, obstruction, diverticulitis, and deaths, have also been described. Recent data suggest that serious lower gastrointestinal (GI) clinical events linked to NSAID use may be as frequent and severe as upper GI complications. Treatment and prevention strategies of NSAID-induced damage to the lower GI tract have not been defined so far. Misoprostol, antibiotics, and sulphasalazine have been proven to be effective in animal models, but they have not been properly tested in humans. Preliminary studies with COX-2 selective inhibitors in healthy volunteers have shown that these drugs are associated with less small bowel damage than traditional NSAIDs plus proton pump initiator, although their longterm effects in patients need to be tested. Post hoc analysis of previous outcome studies with these agents have shown contradictory results in the lower GI tract so far.

A vast majority of ulcers of the stomach and duodenum are due to *H pylori* infection or nonsteroidal anti-inflammatory drug (NSAID) usage. In patients with apparent *H pylori* negative NSAID negative ulcers, it is essential to ensure that the *H pylori* tests are not falsely negative and that the patient is not taking mucosal damaging drugs unknowingly. There are a variety of rare causes of true *H pylori* negative NSAID negative ulcers which need to be considered, including underlying cancer/lymphoma, Crohn's disease, rare infections and the Zollinger Ellison syndrome. Patients with idiopathic ulcers should be maintained on proton pump inhibitor therapy and may require higher doses than traditionally used in *H pylori* positive ulcers.

Despite improved understanding of peptic ulcer disease (PUD) pathogenesis, advances in diagnostic modalities, and the availability of modern pharmalogical, endoscopic and surgical treatments, gastroduodenal ulcer remains a major cause of morbidity and mortality worldwide. The predominant risk factors of this disorder remain *Helicobacter pylori* and ulcerogenic drugs. However, the proportion of idiopathic PUD is increasing worldwide often coinciding with the declining prevalence of *H pylori* infection. PUD heterogeneity worldwide is due to host genetic, bacterial and environmental factors. Variable ages in the acquisition of *H pylori* may influence the distribution of gastric versus duodenal ulcers as has the increasing use of aspirin and non-steroidal anti-inflammatory drugs (NSAIDs). Pharmacogenetics affects the magnitude of PUD risk induced by ulcerogenic drugs such as NSAIDs and also efficacy of proton pump inhibitors. Parietal cell mass and maximal acid output is higher in Western populations but it remains uncertain whether susceptibility to drug-induced PUD is influenced by race. *H pylori* antibiotic resistance also varies throughout the world. This review summarizes the similarities and differences in PUD aetiology, clinical features and treatment between the East and the West. In particular, we focus on the recent publications on the prevalence of *H pylori*, which is declining rapidly in various parts of the world resulting in overlapping prevalence rates in the East and the West.

THE CLINICS ARE NOW AVAILABLE ONLINE!

Access your subscription at:
www.theclinics.com

Preface

Peptic Ulcer Disease

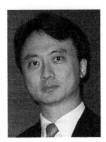

Francis K.L. Chan, MD
Guest Editor

This issue provides an extensive overview of recently published literature on peptic ulcer disease that differ in many respects from the previous issue of the *Gastroenterology Clinics of North America*. A collection of authorities in the field has been assembled to provide focused overviews of new scientific information in key areas. The series begins with an overview of the role of proton-pump inhibitor in the management of upper gastrointestinal bleeding. Controversial issues like pre-endoscopic administration of proton-pump inhibitor and the impact of proton-pump inhibitor therapy on mortality are discussed. Recurrent bleeding and death continue to be a major problem despite advances in therapeutic endoscopy and pharmacotherapy. The authors critically reviewed predictive models of poor outcome from acute upper gastrointestinal bleeding that may identify high-risk patients for timely management. The optimal management strategy for massive peptic ulcer bleeding remains a challenge - endoscopists, surgeons, and interventional radiologists often have divergent views. Leading investigators in the field discuss the options of repeated endoscopic therapy, early surgery, and angiographic embolization in high-risk patients. Other articles provide an authoritative overview of the management of stress-ulcer in critically ill patients and the approach to refractory peptic ulcer disease. In the last decade, nonsteroidal anti-inflammatory drugs (NSAIDs) and low-dose aspirin have gradually replaced *Helicobacter pylori* infection as the major cause of peptic ulcer disease in our aging population. Until recently, gastroenterologists and cardiologists used to have different views on strategies of preventing ulcer complications in patients requiring anti-platelet therapy. Now there is evidence that cyclo-oxygenase (COX)-2 selective and nonselective NSAIDs increase the risk of cardiothrombotic events. How to balance risks and benefits of NSAID use is an important issue for primary care doctors and rheumatologists. Experts in this field have provided critical and updated reviews on these frequently debated issues. The article entitled "Prevention of NSAID-induced ulcer: Looking to the future" provides a comprehensive update of new drugs and novel compounds that carry the potential of reducing gastrointestinal toxicity of NSAIDs.

Gastroenterol Clin N Am 38 (2009) xi–xii
doi:10.1016/j.gtc.2009.04.001
0889-8553/09/$ – see front matter © 2009 Elsevier Inc. All rights reserved.

gastro.theclinics.com

Although not widely recognized, NSAIDs can cause serious complications to the entire gastrointestinal tract. It is therefore relevant to include an updated review of NSAID-associated lower gastrointestinal complications amongst other articles on peptic ulcer disease. With a declining prevalence of *H pylori*, ulcers not associated with *H pylori* or NSAID use (non-NSAID non-*H pylori* ulcer) are increasingly recognized. The author provides an authoritative overview and practical approach to this diagnostic dilemma. Last but not least, a comprehensive review of the differences in peptic ulcer disease between the East and the West can hardly be found elsewhere.

I am grateful to the many experts who contributed to the current issue, and to Kerry Holland at Elsevier for editorial assistance. My goal is to provide the reader with a practical overview and stimulate future work in peptic ulcer disease.

Francis K.L. Chan, MD
Gastroenterology and Hepatology
Department of Medicine and Therapeutics
Chinese University of Hong Kong
30-32 Ngan Shing Street
Hong Kong, China

E-mail address:
fklchan@cuhk.edu.hk (F.K.L. Chan)

The Role of Proton Pump Inhibitors in the Management of Upper Gastrointestinal Bleeding

Grigorios I. Leontiadis, MD, PhD[a],*, Colin W. Howden, MD[b]

KEYWORDS

• Proton pump inhibitor • Peptic ulcer
• Nonvariceal upper gastrointestinal bleeding
• Rebleeding • Mortality • Management

Acute upper gastrointestinal (GI) bleeding is a common emergency, associated with substantial morbidity, mortality, and health care cost. Patients with portal hypertension who bleed from esophageal or gastric varices comprise a small proportion of bleeders,[1] but have worse prognosis and require a different therapeutic approach than patients with nonvariceal bleeding.[2] Peptic ulcer bleeding is the principal cause of nonvariceal upper GI bleeding.[1,3]

Prompt resuscitation and fluid replacement are of major importance[4] especially in severe bleeding. Concurrent major diseases should be carefully monitored and treated; there may be further decompensation following the bleeding episode, and co-morbidity is the major cause of mortality.[3] Endoscopic hemostatic treatment is of established efficacy in patients with nonvariceal upper GI bleeding.[5,6] Proton pump inhibitor (PPI) treatment is widely used as pharmacotherapy in nonvariceal upper GI bleeding, but its effect on mortality is not clear and is difficult to interpret.[7,8]

There was no financial support for this work.

Financial disclosure obligations: Dr Leontiadis has received speaker honoraria and reimbursement for expenses to attend scientific meetings from AstraZeneca, Sanofi-Aventis, GlaxoSmithKline, and Janssen-Cilag. Dr Howden has served as a consultant to TAP Pharmaceuticals Inc, Takeda Global Research and Development, Santarus, Novartis, Otsuka, Biovail, Extera Partners, and KV Pharmaceuticals. He has received speaking honoraria from Santarus, AstraZeneca, and Otsuka. He has received research grant support from AstraZeneca.

[a] Division of Gastroenterology, Department of Medicine, McMaster University Medical Centre, 1200 Main Street West, Suite 4W8B, Hamilton, ON L8N 3Z5, Canada
[b] Division of Gastroenterology, Department of Medicine, Northwestern University Feinberg School of Medicine, 676 N. St. Clair Street, Suite 1400, Chicago, IL 60611, USA
* Corresponding author.
E-mail address: leontia@mcmaster.ca (G.I. Leontiadis).

This article will summarize and critically evaluate the evidence from randomized controlled trials (RCTs) and meta-analyses of RCTs on the role of PPIs in nonvariceal upper GI bleeding, with specific emphasis on peptic ulcer bleeding.

RATIONALE FOR ACID SUPPRESSION PHARMACOTHERAPY

Endoscopic hemostatic therapy reduces but does not eliminate the risk for adverse outcomes in patients with nonvariceal upper GI bleeding.[5,6] Thus, there is room for further improvement in outcomes. Pharmacotherapy is a good candidate for adjuvant therapy, because it does not require any technical skills or specialty training to administer.

Furthermore, there is a biologically plausible underlying principle with regard to acid suppression therapy in this situation. Hemostasis in the stomach and duodenum is antagonized by gastric acid, which inhibits clot formation and promotes clot lysis. In vitro studies have shown that plasma coagulation and platelet aggregation are compromised by 50% in the presence of gastric juice at pH 6.4. At pH 6.0, previously formed platelet aggregates disaggregate; at pH 5.4, plasma coagulation and platelet aggregation are practically abolished; and at pH 4.0, previously formed fibrin clots are dissolved.[9] Pepsin can further inhibit coagulation by promotion of clot lysis in an acidic environment, since its proteolytic activity is maximal at pH 2 and negligible at pH above 5.[9,10] Such findings provided the rationale for rigorous acid suppression treatment attempting to maintain intragastric pH above 6 during the first 1–3 days following a bleeding episode. It is plausible that hydrochloric acid and pepsin can also provoke further bleeding from an ulcer by inducing ongoing tissue damage. However, this mechanism can be easily addressed even with standard doses of histamine H_2-receptor antagonists (H_2RAs) or PPIs; for healing of duodenal and gastric ulcers, maintaining the intragastric pH above 3 and 4 respectively, is adequate.[11–13]

Several RCTs have assessed the efficacy of acid suppression therapy at more than standard doses in nonvariceal upper GI bleeding. These studies had included patients with peptic ulcer bleeding either exclusively or predominantly.

H_2-RECEPTOR ANTAGONISTS IN PEPTIC ULCER BLEEDING

H_2RAs were the first class of acid suppression medications to be tested in this patient population. In 1985 Collins and Langman published a seminal meta-analysis of 27 RCTs that had compared either cimetidine (Tagamet) or ranitidine (Zantac) with placebo in a total of 2670 patients with nonvariceal upper GI bleeding.[14] There were marginally significant reductions in mortality and surgical intervention rates in the H_2RA group, but no evidence of an effect on rebleeding rates. When the analysis was restricted to studies that reported outcomes separately for patients who had bled from gastric and duodenal ulcers, the beneficial effect of H_2RAs was confined to patients with gastric ulcers; H_2RAs significantly reduced mortality, rebleeding and surgical intervention rates in patients with gastric ulcer bleeding, but there was no evidence of an effect on clinical outcomes in patients with duodenal ulcer bleeding.[14] That meta-analysis was updated in 2002 by Levine and colleagues,[15] who pooled 30 RCTs that had compared intravenous cimetidine, ranitidine, or famotidine (Pepcid) with placebo in patients with peptic ulcer bleeding. The meta-analysis found no evidence of an effect of intravenous H_2RAs on mortality (odds ratio [OR] 0.81; 95% confidence intervals [CI] 0.62–1.06), rebleeding (OR 0.86; 95% CI 0.74–1.00), or surgical intervention rates (OR 0.83; 95% CI 0.68–1.00), even though there were trends toward significance in rebleeding and surgical intervention rates. Subgroup analysis showed that H_2RAs significantly reduced rebleeding and surgical interventions in patients with gastric ulcer bleeding, but had no verifiable effect on mortality. As in the previous meta-analysis, H_2RAs did not significantly affect any clinical outcome in patients with duodenal ulcer bleeding.[15]

A planned subgroup analysis of 17 RCTs from a recent Cochrane meta-analysis showed that PPIs compared with H_2RAs significantly reduced rebleeding rates in patients with peptic ulcer bleeding (OR 0.61; 95% CI 0.48–0.78; number needed to treat [NNT] 20; 95% CI 13–34). There was no verifiable difference in mortality and surgical intervention rates.[7,8]

Therefore, there is insufficient evidence to recommend H_2RA treatment for peptic ulcer bleeding. This was also the conclusion of a consensus meeting that recommended against the use of H_2RAs in the management of nonvariceal upper GI bleeding.[4]

PROTON PUMP INHIBITORS IN PEPTIC ULCER BLEEDING
Effects of PPIs on Clinical Outcomes: Evidence From Meta-analyses of Randomized Controlled Trials

A recent Cochrane meta-analysis aimed to evaluate the efficacy of PPIs in treating peptic ulcer bleeding, using evidence from RCTs that had compared PPIs with either H_2RAs or placebo and had been published in November 2004.[7,8] Twenty-four RCTs comprising 4373 patients were included.

The meta-analysis revealed a highly significant and robust reduction in rebleeding rates with PPI treatment. PPIs significantly reduced 30-day rebleeding rates compared with control treatment; unweighted pooled rates were 10.6% and 17.3%, respectively (OR 0.49, 95% CI 0.37–0.65; NNT 13, 95% CI 10–25) (**Fig. 1**). Three-day rebleeding rates were also significantly reduced by PPI treatment (8.3%) compared with control (14.2%); OR 0.39; 95% CI 0.19–0.80; NNT 13, 95% CI 8–34. The reduction of 30-day rebleeding rates remained statistically significant in all predetermined subgroup analyses. That is, PPIs significantly reduced rebleeding independent of methodological quality of the trials, severity of baseline endoscopic signs of recent hemorrhage, type of control treatment (placebo or H_2RA), geographic location of the trials (conducted in Asia or elsewhere), mode of PPI administration (oral or intravenous), dose of PPI (high-dose defined as at least 80 mg bolus followed by an intravenous infusion of 8 mg/h for 72 hours; low-dose defined as any lesser dose intravenous or oral), and whether or not endoscopic hemostatic treatment was given.[7,8]

Nevertheless, there was statistically significant heterogeneity among trials for rebleeding ($P = .04$) and this had to be explained. The abovementioned subgroup analyses provided clues about the effect of population and study characteristics. Two of the subgroup analyses, according to route of administration of PPI and geographic location of trials, resulted in groups of trials that were statistically homogeneous for rebleeding. Moreover, when the influence of predefined study characteristics on the effect of treatment on rebleeding was assessed by metaregression, only the geographic location of the studies had a significant influence: PPIs produced quantitatively greater reductions in rebleeding among RCTs that had been conducted in Asia compared with RCTs that had been conducted elsewhere. The findings of the subgroup analysis and the metaregression not only explained the heterogeneity for the outcome of rebleeding, but also provided indirect evidence of increased efficacy of PPIs for peptic ulcer bleeding in Asian trials.[7,8]

The trials were nonheterogeneous for the other outcomes that were assessed. Surgical interventions were significantly less common with PPI treatment (6.1%) than with control treatment (9.3%); OR 0.61, 95% CI 0.48–0.78; NNT 34, 95% CI 20–50. Further endoscopic hemostatic treatment (after randomization) was also

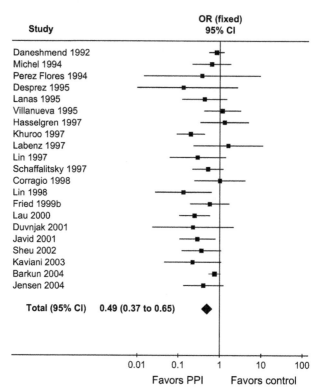

Fig. 1. Forest plot of the OR and the 95% confidence intervals of individual studies and pooled estimate for rebleeding. *Abbreviations:* PPI, proton pump inhibitor; OR, odds ratios; CI, confidence intervals. (*Data from* Leontiadis GI, Sharma VK, Howden CW. Proton pump inhibitor treatment for acute peptic ulcer bleeding. Cochrane Database Syst Rev 2006;(1):CD002094.[7])

reduced with PPIs (5.6%) compared with control treatment (15.7%); OR 0.32, 95% CI 0.20–0.51; NNT 10, 95% CI 8–17.[7,8]

Despite the beneficial effect of PPI treatment on the above outcomes, there was no evidence of an effect on all-cause mortality rates (OR 1.01, 95% CI 0.74–1.40; **Fig. 2**). Unweighted pooled rates were 3.9% for PPI treatment and 3.8% for control treatment. It is plausible that any beneficial or detrimental effect of PPIs on mortality could have been diluted by the inclusion of patients with low-risk in the studies. A planned subgroup analysis was restricted to patients with high-risk endoscopic findings of active bleeding or a nonbleeding visible vessel—the patient population that clinicians are mainly concerned about. In this population PPIs significantly reduced mortality; OR 0.53, 95% CI 0.31–0.91, NNT 50, 95% CI 34–100. Among such patients, the reduction of mortality by PPI treatment remained significant when the analysis was confined to the RCTs that consistently used initial endoscopic hemostatic treatment, which is the accepted standard of care for such patients (OR 0.54, 95% CI 0.30–0.96; NNT 50, 95% CI 34–100), but was not significant among trials that did not consistently do so.[7,8]

Separating the trials according to geographic location was the only other subgroup analysis that showed a statistically significant effect of PPI treatment on mortality. PPIs significantly reduced mortality among trials that had been conducted in Asia (OR 0.35,

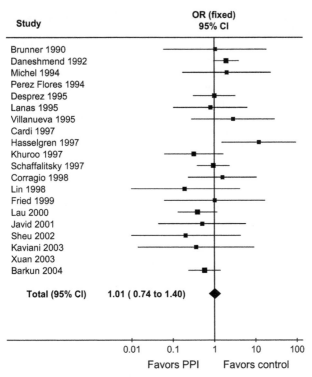

Study	OR (fixed) 95% CI
Brunner 1990	
Daneshmend 1992	
Michel 1994	
Perez Flores 1994	
Desprez 1995	
Lanas 1995	
Villanueva 1995	
Cardi 1997	
Hasselgren 1997	
Khuroo 1997	
Schaffalitsky 1997	
Corragio 1998	
Lin 1998	
Fried 1999	
Lau 2000	
Javid 2001	
Sheu 2002	
Kaviani 2003	
Xuan 2003	
Barkun 2004	
Total (95% CI)	1.01 (0.74 to 1.40)

0.01 0.1 1 10 100

Favors PPI Favors control

Fig. 2. Forest plot of the OR and the 95% CI of individual studies and pooled estimate for mortality. *Abbreviations*: PPI, proton pump inhibitor; OR, odds ratios; CI, confidence intervals. (*Data from* Leontiadis GI, Sharma VK, Howden CW. Proton pump inhibitor treatment for acute peptic ulcer bleeding. Cochrane Database Syst Rev 2006;(1):CD002094.[7])

95% CI 0.16–0.74; NNT 34, 95% CI 20–100), but had no verifiable effect among trials that had been conducted elsewhere (OR 1.36, 95% CI 0.94–1.96). Similarly to the outcome of rebleeding, a higher treatment effect of PPIs in Asian trials was confirmed by metaregression.[7,8]

Funnel plots for mortality, rebleeding and surgical interventions were visually asymmetric, suggesting the presence of publication bias because of some missing small trials with negative results. However, this was only confirmed statistically for the outcome of surgical interventions.[7,8]

There have been three other published meta-analyses of RCTs that have assessed the role of PPIs in peptic ulcer bleeding.[16–18] The most consistent finding of these meta-analyses, which is also in agreement with the Cochrane meta-analysis, is that PPIs compared with H_2RAs or placebo significantly reduce rebleeding rates in patients with peptic ulcer bleeding.

Khuroo and colleagues pooled RCTs on acute nonvariceal upper GI bleeding that had been published till 2002.[18] They found no evidence that PPI treatment compared with H_2RAs or placebo affected all-cause mortality. PPI treatment significantly reduced rebleeding and surgical intervention rates. However, a predetermined subgroup analysis showed that these beneficial effects of PPIs were restricted to trials on patients who had bled from peptic ulcers with active bleeding, nonbleeding visible vessels, or adherent clots. There was no verifiable effect of PPI treatment on rebleeding or surgical intervention rates among trials that had included patients with all causes of nonvariceal upper GI bleeding.[18]

Khuroo and colleagues also reported that all-cause mortality in nonvariceal upper GI bleeding was significantly increased with intravenous PPI treatment, although it was significantly reduced with oral PPI treatment. They also reported that PPI treatment significantly reduced deaths directly caused by bleeding, while it significantly increased deaths caused by associated diseases or of unknown etiology.[18] However, the validity of these analyses on mortality was undermined by several factors: some eligible RCTs were missed, noneligible trials were inadvertently included, and there were mistakes in the data extraction process.[19] When the authors re-extracted raw data and repooled the trials, it was found that PPI treatment marginally reduced "bleeding related" deaths and had no effect on "non–bleeding related" deaths.[19] The fact that the vast majority of published trials did not provide sufficient data to allow for a reliable differentiation of causes of deaths renders even this "corrected" analysis unreliable. It would be very useful if future studies were prospectively designed to categorize causes of death in patients with nonvariceal upper GI bleeding in a systematic way (as only one of the published studies did[20]), but until then it would be premature to draw conclusions regarding any differential effect of PPIs on different causes of death.

Andriulli and colleagues[16] conducted a series of meta-analyses of RCTs published till August 2003 on PPI treatment for peptic ulcer bleeding. It was concluded that PPI treatment, compared with H_2RA or placebo, significantly reduced rebleeding but not surgical intervention or all-cause mortality rates.

The meta-analysis by Bardou and colleagues[17] included RCTs published up to April 2003 that compared PPIs with H_2RAs or placebo in patients with peptic ulcers with active bleeding, non-bleeding visible vessels, or adherent clots. The trials were divided into three groups according to the dose of PPI treatment: high-dose intravenous PPI (40–80 mg bolus followed by intravenous infusion of at least 6 mg/h), high-dose oral PPI (at least twice the standard dosage), and non-high-dose PPI (any other dose of PPI). In each group, trials were further subgrouped according to the control treatment used. PPI treatment significantly reduced rebleeding rates in all comparisons apart from that of high-dose intravenous PPI versus H_2RA. The effect of PPIs on surgical intervention rates was less consistent. Mortality was significantly reduced in the analyses of high-dose intravenous versus placebo and non-high-dose PPI versus placebo. The authors have expressed concerns[21] about the exclusion of two studies[22,23] from the former analysis and the misclassification of another study[24] in the latter analysis. Nevertheless, this was the first meta-analysis that showed that PPIs significantly reduced mortality in a subgroup of patients with high-risk endoscopic stigmata.

Effects of Proton Pump Inhibitors on Clinical Outcomes: Evidence From Recent Randomized Controlled Trials

Since the completion of the most recent of the above meta-analyses,[7,8] two RCTs that had been included in the meta-analysis as abstracts were published in full.[25,26] Furthermore, eight new RCTs that assessed the efficacy of PPI treatment in peptic ulcer bleeding have been published.[27–34] The characteristics and main results of these trials are shown in **Table 1**. PPI treatment produced statistically significant reductions in rebleeding rates in all but 1 trial,[33] did not have a verifiable effect on mortality in any trial, and significantly reduced surgical interventions in one trial.[28] Since these results are consistent with the results of the Cochrane meta-analysis,[7,8] it is unlikely that the inclusion of the above trials will significantly affect the update of the meta-analysis scheduled for 2009. The trial by Sung and colleagues[32] is of particular importance. It had great methodological quality (in fact the protocol had been registered in

Table 1
Key characteristics and findings of randomized controlled trials that have been published since the completion of the Cochrane meta-analysis.[7,8]

| Trial | Participants | Interventions | | Outcomes that Showed Statistically Significant Difference | | |
		PPI	Control	Mortality	Rebleeding	Surgery
Hsu et al, 2004[27]	N = 102; Taiwan	IV bolus	IV bolus H₂RA	No	In favor of PPI	No
Lin et al, 2006[30]	N = 200; Taiwan	IV bolus	IV bolus H₂RA	No	In favor of PPI	No
Zargar et al, 2006[34]	N = 203; India	Continuous IV infusion	Placebo	No	In favor of PPI	No
Khoshbaten et al, 2006[29]	N = 80; Iran	Oral	Continuous IV infusion H₂RA	No	In favor of PPI	No
Wei et al, 2007[33]	N = 70; Taiwan	Oral	Placebo	No	No	No
Hung et al, 2007[28]	N = 153; China (Hong Kong)	Continuous IV infusion; IV bolus	No treatment	No	In favor of PPI	In favor of PPI (continuous IV infusion)
Naumonski-Mihalic et al, 2007[31]	N = 70; Croatia	IV bolus	IV bolus H₂RA	No	In favor of PPI	No
Sung et al, 2008[32]	N = 764; 14 European countries, South Africa, Turkey, China (Hong Kong)	Continuous IV infusion	Placebo	No	In favor of PPI	No

Abbreviations: PPI, proton pump inhibitor; H₂RA, Histamine-2 receptor antagonists; IV, intravenous.

ClinicalTrials.gov and prospectively published[35]), was adequately powered, and was the first trial to use high-dose intravenous esomeprazole (Nexium). Among the 18 RCTs that had compared PPI treatment with H_2RAs or placebo in predominantly Caucasian populations, it is the only trial that has shown a highly significant reduction of rebleeding rates with PPI treatment; 3-day rebleeding rates were 5.9% and 10.3% ($P = .03$) and 30-day rebleeding rates were 7.7% and 13.6% ($P = .01$), respectively.[32] The results of a predetermined analysis confined to Caucasian patients (87% of total population) were very similar to the results from the total study population, which also included Asians, blacks, and others.[36] The only other trial on Caucasian patients that reported that PPIs significantly reduced rebleeding rates is a small trial by Naumov-ski-Mihalic and colleagues,[31] but the statistical significance of this finding is dependent on the statistical test used, and is marginal at best.

Effects of Proton Pump Inhibitors on Clinical Outcomes: Evidence From Observational Studies

The effectiveness of PPI treatment in a "real-life" setting was shown in an analysis of the Canadian Registry of patients with Upper Gastrointestinal Bleeding and Endoscopy by Barkun and colleagues.[3] They analyzed data from 1869 randomly selected patients who underwent endoscopy for nonvariceal upper GI bleeding at 18 community and tertiary care institutions from across Canada between 1999 and 2002. Peptic ulcer was the commonest cause of bleeding (responsible for 55% of episodes). Logistic regression models identified that PPI use was significantly and independently associated with decreased mortality in patients with high-risk endoscopic findings defined as active bleeding, visible vessels, or visible vessels with clots (OR 0.53, 95% CI 0.37–0.77), and decreased rebleeding in all patients regardless of the severity of endoscopic findings (OR 0.18, 95% CI 0.04–0.80). Despite the large sample size and the superior methodological quality of this database analysis, the authors noted that "because of the nature of the study design, these findings should be considered exploratory and require prospective confirmation."[3] These results were confirmed by subsequent meta-analyses of RCTs, as described above.[7,8,17]

Are Proton Pump Inhibitors More Efficacious in Asia?

The suggestion that PPI therapy for peptic ulcer bleeding is more efficacious in trials that had been conducted in Asia than elsewhere originated from a post hoc analysis[37] of the initial Cochrane meta-analysis.[38] The difference in efficacy persisted in the updated Cochrane meta-analysis, as described above.[7,8] PPI treatment compared with H_2RA treatment or placebo significantly reduced mortality among the 8 RCTs that had been conducted in Asia, but had no effect on mortality among the 16 RCTs that had been conducted elsewhere. (One trial had been performed in the US,[39] 14 in Europe, and one predominantly in Europe but also in Canada and South Africa[40]). Although rebleeding rates were significantly reduced by PPI treatment in both subgroups, the reduction was quantitatively greater in the Asian trials. Separating Asian from non-Asian trials eliminated the statistical heterogeneity among trials for rebleeding. Furthermore, the increased efficacy of PPIs in Asian trials was confirmed by metaregression.[7,8] Although the results of subgroup analyses and metaregression should be interpreted cautiously, the above findings seem to be robust.

There are a number of possible explanations for this apparent difference in efficacy. Asian patients seem to have a lesser parietal cell mass and an increased higher prevalence of *Helicobacter pylori* infection and genetically determined slow metabolism of PPIs. All these factors would tend to produce a greater antisecretory effect of PPI therapy in Asian than in non-Asian patients.[37]

The recent trial by Sung and colleagues[32,36] may shed more light on this issue. The outcomes provided by the abstract publications of the trial have shown that PPI therapy is beneficial in Caucasian patients with peptic ulcer bleeding. The full publication of the trial may allow for the comparison of outcomes between Asian and non-Asian patients, which, although less important from a practical point of view, is scientifically interesting.

What is the Optimal Regimen of Proton Pump Inhibitors Treatment for Peptic Ulcer Bleeding?

Omeprazole (Prilosec, Losec) had been the PPI most commonly used in RCTs in peptic ulcer bleeding, followed by pantoprazole (Protonix), esomeprazole and lansoprazole (Prevacid). There is no obvious indication that any one PPI was more efficacious than the others. Metaregression analysis found no evidence that using omeprazole as opposed to another PPI affected the treatment effect regarding mortality, rebleeding, or surgical interventions.[7,8] Three small RCTs have reported clinical outcomes for similar doses of head-to-head comparisons of different PPIs in peptic ulcer bleeding.[41–43] None of these trials has provided conclusive evidence of clinical superiority of any one PPI over another. Therefore, it is reasonable to assume that the effect of PPIs on clinical outcomes of peptic ulcer bleeding is a class effect.

One of the most controversial issues in the management of peptic ulcer bleeding is on the optimal dose and route of administration (intravenous or oral) of PPI treatment. Predetermined subgroup analyses and metaregression from the Cochrane meta-analysis of RCTs showed no evidence that the effects of PPI treatment were dependent on the route of administration or the dose of the PPI.[7,8] A post hoc subgroup analysis found that the reduction in mortality among patients with high-risk endoscopic signs remained significant when the analysis was confined to the four trials[39,40,44,45] that had consistently applied initial endoscopic hemostatic treatment and also used high-dose intravenous PPI treatment (80 mg bolus followed by 8 mg/h for 72 hours); OR 0.46, 95% CI 0.24–0.90; NNT 50, 95% CI 34–100.[8] There was no evidence of an effect on mortality among the trials on patients with high-risk endoscopic signs that had consistently applied initial endoscopic hemostatic treatment but used a lesser dose of intravenous PPI or an oral PPI (OR 1.01, 95% CI 0.26–3.83).[8] Although this post hoc subanalysis suggests that high-dose intravenous PPIs are more efficacious than lower-dose PPIs, the suggestion should be regarded with caution since the comparison is not a direct one. Furthermore, the latter subgroup analysis may have been underpowered.

The authors are aware of at least 16 RCTs that had compared head-to-head different doses and/or routes of administration of PPIs in peptic ulcer bleeding and had reported clinical outcomes. Most of these have undoubtedly been underpowered. An ongoing Cochrane meta-analysis aims to assess the potential differences among various regimens of PPIs using evidence from such RCTs.

Defining the minimum effective dose of PPI will have important cost-saving implications to health care systems. Cost-effectiveness analyses have shown that either oral or intravenous PPI treatment is more effective and less costly than treatment with H_2RAs or placebo following endoscopic hemostatic treatment for peptic ulcer bleeding in the US and Canadian settings.[46,47] However, cost-effectiveness analyses of oral versus intravenous administration of PPIs in the US, Canada, and the UK have yielded conflicting results.[46–48]

Proton Pump Inhibitors for Upper Gastrointestinal Bleeding Before Endoscopy

Since PPIs reduce rebleeding in patients with peptic ulcer bleeding, it might be argued that they should be administered to patients with upper GI bleeding at the time of presentation and while awaiting endoscopy. Since most patients with nonvariceal upper GI bleeding will bleed from a peptic ulcer, this seems a logical and justifiable approach. This issue was addressed by another Cochrane meta-analysis published in 2006[49] that had included four RCTs published in full[20,50-52] and the preliminary results of a fifth RCT by Lau and colleagues[53] which, at that time, was only available as an abstract. These RCTs had studied the efficacy of PPI treatment initiated on admission in patients with upper GI bleeding, after having excluded patients suspected of having variceal bleeding. The patients in the comparator arms had received either an H_2RA[51,52] or placebo.[20,50,53] Endoscopy was performed within 24[20,50,51,53] or 48 hours[52] of admission. Three trials had been conducted in Europe,[20,50,52] one in Turkey[51] and one in China (Hong Kong).[53] Pooling of the trials that reported outcomes for all patients who were randomized (four trials[20,50-52] with 1512 patients in total) showed no evidence of an effect of pre-endoscopic PPI treatment on mortality (OR 1.12; 95% CI 0.72–1.73), rebleeding (OR 0.81; 95% CI 0.61–1.09), requirement for endoscopic hemostatic treatment at subsequent index endoscopy (OR 0.93, 95% CI 0.53–1.64) or surgical intervention rates (OR 0.96, 95% CI 0.68–1.35). There was no detectable heterogeneity among the trials. The effect of pre-endoscopic PPI treatment on the abovementioned outcomes remained nonsignificant when the trials were pooled separately according to the type of control treatment (H_2RA or placebo), the route of PPI administration (intravenous or oral), and the methodological quality of the trials. The only significant effect of pre-endoscopic PPI treatment was a reduction in the proportion of patients with active bleeding, a nonbleeding visible vessel, or an adherent clot found at the index endoscopy; pooled (unweighted) rates were 37.2% on PPI treatment and 46.5% on control treatment; OR 0.67; 95% CI 0.54–0.84.[49]

Following the publication of the above meta-analysis, Lau and colleagues[54] published in full the final results of their RCT, which was the only trial that had used high-dose pre-endoscopic PPI treatment (80 mg intravenous bolus of omeprazole followed by continuous intravenous infusion of 8 mg/h). Their results are in general agreement with those of the meta-analysis of the four previously published trials. PPI treatment before endoscopy compared with placebo did not significantly affect mortality, rebleeding, or surgical intervention rates.[54] Among the 377 patients with peptic ulcer bleeding (60% of study population), pre-endoscopic PPIs accelerated the resolution of stigmata of recent bleeding as assessed at index endoscopy performed at a mean of 15 hours after treatment initiation.[54] The requirement for endoscopic hemostatic treatment at index endoscopy among all patients who were randomized with nonvariceal upper GI bleeding was also significantly reduced by pre-endoscopic PPI treatment compared with placebo (19% versus 28%; $P =$ .007). Subgroup analysis showed that this beneficial effect was driven by, and confined to, patients with bleeding from peptic ulcers; there was no difference in the need for endoscopic therapy among patients with other sources of bleeding.[54]

Hence, is the glass half empty or half full? Does the downstaging of the stigmata of recent bleeding and possibly the reduction of the requirement for endoscopic hemostatic treatment at index endoscopy justify the use of pre-endoscopic PPIs, despite the lack of evidence of an effect on clinical outcomes? Given the efficacy of endoscopic hemostatic treatment and postendoscopic PPI treatment, it is unlikely that an RCT adequately powered to detect a further reduction in rebleeding or mortality will ever be conducted. Analyses of large multicenter databases using propensity score methods to adjust for overt biases may be able to detect such effects,[55] but such studies have yet to be conducted. The two small retrospective observational studies, both from Canada, have produced different results among them. Andrews and colleagues[56] reported that intravenous PPI treatment before endoscopy did not affect clinical outcomes in patients with peptic ulcers with high-risk endoscopic stigmata of recent hemorrhage. Keyvani and colleagues[57] found that pre-endoscopic PPI (which had been administered orally in 91% of the cases) significantly reduced mortality, rebleeding, and surgical intervention rates in patients with nonvariceal upper GI bleeding.

Cost-effectiveness analyses have not been in full agreement among them. Initiation of high-dose intravenous PPI treatment before endoscopy was both marginally more costly and effective than after endoscopy in the US and Canadian settings[58] but was less costly and more effective in Hong Kong.[59]

A consensus meeting stated that "in patients awaiting endoscopy empiric therapy with a high-dose PPI should be considered," although only 40% of the participants accepted this recommendation without reservations.[4]

SUMMARY

Pre-endoscopic administration of PPIs in patients with nonvariceal upper GI bleeding is still of controversial efficacy. It downstages the severity of the endoscopic signs of recent bleeding and may reduce the requirement for endoscopic hemostatic therapy at index endoscopy. However, there is no evidence of an effect on mortality, rebleeding, or surgical intervention rates.

In contrast, the efficacy of PPIs in endoscopically diagnosed peptic ulcer bleeding is supported by high-quality evidence from numerous RCTs and meta-analyses of RCTs. PPIs compared with H_2RAs or placebo consistently reduce rebleeding rates regardless of dose, route of administration, application or not of endoscopic hemostatic treatment, and geographic location. Surgical intervention rates and the need for further endoscopic hemostatic treatment are also reduced by PPI treatment, although the results are not as robust as those for rebleeding. There is no evidence of an overall effect of PPI treatment on all-cause mortality. However, all-cause mortality is reduced among patients with high-risk endoscopic signs and among trials that had been conducted in Asia. The optimal dose and route of PPI administration has yet to be determined.

REFERENCES

1. Rockall TA, Logan RFA, Devlin HB, et al. Incidence of and mortality from acute upper gastrointestinal haemorrhage in the United Kingdom. BMJ 1995;311: 222–6.
2. Garcia-Tsao G, Sanyal AJ, Grace ND, et al. Prevention and management of gastroesophageal varices and variceal hemorrhage in cirrhosis. Am J Gastroenterol 2007;102(9):2086–102.
3. Barkun A, Sabbah S, Enns R, et al. The Canadian Registry on Nonvariceal Upper Gastrointestinal Bleeding and Endoscopy (RUGBE): endoscopic hemostasis and proton pump inhibition are associated with improved outcomes in a real-life setting. Am J Gastroenterol 2004;99(7):1238–46.
4. Barkun A, Bardou M, Marshall JK. Consensus recommendations for managing patients with nonvariceal upper gastrointestinal bleeding. Ann Intern Med 2003; 139(10):843–57.
5. Cook DJ, Guyatt GH, Salena BJ, et al. Endoscopic therapy for acute nonvariceal upper gastrointestinal hemorrhage: a meta-analysis. Gastroenterology 1992; 102(1):139–48.

6. Laine L, McQuaid KR. Endoscopic therapy for bleeding ulcers: an evidence-based approach based on meta-analyses of randomized controlled trials. Clin Gastroenterol Hepatol 2009;7(1):33–47.

7. Leontiadis GI, Sharma VK, Howden CW. Proton pump inhibitor treatment for acute peptic ulcer bleeding. Cochrane Database Syst Rev 2006;(1):CD002094.

8. Leontiadis GI, Sharma VK, Howden CW. Proton pump inhibitor therapy for peptic ulcer bleeding: cochrane collaboration meta-analysis of randomized controlled trials. Mayo Clin Proc 2007;82(3):286–96.

9. Green FJ, Kaplan MM, Curtis LE, et al. Effects of acid and pepsin on blood coagulation and platelet aggregation. A possible contributor to prolonged gastro duodenal mucosal haemorrhage. Gastroenterology 1978;7438–43.

10. Patchett SE, Enright H, Afdhal N, et al. Clot lysis by gastric juice: an in vitro study. Gut 1989;30(12):1704–7.

11. Jones DB, Howden CW, Burget DW, et al. Acid suppression in duodenal ulcer: a meta-analysis to define optimal dosing with antisecretory drugs. Gut 1987; 28(9):1120–7.

12. Howden CW, Jones DB, Peace KE, et al. The treatment of gastric ulcer with antisecretory drugs. Relationship of pharmacological effect to healing rates. Dig Dis Sci 1988;33(5):619–24.

13. Howden CW, Hunt RH. The relationship between suppression of acidity and gastric ulcer healing rates. Aliment Pharmacol Ther 1990;4(1):25–33.

14. Collins R, Langman M. Treatment with histamine H_2 antagonists in acute upper gastrointestinal hemorrhage. Implications of randomized trials. N Engl J Med 1985;313:660–6.

15. Levine JE, Leontiadis GI, Sharma VK, et al. Meta-analysis: the efficacy of intravenous H2-receptor antagonists in bleeding peptic ulcer. Aliment Pharmacol Ther 2002;16(6):1137–42.

16. Andriulli A, Annese V, Caruso N, et al. Proton-pump inhibitors and outcome of endoscopic hemostasis in bleeding peptic ulcers: a series of meta-analyses. Am J Gastroenterol 2005;100:207–19.

17. Bardou M, Toubouti Y, Benhaberou-Brun D, et al. Meta-analysis: proton-pump inhibition in high-risk patients with acute peptic ulcer bleeding. Aliment Pharmacol Ther 2005;21:677–86.

18. Khuroo MS, Khuroo MS, Farahat KL, et al. Treatment with proton pump inhibitors in acute non-variceal upper gastrointestinal bleeding: a meta-analysis. J Gastroenterol Hepatol 2005;20(1):11–25.

19. Leontiadis GI, Sharma VK, Howden CW. Proton pump inhibitors in acute non-variceal upper gastrointestinal bleeding. J Gastroenterol Hepatol 2006;21(11):1763–5.

20. Daneshmend TK, Hawkey CJ, Langman MJ, et al. Omperpazole versus placebo for acute upper gastrointestinal bleeding: randomised double blind controlled trial. BMJ 1992;304:143–7.

21. Leontiadis GI, Sharma VK, Howden CW. Explaining divergent results of meta-analyses on proton pump inhibitor treatment for ulcer bleeding. Gastroenterology 2005;129(5):1804–5.

22. Schaffalitzky De Muckadell OB, Havelund T, et al. Effect of omeprazole on the outcome of endoscopically treated bleeding peptic ulcers. Randomized double-blind placebo-controlled multicentre study. Scand J Gastroenterol 1997; 32(4):320–7.

23. Hasselgren G, Lind T, Lundell L, et al. Continuous intravenous infusion of omeprazole in elderly patients with peptic ulcer bleeding. Scand J Gastroenterol 1997; 32:328–33.

24. Khuroo MS, Yattoo GN, Javid G, et al. A comparison of omeprazole and placebo for bleeding peptic ulcer. N Engl J Med 1997;336(15):1054–8.
25. Jensen DM, Pace SC, Soffer E, et al. Continuous infusion of pantoprazole versus ranitidine for prevention of ulcer rebleeding: a U.S. multicenter randomized, double-blind study. Am J Gastroenterol 2006;101(9):1991–9.
26. Van Rensburg C, Barkun AN, Racz I, et al. Intravenous pantoprazole versus ranitidine for the prevention of peptic ulcer rebleeding: a multicenter, multi-national, randomized trial. Aliment Pharmacol Ther 2009;22:497–507.
27. Hsu PI, Lo GH, Lo CC, et al. Intravenous pantoprazole versus ranitidine for prevention of rebleeding after endoscopic hemostasis of bleeding peptic ulcers. World J Gastroenterol 2004;10(24):3666–9.
28. Hung WK, Li VK, Chung CK, et al. Randomized trial comparing pantoprazole infu-sion, bolus and no treatment on gastric pH and recurrent bleeding in peptic ulcers. ANZ J Surg 2007;77(8):677–81.
29. Khoshbaten M, Fattahi E, Naderi N, et al. A comparison of oral omeprazole and intravenous cimetidine in reducing complications of duodenal peptic ulcer. BMC Gastroenterol 2006;6:2.
30. Lin HJ, Lo WC, Cheng YC, et al. Role of intravenous omeprazole in patients with high-risk peptic ulcer bleeding after successful endoscopic epinephrine injec-tion: a prospective randomized comparative trial. Am J Gastroenterol 2006; 101(3):500–5.
31. Naumovski-Mihalic S, Katicic M, Bozek T, et al. Gastric acid suppression in acute ulcer bleeding in patients with comorbid illnesses. Gut 2007;56(Suppl 3):A234.
32. Sung JJY, Barkun A, Kuipers EJ, et al. Intravenous esomeprazole for prevention of peptic ulcer re-bleeding: a multinational, double-blind, placebo controlled randomised study. Gut 2008;57(Suppl II):A70.
33. Wei KL, Tung SY, Sheen CH, et al. Effect of oral esomeprazole on recurrent bleeding after endoscopic treatment of bleeding peptic ulcers. J Gastroenterol Hepatol 2007;22(1):43–6.
34. Zargar SA, Javid G, Khan BA, et al. Pantoprazole infusion as adjuvant therapy to endoscopic treatment in patients with peptic ulcer bleeding: prospective randomized controlled trial. J Gastroenterol Hepatol 2006;21(4):716–21.
35. Sung JJY, Mossner J, Barkun A, et al. Intravenous esomeprazole for prevention of peptic ulcer re-bleeding: rationale/design of peptic ulcer bleed study. Aliment Pharmacol Ther 2008;27(8):666–77.
36. Barkun A, Sung JJY, Kuipers Ernst, et al. Intravenous esomeprazole fro preven-tion of peptic ulcer re-bleeding in a predominantly Caucasian population: results on clinical benefits and hospital resource use. Gut 2008;57(Suppl 2):A70.
37. Leontiadis GI, Sharma VK, Howden CW. Systematic review and meta-analysis: enhanced efficacy of proton-pump inhibitor therapy for peptic ulcer bleeding in Asia - a post hoc analysis from the Cochrane Collaboration. Aliment Pharmacol Ther 2005;21(9):1055–61.
38. Leontiadis GI, Sharma VK, Howden CW. Systematic review and meta-analysis of proton pump inhibitor therapy in peptic ulcer bleeding. BMJ 2005;330(7491): 568–70.
39. Jensen DM, Pace SC, Soffer EF, et al. Lower rebleeding rates in high risk patients treated with IV pantoprazole than IV ranitidine after endoscopic hemostasis in a randomized controlled US study. Am J Gastroenterol 2004;99:S296.
40. Barkun A, Racz I, van Rensburg C, et al. Prevention of peptic ulcer rebleeding using continuous infusion of pantoparzole vs ranitidine: a multicenter,

multinational, randomized, double-blind, parallel-group comparison. Gastroenterology 2004;126(4 Suppl 2):A78.

41. Chilovi F, Piazzi L, Zancanella L, et al. Intravenous omeprazole and pantoprazole after endoscopic treatment of bleeding peptic ulcers. Gastrointest Endosc 2003; 57:AB150.

42. Chahin NJ, Meli M, Zaca F. Endoscopic injection plus continuous intravenous pantoprazole vs endoscopic injection plus continuous intravenous omeprazole for the treatment of upper nonvariceal bleeding. Can J Gastroenterol 2006; 20(Suppl A):112.

43. Zhonglin Y, Sanren L, Huiji W. Effectiveness and safety of pantoprazole i.v. and omeprazole i.v. in the treatment of patients with peptic ulcer bleeding. J Gastroenterol Hepatol 2002;17:A257.

44. Lau JYW, Sung JJY, Lee KKC, et al. Effect of intravenous omeprazole on recurrent bleeding after endoscopic treatment of bleeding peptic ulcers. N Engl J Med 2000;343(5):310–6.

45. Lin HJ, Lo WC, Lee FY, et al. A prospective randomized comparative trial showing that omeprazole prevents rebleeding in patients with bleeding peptic ulcer after successful endoscopic therapy. Arch Intern Med 1998;158(1):54–8.

46. Barkun AN, Herba K, Adam V, et al. The cost-effectiveness of high-dose oral proton pump inhibition after endoscopy in the acute treatment of peptic ulcer bleeding. Aliment Pharmacol Ther 2004;20:195–202.

47. Spiegel BM, Dulai GS, Lim BS, et al. The cost-effectiveness and budget impact of intravenous versus oral proton pump inhibitors in peptic ulcer hemorrhage. Clin Gastroenterol Hepatol 2006;4(8):988–97.

48. Leontiadis GI, Sreedharan A, Dorward S, et al. Systematic reviews of the clinical effectiveness and cost-effectiveness of proton pump inhibitors in acute upper gastrointestinal bleeding. Health Technol Assess 2007;11(51):iii–iv, 1–164.

49. Dorward S, Sreedharan A, Leontiadis GI, et al. Proton pump inhibitor treatment initiated prior to endoscopic diagnosis in upper gastrointestinal bleeding. Cochrane Database Syst Rev 2006;(4):CD005415.

50. Hawkey GM, Cole AT, McIntyre AS, et al. Drug treatments in upper gastrointestinal bleeding: value of endoscopic findings as surrogate end points. Gut 2001; 49(3):372–9.

51. Hulagu S, Demirturk L, Gul S, et al. The effect of omeprazole or ranitidine intravenous on upper gastrointestinal bleeding. Endoscopi Journal 1995;2:35–42.

52. Wallner G, Ciechanski A, Wesolowski M, et al. Treatment of acute upper gastrointestinal bleeding with intravenous omeprazole or ranitidine. European Journal of Clinical Research 1996;8:235–43.

53. Lau JY, Leung WK, Wu JC, et al. Early administration of high dose intravenous omeprazole prior to endoscopy in patients with upper gastrointestinal bleeding: a double blind placebo controlled randomized trial. Gastroenterology 2005; 128(Suppl 4):A347.

54. Lau JY, Leung WK, Wu JC, et al. Omeprazole before endoscopy in patients with gastrointestinal bleeding. N Engl J Med 2007;356(16):1631–40.

55. Braitman LE, Rosenbaum PR. Rare outcomes, common treatments: analytic strategies using propensity scores. Ann Intern Med 2002;137(8):693–5.

56. Andrews CN, Levy A, Fishman M, et al. Intravenous proton pump inhibitors before endoscopy in bleeding peptic ulcer with high-risk stigmata: a multicentre comparative study. Can J Gastroenterol 2005;19(11):667–71.

57. Keyvani L, Murthy S, Leeson S, et al. Pre-endoscopic proton pump inhibitor therapy reduces recurrent adverse gastrointestinal outcomes in patients with

acute non-variceal upper gastrointestinal bleeding. Aliment Pharmacol Ther 2006;24(8):1247–55.

58. Al-Sabah S, Barkun AN, Herba K, et al. Cost-effectiveness of proton-pump inhibition before endoscopy in upper gastrointestinal bleeding. Clin Gastroenterol Hepatol 2008;6(4):418–25.

59. Tsoi KK, Lau JY, Sung JJ. Cost-effectiveness analysis of high-dose omeprazole infusion before endoscopy for patients with upper-GI bleeding. Gastrointest Endosc 2008;67(7):1056–63.

Predicting Poor Outcome from Acute Upper Gastrointestinal Hemorrhage

Philip W.Y. Chiu, MD*, Enders K.W. Ng, MD

KEYWORDS

- Acute non-variceal upper GI hemorrhage
- Acute variceal hemorrhage • Prediction • Mortality
- Rebleeding

Acute upper gastrointestinal (GI) hemorrhage is one of the commonest causes for hospitalization worldwide. In the United States, there are 250,000 to 300,000 hospital admissions and 15,000 to 30,000 deaths each year resulting from acute upper GI hemorrhage.[1,2] In England it is a common medical emergency with an annual incidence of 100 per 100,000.[3,4] Two meta-analyses conducted in the 1990s confirmed that endoscopic therapy is effective in achieving primary hemostasis.[3,4] The shift of management from operation theater to endoscopy suite has not changed the rate of mortality over the past 20 years. The reported mortality for patients with bleeding peptic ulcer still amounts to 15%.[2,5–7] Several hypotheses may account for the lack of improvement in the mortality resulting from bleeding peptic ulcer. Coinciding with the decline in the prevalence of *Helicobacter*-related peptic ulcer, the incidence of aspirin-related or other nonsteroidal antiinflammatory drug (NSAID)–related ulcer disease is on the rise.[8] Patients taking aspirin or other NSAIDs are usually in the older age group and have a background of severe comorbidities such as ischemic heart disease.[9] They are more vulnerable to a physiologic challenge from an acute bleeding episode. One of the potential directions toward improvement in the management of acute GI bleeding is to identify those at risk for adverse outcomes, which may improve the initial triage, timing of primary endoscopic hemostasis, and postendoscopic management.[9–11] Two adverse outcomes generally considered as significant for acute upper GI hemorrhage are rebleeding and mortality, and numerous clinical risk models have been developed to predict these outcomes. The following section focuses on a review of the reported predictive models in the literature on mortality and rebleeding for acute upper GI hemorrhage.

Department of Surgery, Institute of Digestive Disease, Prince of Wales Hospital, The Chinese University of Hong Kong, Hong Kong, China
* Corresponding author.
E-mail address: philipchiu@surgery.cuhk.edu.hk (P.W.Y. Chiu).

Gastroenterol Clin N Am 38 (2009) 215–230
doi:10.1016/j.gtc.2009.03.009
0889-8553/09/$ – see front matter © 2009 Elsevier Inc. All rights reserved.

gastro.theclinics.com

PREDICTION OF MORTALITY FOR ACUTE NONVARICEAL UPPER GI HEMORRHAGE

Rockall and colleagues[12] developed a well known prediction score for mortality from a prospective multicenter study of 4185 cases of acute upper GI hemorrhage. These included diagnosis of various etiologies, such as bleeding peptic ulcers, varices, esophagitis, Mallory-Weiss syndrome, and malignancy. This predictive scoring was subsequently accredited in another cohort of 1625 patients. The Rockall score consisted of age, shock, major comorbidities, the endoscopic diagnosis, and the presence of major stigmata of recent hemorrhage (SRH). All these factors were then combined and the significance of each factor was weighted according to their representation in the multivariate analysis (**Table 1**). These showed that the risk for mortality increased when the score increased. The Rockall score was further validated in a Dutch group's multicenter prospective cohort on prediction of both mortality and rebleeding in 951 patients.[18] On analysis with the receiver-operator characteristics (ROC) curve for prediction of mortality, it showed an area-under-curve (AUC) of 0.73 in the Dutch sample and an AUC of 0.81 in the Rockall sample. This confirmed that Rockall score is satisfactory in predicting mortality among patients with acute upper GI hemorrhage. However, the prediction of rebleeding did not seem to fit in both groups of patients. As Rockall score was initially designed to evaluate the risk for mortality, it may not perform as well to predict rebleeding. Another study enrolled 211 patients who were prospectively collected in two randomized controlled trials, and they were retrospectively evaluated on the prediction of clinical outcomes using Rockall score.[19] The authors found that those with a Rockall score of more than seven had a significantly higher risk for rebleeding and mortality. The study was limited by the sample size and retrospective nature. Zimmerman and colleagues[13] analyzed the prognostic factors among 321 patients with acute upper GI hemorrhage from 1988 to 1991. Multivariate analysis showed that age older than 75 years, blood in stomach, high serum creatinine and aminotransferase, and persistent or recurrent bleeding were significant factors that predicted mortality. In this study, there was no validation cohort to reply and confirm the predictive power of these factors. Moreover, there was a high rate of 18% rebleeding after endoscopic therapy and adjuvant high-dose proton pump inhibitor (PPI) therapy was not used as postendoscopic treatment.[20]

Blatchford and colleagues[5] conducted a regional audit in the west of Scotland on the epidemiology and clinical outcomes of patients who were admitted to 19 regional hospitals with a complaint of acute upper GI hemorrhage. The overall incidence was 172 per 100,000 per annum, and it was 67% more than the peak incidence reported in the United Kingdom. In 6 months the mortality was 8.1% among 1882 patients in the study group. Multiple logistic regression showed that age, uremia, diastolic hypotension, cardiac and hepatic failure, pre-existing malignancy, major pre-existing diseases such as rheumatoid arthritis or inflammatory bowel disease, and presentation with hematemesis or syncopy were associated with increased risk of fatality. Klebl and colleagues[14] reported a retrospective review of 454 patients with upper GI bleeding from 1992 to 1999. The main cause of upper GI hemorrhage in this group is still peptic ulcer, followed by varices and gastritis. Multivariate analysis showed that in-hospital bleeding, coagulopathy, renal disease, use of corticosteroid, cardiovascular disease, and diabetes mellitus were risk factors for mortality. The mortality rate in this group amounts to 26.5%, and 66.3% of these patients needed intensive care. The authors also analyzed the Rockall score for these patients and found that the mean Rockall score was 6.6 ± 1.3. This cohort most likely represented a selected group of patients who were at high risk and managed in a tertiary referral center. These risk factors identified were mostly related to significant comorbidities and background illnesses. Imperiale and colleagues[15] derived and internally validated several clinical prediction rules for risk stratification of patients with acute upper GI bleeding in a prospective cohort involving Veterans Affairs Medical Centers in Durham, Indianapolis, and Seattle. The adverse outcomes were defined as: (1) GI hemorrhage–specific outcomes (rebleeding, need for surgery or hospital death) and (2) GI bleeding–specific outcomes plus new or worsening comorbidity. From a total of 391 patients enrolled, the rate of rebleeding was 4.6% and the overall mortality was 3.1%. From the derivation cohort, several factors were identified from multiple logistic regressions as predictors which included stigmata of recent hemorrhage, APACHE II score greater than 11, diagnosis of esophageal varices, and unstable comorbidity at hospital admission. These factors were then combined to classify the validation cohort into low-, intermediate-, and high-risk for adverse outcomes. The c-statistic for prediction of GI hemorrhage–specific outcomes was 0.83. This study defined outcomes as GI hemorrhage–specific outcomes, including rebleeding, need for surgery, or hospital death. Hence this model was not specific for predicting mortality. Moreover, the population from which this risk model was derived was US veterans, which led to a 99% preponderance of men. APACHE score had been studied by several other groups for risk assessment and prediction of death in acute upper GI hemorrhage.[21–23] Wang and colleagues[22] used APACHE II to differentiate patients at high risk with bleeding gastric ulcers. It was found that the mortality rate was 58% for those with an APACHE score of 15 or greater as compared with 5% for those with a score less than 15. The patients included in this study were those who had failed endoscopic treatment. Hence they represented a selected high-risk group of severe hemorrhage requiring surgical interventions, and their outcomes were expected to be poor. There may also be a logistic issue in clinical application of this risk model, as APACHE score will usually be available after the completion of the clinical management process. Marmo and colleagues[16] reported a prospective multicenter study from Italy on patients with upper GI hemorrhage. Among a prospectively recruited cohort of 1020 patients, they showed an overall mortality of 4.5% and a rebleeding rate of 3.2%. Regression analysis showed that advanced age, presence of severe comorbidity, low hemoglobin levels at presentation, and worsening health status were independent factors that predicted 30-days mortality. The authors used a computer linked system for collection of data with independent data validation from a random set of samples for quality assurance. Ninety-seven percent of patients in this cohort received PPIs after endoscopic hemostasis. The use of H2 receptor antagonist was associated with a significantly increased 30-days mortality (15% versus 4%) while use of PPIs showed a protective effect with an absolute risk reduction of 11.5%. Leontiadis and colleagues[24] reported a systematic review on the use of PPIs after endoscopic therapy for bleeding peptic ulcer and showed that PPIs significantly reduce rebleeding and need for surgery. The focus was on identification of risk factors for bleeding peptic ulcer–related mortality among 3220 patients as derivation cohort, and 634 patients as evaluation cohort.[17] On multivariate analysis, age older than 70 years, presence of listed comorbidities, more than one comorbidity, hematemesis, initial systolic blood pressure <100 mmHg, and in-hospital bleeding were independent pre-endoscopic predictors, whereas rebleeding and need for surgery were postendoscopic predictors for in-hospital mortality. The resulting factors were grouped to a score and validated in a separate cohort of 634 prospective patients. The authors found that the risk for mortality increased when the composite score was ≧3. The model was limited by the fact that only people of Chinese ethnicity were included. Validation would be

Table 1
Summary of the reported predictive factors for mortality in acute upper gastrointestinal bleeding

	Rockall et al (1995)[12]	Zimmerman et al (1995)[13]	Blatchford et al (1997)[5]	Klebl et al (2005)[14]	Imperiale et al (2007)[15]	Marmo et al (2008)[16]	Chiu et al (2008)[17]
Age	2.8 (2.14–3.67)	12.7 (1.9–84.4)	4.5 (2.0–10)			4.7 (2.3–7.0)	1.47 (1.09–1.98)
ASA						7.24 (4.0–10.4)	
APACHE II					3.11 (1.13–8.57)		
No. of comorbidities	—						1.70 (1.23–2.36)
Type of comorbidities	—				5.25 (2.34–11.79)		4.12 (2.65–6.39)
Cardiac failure	7.73 (5.68–10.5)		9.4 (3.2–28)				
Ischemic heart disease	4.3 (3.17–5.81)						
Liver cirrhosis/failure	8.65 (6.01–12.5)		43 (14–133)			11.01 (7.5–14.5)	
Renal disease/failure	10.3 (6.96–15.3)			2.4 (1.3–4.2)		5.29 (2.8–7.8)	
Diabetes mellitus				0.5 (0.3–1.1)			
Disseminated malignancy	11.7 (8.28–16.6)		3.8 (1.8–8.1)			9.81 (7.3–12.3)	
Hematological malignancy	6.23 (3.91–9.94)						
Coagulopathy				3.2 (1.8–5.7)			
Systolic blood pressure			9.8 (5.1–19)				2.24 (1.65–3.05)
Tachycardia	2.17 (1.73–2.71)		0.6 (0.43–0.91)				
Presentation of shock	3.37 (2.58–4.39)						

In-hospital bleeding			4.8 (2.5–9.2)	2.46 (1.78–3.39)
Hematemesis		2.0 (1.1–3.5)		1.45 (1.02–2.05)
Syncope		3.0 (1.3–7.0)		
Corticosteroid usage			2.2 (1.0–4.3)	
Hemoglobin	1.94 (1.61–2.33)	3.8 (2.4–6.2)		4.7 (2.3–7.0)
Urea		18 (5.3–59)[a]		
Creatinine level	14.8 (2.6–83.5)	5.8 (3.2–11)[b]		
Aminotransferase	20.2 (2.9–140.4)			
Diagnosis at endoscopy	3.93 (2.8–5.5)[c]		3.85 (1.31–11.3)	
SRH	3.97 (3.08–5.1)		5.28 (1.89–14.8)	
Blood in stomach	18.9 (1.8–203.7)			
H pylori	-			0.20 (0.13–0.33)
Rebleeding	6.24 (5.15–7.56)	57.3 (7.2–453.9)		1.63 (1.09–2.41)
Surgery				4.60 (2.95–7.19)

[a] Urea ≥ 25 mmol/L.
[b] Creatinine ≥ 200 mmol/L.
[c] Diagnosis at endoscopy is malignancy.

necessary if this predictive score is to apply to acute upper GI hemorrhage and other ethnicities.

Table 1 summarizes the reported predictive factors for mortality in patients presenting with acute upper GI bleeding. Each of the identified predictive factors was represented by the odds ratio and the 95% confidence interval. The most frequently reported factors included old age, presence of significant comorbidity including cardiac disease, liver and renal failure, disseminated malignancy, presentation with shock (in terms of low systolic blood pressure or tachycardia), in-hospital bleeding, low hemoglobin, diagnosis at endoscopy, presence of SRH, and development of rebleeding. These factors can be arbitrarily subclassified into pre-endoscopic and post-endoscopic factors. Pre-endoscopic factors such as advanced age and significant comorbidities coupled with a severe episode of bleeding represented by significant hemodynamic changes or anemia upon presentation, lead to high mortality. A retrospective review from the authors' institute from a cohort of 10,428 patients who presented with peptic ulcer bleeding showed that the majority of the mortality was because of non–bleeding-related death, including multiorgan failure, pulmonary conditions, or terminal malignancy.[25] The clinical applications of these predictive factors were explored in another study which developed the Cedars-Sinai Medical Center predictive index based on an explicit review of the reported risk factors in the literature.[26] The score includes clinical and endoscopic predictors including a predefined list of significant comorbidities, advanced age, endoscopic diagnosis, and evidence of active bleeding. Among a cohort of 500 patients, it was found that the application of this predictive score will allow a significantly shorter hospital stay with minimal complication.

PREDICTION OF MORTALITY FOR ACUTE VARICEAL HEMORRHAGE

Most of the prediction factors for mortality among patients with nonvariceal upper GI hemorrhage were reviewed. Liver failure and cirrhosis were reported in several studies as important comorbidities to predict mortality. For patients with a background of liver cirrhosis presenting with acute variceal hemorrhage, the risk for mortality can be up to 50%.[14,15] Lecleire and colleagues[27] prospectively studied patients from four French geographic areas, with or without liver cirrhosis, who presented with acute upper GI hemorrhage. Variceal bleeding served as the most common cause (59.1%) for patients with cirrhosis, whereas bleeding peptic ulcer was the commonest diagnosis (41.8%) for patients without cirrhosis. Six independent predictors for mortality were identified for both groups, which included decreased prothrombin level, coexisting digestive carcinoma, use of corticosteroid, occurrence of upper GI hemorrhage in an inpatient, hematemesis, and age over 60 years (**Table 2**). The prothrombin level directly correlated with the severity of liver cirrhosis. Le Moine derived predictive factors for early mortality in patients who had cirrhosis with bleeding varices among 121 patients. Three independent prognostic indicators were identified including encephalopathy, prothrombin time, and amount of blood transfused.[29] The authors compared the predictive power of these factors to the Child-Pugh grading and found that the composite model achieved a better prediction. Two of the factors within the Child-Pugh grading, namely encephalopathy and prothrombin time, are important predictors for mortality. Sakaki and colleagues reviewed 98 patients who were on long-term endoscopic sclerotherapy and presented with acute variceal hemorrhage. It was found that the presence of hepatocellular carcinoma, bilirubin and albumin levels, and time to reach hospital were independent predictive factors for mortality. The conclusion coincided with the previous report that remnant hepatic function was an important prognostic indicator. Gatta and

Table 2
Summary of the reported predictive factors for mortality in acute variceal bleeding

	Garden et al (1985)[28]	Le Moine et al (1992)[29]	Lee et al (1992)[30]	Gatta et al (1994)[31]	Sakaki et al (1998)[32]	Lecleire et al (2005)[32]
Age >60						1.83 (1.07–3.13)[a]
Gender				0.386 (0.043)		
Encephalopathy	<0.001[b]	−2.748 (<0.01)				
GCS			1.3[c]			
Hepatocellular carcinoma				−0.842 (0.004)	0.968 (0.0027)	4.54 (2.07–9.95)[a]
Ascites				−0.306 (<0.001)		
In-hospital bleeding						3.55 (1.92–6.58)[a]
Hematemesis				0.405 (0.037)		2.66 (1.46–4.84)[a]
Corticosteroid usage						3.80 (1.32–10.9)[a]
Time to hospital					1.931 (0.0001)	
Shock			3.7[c]			
Blood transfusion (units)	0.005[b]	−0.310 (<0.05)	6.1[c]			
Bilirubin				−0.010 (0.001)	1.463 (0.0001)	
Prothrombin time/INR		0.102 (<0.01)	1.9[c]	0.036 (0.013)		7.93 (4.58–13.7)[a]
Albumin					−1.068 (0.0033)	
Urea	0.05[b]					
Creatinine level	0.001[b]			−0.016 (<0.001)		
Varices as source of bleeding				−0.442 (0.020)		
Endoscopic sclerotherapy (volume of sclerosant injected)			1.2[c]			

[a] odds ratio with 95% confidence intervals.
[b] only P value was provided.
[c] odds ratio only.

colleagues[31] developed and validated a prognostic index on the basis of risk factors identified from 268 patients with cirrhosis. These factors included gender, presentation with hematemesis, serum creatinine, ascites, hepatocellular carcinoma, serum bilirubin, prothrombin index, and bleeding varices. This prognostic index was significantly better than Child-Pugh score and the Garden prognostic index in predicting mortality among patients with upper GI bleeding and cirrhosis.[28] Afessa and Kubilis[33] compared the Child-Pugh grading, Garden' score, Gatta's score, and APACHE II score in predicting the clinical outcomes for patients with cirrhosis and acute upper GI bleeding. Among 85 patients, the in-hospital mortality rate was 21% and the intensive care unit (ICU) admission rate was 71%. Child-Pugh grading showed an area-under-curve (AUC) of 0.76, which was similar to Garden's (AUC of 0.70) and Gatta's scores (AUC of 0.71). Although APACHE II achieved a similar AUC of 0.78, it tended to overestimate the risk for mortality. The new APACHE III system may improve the deficiency of APACHE II in predicting the outcome for patients with cirrhosis as its components include liver function.[33] Among 101 patients with liver cirrhosis and esophageal variceal bleeding requiring ICU admission, total volume of ethanolamine injection during sclerotherapy, multiple blood transfusions, Glasgow Coma Scale (GCS), international normalized ratio (INR), and the presence of shock on admission were independent predictors for mortality.[30] In this study, neither the APACHE II nor Child-Pugh grading was an independent predictor for mortality. The authors commented that both Child-Pugh and APACHE II were not predictors despite showing a difference in the outcomes by univariate analysis, GCS having a strong predictive value on multivariate analysis. GCS probably reflected the severity of hepatic encephalopathy as urea or creatinine levels showed the severity of hepatorenal syndrome.

PREDICTION OF REBLEEDING/THERAPEUTIC FAILURE FOR ACUTE UPPER GASTROINTESTINAL HEMORRHAGE

Rebleeding is one of the important predictive factors for mortality.[7,12,17] Prevention of rebleeding aims to reduce the risk of mortality. Strategies to prevent rebleeding can be divided into improvement in the primary endoscopic hemostasis, management before endoscopic hemostasis, and enhancement of the post-endoscopic management.[20,34–36] By recognizing the predictive factors for rebleeding, it is possible to stratify patients' risk levels, and resources can be allocated for more intensive clinical management of patients at high risk. There are numerous studies reporting predictive factors for rebleeding, and the following section summarizes the findings.

Before the era of primary endoscopic hemostasis, the importance of predicting continuous and recurrent bleeding was to select patients for early surgical intervention. Storey and colleagues[37] showed that endoscopic SRH were an important factor to predict further bleeding. Clason and colleagues[38] reported on the clinical factors to predict rebleeding in 326 patients with acute upper GI hemorrhage. Age older than 60 years, decreased hemoglobin, and presence of endoscopic stigmata predicted further hemorrhage. Endoscopic SRH appeared to be the significant factor to predict rebleeding before the era of endoscopic treatment.[39] The effect of SRH in predicting further bleeding, however, may not be consistent, as the natural history could be changed by endoscopic treatment. Moreover, a wide inter-observer variation would further compromise the usefulness of SRH.[40]

Saeed and colleagues[41] derived a prediction score to stratify patients with acute upper GI hemorrhage into high or low risk for rebleeding among 80 patients in a prospective randomized trial. The prediction model consisted of pre-endoscopic and endoscopic scores. The pre-endoscopic score included age, number of illnesses, and severity of illnesses, whereas the postendoscopic score included site and the stigmata of hemorrhage. It was found that those who developed rebleeding had a pre-endoscopic score of ≥ 6 and postendoscopic score of ≥ 11. Using the Baylor score to select patients for second-look endoscopy, they were able to show a significant reduction in rebleeding as compared with those managed conservatively.[42] The number of samples recruited to develop and validate the Baylor score is, however, limited. Moreover, the predictive factors were not identified using multivariate analysis. Villanueva and colleagues[43] studied the risk factors to predict therapeutic failure after endoscopic hemostasis in a cohort of 233 patients with bleeding peptic ulcers. The factors identified from stepwise logistic regression included location of the ulcer at posterior and superior walls of the duodenal bulb, ulcer size, and presence of associated diseases. A prognostic score developed from these factors was validated with a prospective cohort of 88 patients, which yielded a sensitivity and specificity of 75.2%. Lin and colleagues[44] studied the risk factors for rebleeding among 140 patients with bleeding peptic ulcers having a visible vessel. On multivariate analysis, coffee ground–like material or blood in the stomach and ulcer size greater than 2 cm emerged as independent factors to predict rebleeding. This study aimed at clarifying various appearances of endoscopic stigmata and definition of visible vessel, and the patient group was selected to be those with nonbleeding visible vessels alone. Park and colleagues[56] reported a prospective cohort of 135 patients with acute upper GI bleeding and found that tachycardia, ulcer location, and obesity were independent factors to predict rebleeding. The authors, however, did not report the resulting odds ratio or P values from the logistic regression. Brullet and colleagues[45,46] reported the factors to predict rebleeding after endoscopic therapy for gastric and duodenal ulcers in 2 separate articles. Multivariate analysis showed that for both gastric and duodenal ulcers presence of shock and ulcer size larger than 2 cm were common risks factors for rebleeding, whereas active bleeding at endoscopy and high lesser-curvature ulcers were additional risk factors for rebleeding in gastric ulcers. High lesser-curvature ulcers were shown to be a significant risk factor for rebleeding which could be related to the difficult anatomic location for successful endoscopic therapy and the close proximity of this ulcer to the left gastric artery.[47,48] Chung and colleagues[49] found that on multivariate analysis among 143 patients with bleeding peptic ulcers, arterial spurter was the single independent factor to predict rebleeding. In this study, the location of the ulcer at lesser curvature and posterior duodenal bulb and ulcer larger than 2 cm in size were important risk factors for rebleeding in univariate analysis though not statistically significant on multivariate analysis. Thomopoulos and colleagues[50] reported from a cohort of 427 patients with bleeding peptic ulcers that shock on admission, active spurter on endoscopy, and posteriorly located duodenal ulcer were important factors to predict failure of endoscopic hemostasis. Another prospective study from Italy analyzed the factors that predict rebleeding among 738 patients with bleeding peptic ulcers.[51] Multivariate analysis showed that liver cirrhosis, recent surgery, shock, hematemesis, endoscopic stigmata of Forrest I, IIa, and IIb, ulcer size, and site were significant factors to predict rebleeding. In this cohort, only patients with bleeding peptic ulcers were recruited and the management included endoscopic hemostasis for Forrest I, IIa, and IIb lesions, postendoscopic omeprazole given as a bolus, and a routine second endoscopy 48 hours afterwards. Numerous studies recognized that significant SRH were factors to predict rebleeding.[46,50–52] This could reflect that significant stigmata represented important factors to predict rebleeding, or the possibility of inadequate primary endoscopic therapy to achieve perfect hemostasis. Most of these studies employed the endoscopic techniques of monotherapy. Calvet and colleagues summarized the results of 16 randomized trials between

1990 and 2000 comparing injection of epinephrine alone against addition of a second treatment for ulcer hemostasis. Addition of a second therapy significantly reduced rebleeding (18.4% to 10.6%) and need of surgery (11.3% to 7.6%).[35] The current standard treatment for endoscopic hemostasis of bleeding peptic ulcer should be dual therapy combining injection and thermal or mechanical therapy. Swain and colleagues[53] studied specimens of gastrectomies for uncontrolled bleeding peptic ulcer in 27 patients. 96% of these ulcers with visible vessel identified during endoscopy showed the same vessel upon histologic examination. Most of these vessels were shown either protruded above the ulcer crater or a clot in continuity with a breach in the vessel wall. Lau and colleagues[54] studied the evolution of SRH on consecutive endoscopic re-examination among 778 patients with bleeding peptic ulcers. The prevalence of numerous stigmata showed a downgrading trend from day 1 to day 3. The overall rebleeding risk was 9.9%, 4.9%, and 2.7% on days 1, 2, and 3 respectively. Hence a successful hemostasis for bleeding peptic ulcers should persist for at least 72 hours. The authors reviewed 3386 patients admitted with bleeding peptic ulcers treated by endoscopic therapy.[55] On multivariate analysis, hypotension, hemoglobin less than 10 g/dL, fresh blood in stomach, active bleeding ulcer, and large ulcers were independent factors to predict rebleeding. In 2008, Elmunzer and colleagues[52] performed a systematic review to summarize numerous factors to predict recurrent hemorrhage after endoscopic therapy for patients with bleeding peptic ulcers. A thorough search in Medline and Embase with independent review from two investigators selected prospective studies that addressed the issue of identifying factors that predict rebleeding after endoscopic hemostasis with a multivariate analysis. The studies which were included in this systematic review were mostly discussed in the last section.[41,43,45,49–51,55–57] On pooling data, the authors found that the overall rate of successful primary hemostasis was 92.3% with a rebleeding rate of 16.4%. Independent risk factors for ulcer rebleeding after endoscopic therapy included (1) hemodynamic instability; (2) comorbid illnesses; (3) active bleeding; (4) large ulcer size; (5) posterior duodenal ulcer; and (6) lesser curvature ulcer.

PREDICTORS FOR ULCER REBLEEDING DIFFER FROM THOSE FOR MORTALITY IN ACUTE UPPER GASTROINTESTINAL BLEEDING

There is a difference in the characteristics of the factors that predict ulcer rebleeding and mortality for acute upper GI hemorrhage (see **Table 1**; **Table 3**). Predictors for recurrent bleeding are usually those related to the severity of hemorrhage and the characteristics of ulcer, whereas those for mortality are more attributed to physical status and comorbidity of the patient. Although age and various types of comorbidities were frequently factors to predict mortality, scarcely were these risk factors for rebleeding in acute upper GI hemorrhage. Most of the predictive models for mortality were developed from a cohort of patients with acute upper GI bleeding regardless of the cause of hemorrhage. Hence diagnosis at endoscopy served as one of the predictive factors. Most studies addressing the prediction of rebleeding were built from a cohort of patients with bleeding peptic ulcers. This might partly explain the issue of differences in the predictive factors for rebleeding and mortality. A consensus guideline on management of non-variceal upper GI bleeding recommends risk stratification at patient presentation for triaging cases with high and low risk for rebleeding and death.[58] Most experts agreed that the risk factors for mortality included age older than 60 years; shock; poor overall health status; comorbid illnesses; continued bleeding or rebleeding; fresh red blood on rectal examination, in the emesis or in the nasogastric aspirate; onset of bleeding while hospitalized for another reason; sepsis; or elevated urea, creatinine, or

Table 3
Summary of the reported predictive factors for rebleeding in acute upper gastrointestinal bleeding

	Villanueva et al (1993)[43]	Lin et al (1994)[44]	Brullet et al (1996)[46]	Brullet et al (1991)[47]	Chung et al (2001)[49]	Thomopoulos et al (2001)[50]	Guglielmi et al (2002)[51]	Wong et al (2002)[55]
Comorbidity	0.012[a]							
Liver cirrhosis							2.30 (1.0–5.29)	
Recent surgery							2.50 (1.19–5.28)	
Hematemesis							1.57 (0.94–2.61)	
Shock			2.38 (0.86–6.56)	3.53 (1.27–4.10)		2.31 (1.33–6.97)	3.68 (1.99–6.81)	2.21 (1.40–3.48)
Hb < 10 g/dL								1.87 (1.18–2.96)
Coffee ground fluid		3.54 (1.41–8.85)						
Blood in stomach		11.53 (2.83–47.1)						2.15 (1.40–3.31)
Active bleeding			2.98 (1.12–7.91)		6.48 (1.88–22.5)	2.45 (1.51–3.93)		1.65 (1.07–2.56)
Visible vessel							10.6 (2.39–46.98)	
Adherent clot							11.3 (2.47–51.64)	
Ulcer size	0.011[a]	5.24 (0.82–33.6)	3.64 (1.34–9.89)	2.29 (1.13–10.9)			4.61 (2.20–9.64)	1.80 (1.15–2.83)
Posterior duodenal bulb	0.004[a]					2.48 (1.37–7.01)	1.19 (0.49–2.9)	
High lesser-curve ulcer			2.79 (1.01–7.69)				2.56 (1.12–5.83)	

[a] P values.

serum aminotransferase levels. Although these coincided with most of the factors reviewed, concerns about generalizability of various predictive models and insufficient external validation remained. There is a wide variation in the quality of study and older studies predated modern resuscitation and endoscopic management.

POTENTIAL MANAGEMENT OF STRATIFIED PATIENTS WITH ACUTE UPPER GASTROINTESTINAL HEMORRHAGE

Several strategies may be applied to those stratified as high-risk with a view to prevent catastrophic events for acute upper GI bleeding. Baradarian and colleagues[10] reported that early aggressive resuscitation reduced the days in the ICU , surgical intervention, and mortality from upper GI bleeding. Early endoscopy within 24 hours after admission would also be performed for those categorized as high-risk. A randomized controlled trial confirmed that early endoscopic therapy reduced transfusion requirements and length of hospital stay.[59,60] Although selective second-look endoscopy reduces rebleeding in high-risk patients, a routine practice is not recommended because of the high cost and the pressure on endoscopists' workload.[28,56,58] The use of high-dose adjunctive intravenous PPIs would certainly be justified in these patients with high risk.[20] Outpatient management for those categorized as low-risk may be another approach to reduce hospital admissions and allow better resource allocation.[52] A recent multicenter study calculated the Glasgow-Blatchford bleeding score (GBS) for 676 patients who presented with acute upper GI hemorrhage to predict the need for hospital-based interventions including transfusion, endoscopic treatment, or surgery.[61] The GBS was shown to be better in predicting need for intervention or death as compared with the Rockall score. Twenty-two percent of patients from another validation cohort were classified as low-risk, and 68% of these were managed as outpatient without adverse events. Cooper and colleagues[62] studied a retrospectively identified cohort of patients from Medicare who had acute upper GI hemorrhage managed as outpatients. Almost 40% of these patients were managed as outpatient, with an excessive 30-day mortality of 6.3% as compared with 8.0% for those managed as inpatients. This suggested that more stringent criteria of selection and prospective validation of these models may be necessary before application to stratify patients for outpatient management.[62]

SUMMARY

In conclusion, numerous prediction models identified pre-endoscopic and endoscopic risk factors for adverse clinical outcomes in patients with acute upper GI hemorrhage. The risk factors for mortality are different from those of rebleeding. Predictors for rebleeding are usually related to the severity of the bleeding and characteristics of the ulcer, whereas advanced age, physical status of the patient, and co-morbidities are important predictors for mortality in addition to those for rebleeding. Future studies should focus on validation of these predictors in a prospective cohort and application of these prediction models to guide clinical management in patients with acute upper GI hemorrhage.

REFERENCES

1. Gilbert DA. Epidemiology of upper gastrointestinal bleeding. Gastrointest Endosc 1990;36(Suppl):S8–13.
2. Rockall TA, Logan RFA, Devlin HB, et al. Incidence of and mortality from acute upper gastrointestinal hemorrhage in the UK. Br Med J 1995;311:222–6.

3. Cook DJ, Guyatt GH, Salena BJ, et al. Endoscopic therapy for acute non-variceal upper gastrointestinal hemorrhage: a meta-analysis. Gastroenterology 1992;102: 139–48.
4. Sacks HS, Chalmers TC, Blum AL, et al. Endoscopic hemostasis: an effective therapy for bleeding peptic ulcer. JAMA 1990;264(4):494–9.
5. Blatchford O, Davidson LA, Murray WR, et al. Acute upper gastrointestinal hemorrhage in west of Scotland: case ascertainment study. Br Med J 1997; 315:510–4.
6. Longstreth GF. Epidemiology of hospitalization for acute upper gastrointestinal hemorrhage: a population-based study. Am J Gastroenterol 1995;90(2): 206–10.
7. van Leerdam ME, Vreeburg EM, Rauws EA, et al. Acute upper GI bleeding: did anything change? Time trend analysis of incidence and outcome of acute upper GI bleeding between 1993/1994 and 2000. Am J Gastroenterol 2003;98(7): 1494–9.
8. Graham DY, Chan FK. NSAIDs, Risks and Gastroprotective strategies: Current status and future. Gastroenterology 2008;134:1240–57.
9. Chan FK, Leung WK. Peptic ulcer disease. Lancet 2002;360:933–41.
10. Baradarian R, Ramdhaney S, Chapalamadugu R. Early intensive resuscitation of patients with upper gastrointestinal bleeding decreases mortality. Am J Gastroenterol 2004;99:619–22.
11. Adamopoulos AB, Baibas NM, Efstathiou SP, et al. Differentiation between patients with acute upper gastrointestinal bleeding who need early urgent upper gastrointestinal endoscopy and those who do not. A prospective study. Eur J Gastroenterol Hepatol 2003;15(4):381–7.
12. Rockall TA, Logan RFA, Devlin HB, et al. Risk assessment after acute upper gastrointestinal hemorrhage. Gut 1996;38:316–21.
13. Zimmerman J, Siguencia J, Tsvang E, et al. Predictors to mortality in patients admitted to hospital for acute upper gastrointestinal hemorrhage. Scand J Gastroenterol 1995;30:327–31.
14. Klebl F, Bregenzer N, Schofer L, et al. Risk factors for mortality in severe upper gastrointestinal bleeding. Int J Colorectal Dis 2005;20:49–56.
15. Imperiale T, Dominitz J, Provenzale DT, et al. Predicting poor outcome from acute upper gastrointestinal hemorrhage. Arch Intern Med 2007;167:1291–6.
16. Marmo R, Koch M, Cipolletta L, et al. Predictive factors of mortality from non-variceal upper gastrointestinal hemorrhage: a multicenter study. Am J Gastroenterol 2008;103:1639–47.
17. Chiu PW, Ng EK, Cheung FK, et al. Predicting mortality in patients with bleeding peptic ulcers after therapeutic endoscopy. Clin Gastroenterol Hepatol 2009;7: 311–6.
18. Vreeburg EM, Terwee CB, Snel P, et al. Validation of the Rockall risk scoring system in upper gastrointestinal bleeding. Gut 1999;44(3):331–5.
19. Church NI, Palmer KR. Relevance of the Rockall score in patients undergoing endoscopic therapy for peptic ulcer hemorrhage. Eur J Gastroenterol Hepatol 2001;13:1149–52.
20. Lau JYW, Sung JJY, Lee KKC, et al. Effect of intravenous omeprazole on recurrent bleeding after endoscopic treatment of bleeding peptic ulcer. N Engl J Med 2000;343:310–6.
21. Gorad DA, Newton M, Burnham WR. APACHE II scores and deaths after upper gastrointestinal endoscopy in hospital inpatients. J Clin Gastroenterol 2000;30: 392–6.

22. Wang BW, Mok KT, Chang HT, et al. APACHE II score: a useful tool for risk assessment and an aid to decision-making in emergency operation for bleeding gastric ulcer. J Am Coll Surg 1998;187:287–94.

23. Schein M, Gecelter G. APACHE II score in massive upper gastrointestinal hemorrhage from peptic ulcer: prognostic value and potential clinical applications. British Journal of Surgery 1989;76(7):733–6.

24. Leontiadis GI, Sharma VK, Howden CW. Proton pump inhibitor treatment for acute peptic ulcer bleeding [review]. Cochrane Database Syst Rev 2006;(1):CD002094.

25. Sung JJY, Tsoi KKF, Ma TKW, et al. Causes of mortality in patients with peptic ulcer bleeding: a prospective cohort study of 10,428 cases. Gastrointest Endosc 2008;67(5):AB88.

26. Hay JA, Lyubashevsky E, Elashoff J, et al. Upper gastrointestinal hemorrhage clinical guideline – determining the optimal hospital length of stay. Am J Med 1996;100:313–22.

27. Lecleire S, Di Fiore F, Merle V, et al. Acute upper gastrointestinal bleeding in patients with liver cirrhosis and in noncirrhotic patients – epidemiology and predictive factors of mortality ina prospective multicenter population based study. J Clin Gastroenterol 2005;39(4):321–7.

28. Garden OJ, Motyl H, Gilmour WH, et al. Prediction of outcome following acute variceal hemorrhage. Br J Surg 1985;72(2):91–5.

29. Le Moine O, Adler M, Bourgeois N, et al. Factors related to early mortality in cirrhotic patients bleeding from varices and treated by urgent sclerotherapy. Gut 1992;33:1381–5.

30. Lee HL, Hawker FH, Selby W, et al. Intensive care treatment of patients with bleeding esophageal varices: results, predictors of mortality, and predictors of the adult respiratory distress syndrome. Crit Care Med 1992;20:1555–63.

31. Gatta A, Merket C, Amodio P, et al. Development and validation of a prognostic index predicting death after upper gastrointestinal bleeding in patients with liver cirrhosis: a multicenter study. Am J Gastroenterol 1994;89(9):1528–36.

32. Sakaki M, Iwao T, Oho K, et al. Prognostic factors in cirrhotic patients receiving long-term sclerotherapy for the first bleeding from esophageal varices. Eur J Gastroenterol Hepatol 1998;10(1):21–6.

33. Afessa B, Kubilis PS. Upper gastrointestinal bleeding in patients with hepatic cirrhosis: clinical course and mortality prediction. American Journal of Gastroenterology 2000;95:484–9.

34. Chiu PWY, Lam CYW, Lee SW, et al. Effect of scheduled second therapeutic endoscopy on peptic ulcer rebleeding: a prospective randomized trial. Gut 2003;52:1403–7.

35. Calvet X, Vergara M, Brullet E, et al. Addition of a second endoscopic treatment following epinephrine injection improves outcome in high risk bleeding ulcers. Gastroenterology 2004;126:441–50.

36. Lau JYW, Leung WK, Wu JCY, et al. Omeprazole before endoscopy in patients with gastrointestinal bleeding. N Engl J Med 2007;356:1631–40.

37. Storey DW, Bown SG, Swain P, et al. Endoscopic prediction of recurrent bleeding in peptic ulcers. N Engl J Med 1981;305:915–6.

38. Clason AE, Macleod DAD, Elton RA. Clinical factors in the prediction of further hemorrhage or mortality in acute upper gastrointestinal hemorrhage. Br J Surg 1986;73:985–7.

39. Foster DN, Miloszewski KJA, Losowsky MS. Stigmata of recent hemorrhage in diagnosis and prognosis of upper gastrointestinal bleeding. Br Med J 1978;1:1173–7.
40. Lau JYW, Sung JJY, Chan ACW, et al. Stigmata of hemorrhage in bleeding peptic ulcers: an interobserver agreement study among international experts. Gastrointest Endosc 1997;46(1):33–6.
41. Saeed ZA, Winchester CB, Michaletz PA, et al. A scoring system to predict rebleeding after endoscopic therapy of nonvariceal upper gastrointestinal hemorrhage with a comparison of heat probe and ethanol injection. Am J Gastroenterol 1993;88:1842–9.
42. Saeed ZA, Cole RA, Ramirez FC, et al. Endoscopic retreatment after successful initial hemostasis prevents ulcer rebleeding: a prospective randomized trial. Endoscopy 1996;28:288–94.
43. Villanueva C, Balanzo J, Espinos JC, et al. Prediction of therapeutic failure in patients with bleeding peptic ulcer treated with endoscopic injection. Dig Dis Sci 1993;38(11):2062–70.
44. Lin HJ, Perng CL, Lee FY, et al. Clinical courses and predictors for rebleeding in patients with peptic ulcers and non-bleeding visible vessels: a prospective study. Gut 1994;35:1389–93.
45. Brullet E, Campo R, Calvet X, et al. Factors related to the failure of endoscopic injection therapy for bleeding gastric ulcer. Gut 1996;39(2):155–8.
46. Brullet E, Calvet X, Campo R, et al. Factors predicting failure of endoscopic injection therapy in bleeding duodenal ulcer. Gastrointest Endosc 1996;43(2):111–6.
47. Brullet E, Campo R, Bedos G, et al. Site and size of bleeding peptic ulcer. Is there any relation to the efficacy of hemostatic sclerotherapy? Endoscopy 1991;23:73–5.
48. Chong CCN, Chiu PWY, Ng EKW. Multibend endoscope facilitates endoscopic hemostasis for bleeding gastric ulcer at high lesser curvature. Journal of Laparoendoscopic and Advanced Surgical Techniques 2008;18(6):837–9.
49. Chung IK, Kim EJ, Lee MS, et al. Endoscopic factors predisposing to rebleeding following endoscopic hemostasis in bleeding peptic ulcers. Endoscopy 2001;33(11):969–75.
50. Thomopoulos K, Mitropoulos J, Katsakoulis E, et al. Factors associated with failure of endoscopic injection haemostasis in bleeding peptic ulcers. Scand J Gastroenterol 2001;36(6):664–8.
51. Guglielmi A, Ruzzenente A, Sandri M, et al. Risk assessment and prediction of rebleeding in bleeding gastroduodenal ulcer. Endoscopy 2002;34(10):778–86.
52. Elmunzer BJ, Young SD, Inadomi JM, et al. Systematic review of the predictors of recurrent hemorrhage after endoscopic hemostatic therapy for bleeding peptic ulcers. Am J Gastroenterol 2008;103:2625–32.
53. Swain CP, Storey DW, Bown SG, et al. Nature of the bleeding vessel in recurrently bleeding gastric ulcer. Gastroenterology 1986;90:595–608.
54. Lau JYW, Chung SC, Leung JW, et al. Evolution of stigmata of hemorrhage in bleeding peptic ulcers: a sequential endoscopic study. Endoscopy 1998;30(6):570–4.
55. Wong SKH, Yu LM, Lau JYW, et al. Prediction of therapeutic failure after adrenaline injection plus heater probe treatment in patients with bleeding peptic ulcer. Gut 2002;50:322–5.
56. Park KG, Steele RJ, Mollison J, et al. Prediction of recurrent bleeding after endoscopic hemostasis in non-variceal upper gastrointestinal hemorrhage. Br J Surg 1994;81:1465–8.

57. Choudari C, Rajgopal C, Elton R, et al. Factors predicting failure of endoscopic therapy for bleeding peptic ulcer: an analysis of risk factors. Am J Gastroenterol 1994;89:1968–72.

58. Barkun A, Bardou M, Marshall JK. Consensus recommendtations for managing patients with nonvariceal upper gastrointestinal bleeding. Ann Intern Med 2003;139:843–57.

59. Da Silveira EB, Lam E, Martel M, et al. The importance of process issues as predictors of time to endoscopy in patients with acute upper GI bleeding using the RUGBE data. Gastrointest Endosc 2006;64(3):299–309.

60. Lin HJ, Wang K, Perng CL, et al. Early or delayed endoscopy for patients with peptic ulcer bleeding. A prospective randomized study. J Clin Gastroenterol 1996;22(4):267–71.

61. Stanley AJ, Ashley D, Dalton HR, et al. Outpatient management of patients with low risk upper gastrointestinal hemorrhage: multicenter validation and prospective evaluation. Lancet 2009;373(3):42–7.

62. Cooper GS, Kou TD, Wong RCK. Outpatient management of nonvariceal upper gastrointestinal hemorrhage: unexpected mortality in medicare beneficiaries. Gastroenterology 2009;136:108–14.

Management of Massive Peptic Ulcer Bleeding

Frances K.Y. Cheung, FRCS, James Y.W. Lau, MD

KEYWORDS
- Bleeding peptic ulcer • Endoscopy • Surgery
- Angiographic embolization

In an old surgical series, massive bleeding from a peptic ulcer has been defined as blood loss of such a magnitude that the patient is either in shock or bleeding actively and being treated for shock.[1] Blood transfusion would be required not simply to correct anemia but to restore or maintain vital signs. There are also signs of active bleeding from the upper gastrointestinal tract as indicated by hematemesis and melena or passage of blood per rectum, associated with continuing bloody aspirate after gastric lavage. In another study of massive bleeding in duodenal ulcer, Gardner and Baronofsky[2] defined massive bleeding as a recent episode of melena or hematemesis and hemoglobin of 8 g/dL or less or a fall in blood pressure.

Mortality in patients with massive bleeding is unacceptably high. They merit intensive monitoring and aggressive treatment. The National United Kingdom Audit conducted in 1993 was a population-based, multicenter, prospective observational study in 4185 patients presenting with acute upper gastrointestinal bleeding.[3] The Audit reported a crude mortality of 14%. In the cohort, there were 2071 patients with peptic ulcer presenting with acute hemorrhage. In the 251 patients (12%) that came to surgery, mortality was 24%.

CLINICAL ASSESSMENT AND PREPARATION OF PATIENTS

Patients with upper gastrointestinal bleeding require prompt assessment and volume resuscitation. Hematemesis, passage of fresh melena, shock, and a low hemoglobin level signify significant ongoing bleed or a recent significant bleed. Endotracheal intubation should be considered in patients with active hematemesis, unstable vital signs, or altered mental state to minimize the risk of aspiration pneumonia.[4] Coagulopathy exacerbates bleeding and should be corrected with blood products. Massive bleeding mandates emergency endoscopy. Emergency endoscopy is performed as soon as the patient is stabilized after initial resuscitation. In patients with exigent bleeding,

Department of Surgery, Prince of Wales Hospital, Chinese University of Hong Kong, Shatin, New Territories, Hong Kong, China
E-mail address: laujyw@surgery.cuhk.edu.hk (J.Y.W. Lau).

Gastroenterol Clin N Am 38 (2009) 231–243
doi:10.1016/j.gtc.2009.03.003
0889-8553/09/$ – see front matter © 2009 Elsevier Inc. All rights reserved.

gastro.theclinics.com

endoscopy can be performed during resuscitation. A more liberal policy in emergency endoscopy should be offered to elderly patients and patients with comorbid illnesses, because they tolerate blood loss poorly and are more likely to suffer from organ dysfunctions consequent to hypotension.

ENDOSCOPIC TREATMENT

Endoscopic therapy remains the first treatment modality in the management of bleeding peptic ulcers, even in those presenting with massive bleeding. Endoscopy allows the bleeding source to be localized and excludes varices as the cause of upper gastrointestinal bleeding, as the management is different from that of ulcer bleeding. As endoscopic signs or stigmata of bleeding are prognostic, an early endoscopy enables clinicians to risk-stratify patients. More importantly, endoscopic therapy improves outcomes in patients with actively bleeding ulcers and ulcers with a visible vessel. Sacks and colleagues[5] performed a meta-analysis of 25 randomized controlled trials that compared endoscopic hemostasis to standard treatment. The systematic review showed that endoscopic therapy reduced the risk of recurrent and continued bleeding (69% relative reduction), emergency surgery (62% relative reduction), and mortality (30% relative reduction). Cook and colleagues[6] analyzed data from 30 trials and concluded that endoscopic therapy significantly reduced the rate of rebleeding, surgery, and mortality. The effects were greatest in patients with active bleeding ulcers or nonbleeding, visible vessels. There is also recent evidence to suggest that endoscopic treatment of adherent clots is beneficial. Kahi and colleagues[7] performed a meta-analysis pooling results of six clinical trials with 240 randomized patients (two in abstract form only) and concluded that endoscopic therapy would be more effective in preventing recurrent bleeding when compared with medical therapy alone (rate of recurrent bleeding, 8.2% vs 24.7%).

We now have evidence that the addition of a second modality to injection therapy further improves patients' outcomes. A Cochrane systematic review pooled data from 17 trials that compared epinephrine injection to epinephrine injection and a second treatment method in 1763 high-risk patients.[8] The addition of a second treatment conferred a reduction in rate of recurrent bleeding from 18.8% to 10.4%, emergency surgery from 10.8% to 7.1%, and mortality from 5% to 2.5%, regardless of which second procedure was applied. We favor the use of hemoclips or a 3.2-mm heater probe. We believe that firm tamponade of the bleeding artery and its coaptive coagulation with a contact thermal probe produce secure hemostasis. The use of hemoclips is closer to surgical ligature in hemostasis. We performed a pooled analysis of 15 randomized trials that compared hemoclips to the use of a heater probe in nonvariceal bleeding.[9] The rate of definitive hemostasis was high with either treatment modalities (81.5% vs 81.2%, respectively). There was no difference in the rate of recurrent bleeding, surgery, and death. In clinical practice, successful placement of clips is particularly difficult in fibrotic ulcer with a tangential position, where many difficult ulcers occur. In a randomized trial, 10% of patients randomized to a hemoclip group did not receive hemoclip placement due to technical failure.[10] The use of either modality should not be mutually exclusive.

WHAT IS THE LIMIT TO ENDOSCOPIC THERAPY?

A big bleed is often consequent to a big eroded artery. Blood flow is proportional to the fourth power of the vessel diameter; a small increase in diameter would greatly increase flow. Swain and colleagues[11] studied 27 gastrectomy specimens in patients who underwent urgent surgery for bleeding gastric ulcers. He used thin-barium angiography to study the bleeding artery underneath these ulcers. The study predated the widespread use of endoscopic therapy. It was not entirely clear if the ulcers studied had been treated by endoscopic means. The bleeding artery had a mean external diameter of 0.7 mm (0.1–1.8 mm). In 13 ulcers, the arteries were subserosal and were technically outside the stomach wall. The other bleeding arteries were smaller than 1 mm in size and were submucosal in disposition. In about half of the arteries, there were aneurysmal dilations at the bleeding point. Larger penetrating ulcers are more likely to erode into larger subserosal arteries.[12] Swain and colleagues[13] published only in an abstract the size of arteries in patients who died after a major bleed from their peptic ulcers. The mean diameter of the bleeding artery was 3.75 mm.

In a canine mesenteric artery model, Johnston and colleagues[14] studied the limits of endoscopic thermocoagulation in securing hemostasis. The authors emphasized the need for firm compression onto the artery by a contact probe. Due to the limit in the size of the endoscope channel, a 3.2-mm contact thermal probe is arguably the best available hemostatic device. The use of a 3.2-mm contact thermocoagulation device was shown to consistently seal arteries up to 2 mm in size. Findings of an in vitro model in a real clinical situation may not be as applicable as conditions are often less ideal.

Elmunzer and colleagues[15] systematically reviewed 10 prospective series that evaluated predictive factors for endoscopic failure (Table 1). Two of them employed epinephrine injection as a single modality of therapy. Most commonly identified preendoscopic factors were hemodynamic instability and the presence of comorbid illnesses. During endoscopy, active bleeding, large ulcer size, location of ulcer at posterior bulbar duodenum, and lesser curve were identified as predictors for endoscopic failure. The author remarked that on the basis of consistency and statistical strength, hemodynamic instability, active bleeding, large ulcer size, and posterior duodenal location appear to be the most important predictors of recurrent bleeding. Larger ulcers located at the posterior bulbar duodenum and lesser curve are likely to erode into large arterial complexes—the gastroduodenal artery complex and the left gastric artery proper or its branches. The arteries are often sizable. Bleeding from these arteries exceeds the limit of what endoscopic devices can secure.

ROLE AND TIMING OF SURGERY

Surgery remains the commonest salvage method for the few patients in whom bleeding cannot be controlled at endoscopy. In the published literature, surgery is often defined as an end point to trials evaluating endoscopic therapy. The rate of operative intervention has decreased dramatically over the years with the advent of endoscopic therapy. Nonetheless, surgery has an important gate-keeping role, and it often represents the last defense against exsanguination.

As aforementioned, the operative mortality following failed endoscopic therapy is substantial, ranging from 15% to 25%.[16,17] There are several reasons. First, unsuccessful endoscopic therapy leads to more blood loss and patients are left in a poorer shape after episodes of hypotension. Operative mortality increases with number of episodes of recurrent bleeding and endoscopic attempts. Second, we are managing an aging population with bleeding. Third, ulcers not amenable to endoscopic treatment are "difficult" ulcers. These are large chronic ulcers in difficult positions. Following the near extinction of elective ulcer surgery, experience in dealing with these difficult ulcers is patchy. How to decide on the optimal timing of operation in the right patient remains a challenging clinical decision.

Table 1
Independent predictors of rebleeding after endoscopic therapy

Predictor	Study	% Rebleeding in Entire Study Population	% Rebleeding in Patients With Predictor	% Rebleeding in Patients Without Predictor	Odds Ratio (95% CI)
Hemodynamic instability	Guglielmi	20 (86/429)	41.1 (30/73)	14.8 (54/366)	3.68 (1.99–6.81)
	Wong[a]	8.3 (94/1,128)	19.2 (35/182)	6 (56/946)	2.21 (1.40–3.48)
	Thomopolous[a]	22 (86/390)	47.1 (24/51)	16(54/339)	2.31 91.33–6.97)
	Brullet (DU)[a]	16.7 (17/102)	32.0 (8.25)	12.3(10/81)	3.53 (1.27–4.1)
	Park	20 (25/127)	NR	NR	NR
Comorbid illness	Villanueva	24.5 (57/233)	36.5 (42/115)	12.7 (15/118)	NR
	Saeed	12 (8/69)	NR	NR	Likelihood ratio 7.63, P = 0.005
Active bleeding	Guglielmi	20 (86/829)	20.3 (39/192)	18 (45/247)	14.47 oozing, 13.38 spurting
	Wong[a]	8.3 (94/1,128)	12.1 (71/587)	4.2 (23/541)	1.65 (1.07–2.56)
	Chung	25.2 (35/139)	NR	NR	6.48 (1.88–22.49)
	Thomopolous[a]	22 (86/390)	48.9 (46/94)	10.8 (32/296)	2.45 (1.51–3.93)
	Brullet (GU)[a]	13.1 (23/175)	26 (13/50)	8 (10/125)	2.98 (1.12–7.91)

Large ulcer size (≥ 2 cm)	Guglielmi	20 (86/429)	31.3 (40/128)	14.1 (44/311)	4.61 (2.20–9.64)
	Wong[a]	8.3 (94/1,128)	14.8 (36/244)	6.6 (58/884)	1.80 (1.16–2.83)
	Brullet[a] (GU)	13.1 (23/175)	23.9 (16/67)	6.5 (7/108)	3.64 (1.34–9.89)
	Brullet[a] (DU)	16.7 (17/102)	36.3 (8/22)	12 (10/84)	2.29 (1.13–10.9)
Large ulcer size (>1 cm)	Villanueva	24.5 (57/233)	42.0 (34/81)	15.1 (23/152)	NR
Posterior duodenal ulcer	Thomopolous[a]	22 (86/390)	43.2 (16/37)	17.6 (62/353)	2.48 (1.37–7.01)
	Park	20 (25/127)	44 (11/25)	13.7 (14/102)	NR
	Villanueva	24.5 (57/233)	57.1 (20/35)	18.7 (37/198)	NR
Lesser gastric curve ulcer	Brullet[a] (GU)	13.1 (23/175)	22.9 (16/70)	6.7 (7/105)	2.79 (1.01–7.69)
	Park	20 (25/127)	35 (7/20)	16.8 (18/107)	NR

Abbreviations: DU, Duodenal ulcer; GU, Gastric ulcer; NR, Not reported.

* CI = 3.27–64.05.

** CI = 2.69–66.66.

[a] Percentage of patients experiencing rebleeding was not available. Percentage of patients experiencing overall failure (defined as the failure to achieve initial hemostasis and recurrent hemorrhage) is reported.

Data from Elmunzer BJ, Young SD, Inadomi JM, et al. Systematic review of the predictors of recurrent hemorrhage after endoscopic hemostatic therapy for bleeding peptic ulcers. Am J Gastroenterol 2008;103:2625–32.

The timing of surgery was a subject of intense debate in the 1980s when endoscopic therapy was not available or widespread. There were two randomized studies. The Birmingham trial randomized 104 patients with bleeding peptic ulcer to early or delayed surgery.[18] Criteria for early surgery were four units of blood or plasma expander needed to correct acute blood loss in 24 hours, one rebleed, and endoscopic stigmata or one previous bleed with 2 years of dyspepsia. Criteria for surgery in the delayed group were eight units of blood or plasma expander in 24 hours, two rebleeds, and persistent bleeding requiring 12 units of blood in 48 hours or 16 units in 72 hours. In patients younger than 60 years of age, there was no death in either group, but the early surgery policy led to an unacceptably high operation rate (52% in the early and 5% in the delayed group). For those older than 60 years of age, the operation rate was 62% in the early group and 27% in the delayed group. There were three deaths in 48 patients (6%) in the early group and seven deaths in 52 patients (13%) in the delayed group. On an intention-to-treat analysis, there was no statistical difference. There was subgroup difference in favor of early surgery in elderly patients with bleeding gastric ulcers only on per protocol analysis (0 in 19 of the early group vs 5 in 21 of the delayed group, $P<.01$). The trial was criticized for allowing ongoing bleeding in elderly patients. Saperas and colleagues[19] randomized 69 patients older than 50 years of age in whom emergency endoscopy showed nonarterial bleeding or signs of recent hemorrhage without a visible vessel to receive either immediate surgery or expectant management. In the latter group, 23 of 34 (68%) patients had no further bleeding, whereas 11 patients were operated upon for further bleeding. Mortality in those who underwent surgery was 14.7% (5 in 34 patients) and 2.9% (1 in 34 patients) in patients who were managed expectantly. The outcome of both trials leads us to conclude that a routine policy offering early surgery should not be instated particularly when no major endoscopic stigma is evident as shown in the second trial. It is, however, difficult to interpret both trials in the context of endoscopic therapy. Endoscopic therapy should be attempted in patients with massive bleeding from a peptic ulcer. Often endoscopic hemostasis is possible. In patients in whom exigent bleeding cannot be controlled at endoscopy, surgery is clearly indicated. Whether to consider a second endoscopic attempt or immediate surgery in patients in whom bleeding recurs after initial endoscopic control is more controversial. Such patients are often elderly and at high surgical risk, and they are likely to benefit if endoscopy is repeated with satisfactory results. Conversely, the hypotension and delay in reestablishing hemostasis from repeated but unsuccessful endoscopic attempts are likely to adversely affect their survival. We compared endoscopic retreatment with surgery in patients in whom bleeding recurred after initial endoscopic control.[20] In a 40-month period 1169 patients with bleeding peptic ulcers were treated by epinephrine injection followed by thermocoagulation to the vessel by a 3.2 mm heater probe. Hemostasis was not achieved in 17 patients, and they went directly to surgery. The rate of recurrent bleeding after endoscopic hemostasis was 8.7%. Ninety-two (mean age, 65 years; 76% men) were randomized; 48 were allocated to endoscopic retreatment and 44 to surgery. With intention-to-treat analysis, the endoscopic retreatment and surgery groups did not differ in mortality at 30 days (10% vs 18%, $P = .37$), duration of hospitalization (median, 10 vs 11 days; $P = .59$), need for or length of intensive care unit stay (5 vs 10 patients; median, 59 days for both; $P=.16$), or units of blood transfused (median, 8 vs 7 units $P = .27$). Patients who underwent surgery were more likely to have complications (7 vs 16; $P = .03$). Endoscopic retreatment was able to control bleeding in three-quarters of patients. In a logistic regression analysis of a small subgroup of patients, ulcers measuring 2 cm or more and hypotension at rebleeding were two independent factors predicting failure with endoscopic retreatment. Findings from this trial led us to conclude that we can be selective in offering treatment to patients during their first rebleed. Cases of recurrent bleeding after initial endoscopic hemostasis can be broadly divided into those with suboptimal primary endoscopic treatment and those with arteries deemed to fail endoscopic treatment. Endoscopic retreatment is often successful and worthwhile in smaller ulcers. The pertinent message to the subgroup analysis is that initial control in ulcers predicted to fail may represent a window of opportunity for more aggressive treatment before its first bleed. Our clinical trial should prompt us to investigate the role of early intervention after initial endoscopic hemostasis in selected high-risk ulcers.

Imhof and colleagues[21] reported results of a multicenter trial comparing endoscopic fibrin glue injection with early elective surgery in peptic ulcer patients with arterial bleeding or a visible vessel of 2 mm or more. After initial endoscopic control of bleeding, patients were randomized to repeated fibrin glue injection or early elective surgery. With an intention-to-treat analysis, bleeding recurred in 50% (16 of 33) of the patients in the endoscopic group and 4% (3 of 28) in the early surgical group. Mortality (two in each group) between groups, however, did not differ. We can only conclude from the trial that surgery is more definitive in hemostasis. In a prospective series using the concept of early elective surgery following endoscopic control in patients with arterial bleeding and a visible vessel of 2 mm or more in size, Imhof and colleagues[22] reported an admirable overall operative mortality of 5%, whereas the mortality of a historical control group in which patients were treated conservatively was 14%.

Indeed, good results can be achieved with early surgery with adherence to defined protocols in dedicated units. Bender and colleagues[23] operated on patients with shock on admissions, age greater than 65 years, ulcer size greater than 2 cm, or with stigmata of recent hemorrhage and previous admission for ulcer complication. About 66 patients (mean age, 58 years) were included in a 5-year period with no mortality. Mueller and colleagues operated on patients with spurting hemorrhage, nonbleeding visible vessels on posterior duodenal ulcers, blood transfusion greater than 6 units in the first 24 hours, and rebleeding in 48 hours. In a consecutive series of 157 patients, the 30-day mortality was 7%.[24]

Data from surgical units dedicated to the management of bleeding peptic ulcers support the use of early elective surgery in selected high-risk patients. There was probably publication bias, as the mean age in some of these series was low. These series were mostly uncontrolled trials.

TYPES OF SURGERY

The type of surgery to use has also been a subject of debate. In the presence of powerful proton pump inhibitor and *Helicobacter pylori* eradication, the aim of emergency surgery is no longer to cure ulcer diathesis but to secure bleeding. Acid reduction surgery is therefore unnecessary. Two randomized studies published in the 1980s, however, supported a more aggressive approach in surgical management. In a multicenter, randomized, controlled trial reported by Poxon and colleagues,[25] comprising 137 patients with bleeding peptic ulcer, patients were randomized to simple intraluminal ligature, plication, or conventional surgery (ulcer excision with either vagotomy and pyloroplasty or gastrectomy). H_2 antagonist was used after surgery. Eight patients were excluded from the study due to misdiagnosis or loss of data. Recurrent bleeding occurred in 6 of the 62 patients who underwent simple plication, whereas none rebled after conventional surgery. The trial was aborted because of a high rate of fatal rebleeding in those randomized to simple intraluminal ligature or plication alone. A total of 29 patients died—16 (26%) after conservative surgery and 13 (19%), after conventional operations.

The French Association of Surgical Research trial was a multicenter study that randomized only patients with bleeding bulbar duodenal ulcers.[26] Of 202 eligible patients, 120 entered the study. They were randomly assigned to oversewing plus vagotomy and drainage or partial gastrectomy. The more aggressive approach of gastric resection was accompanied by a lower rebleeding rate (3% vs 17%). Gastric resection was, however, associated with a higher duodenal leak rate (13% vs 3%). On intention-to-treat analysis, the duodenal leak rate, however, was similar between two groups when leak following reoperation for recurrent bleeding in the vagotomy was taken into account (12% vs 13%). The overall mortality was high (22% in vagotomy group and 23% in gastric resection group). Duodenal stump leak is one of the main complications, either in the gastrectomy group or in the patients who rebleed in simple placation group and require conversion to gastrectomy. The authors suggested that when a gastric resection is required, a Billroth type I reconstruction avoiding closure of a duodenal stump is more desirable. A proper ligation of the gastroduodenal artery complex is necessary to avoid recurrent bleeding when a vagotomy and pyloroplasty are considered.

Findings from these two clinical trials suggested that a more aggressive approach would be warranted. They also underlie the fact that a great amount of surgical exper- tise is required in managing these ulcers. The extinction of elective ulcer surgery also means that there is atrophy in skills in managing these difficult ulcers. Surgeons with experience in dealing with these ulcers should be identified and be an integral member of a bleeding team.

ANGIOGRAPHIC THERAPY—A LESS INVASIVE OPTION?

In the 1970s, angiographic therapy was proposed as an alternative to surgery for massive peptic ulcer bleeding before the advent of therapeutic endoscopy.[27,28] Signif- icant advances have since been made in catheter and guidewire technology. We now have finer microcatheter systems and safer embolization materials such as microcoils. Ischemic complications are less seen today, and vessel occlusion is more long lasting. Ulcers that fail endoscopic hemostasis often erode into large arterial complexes— a lesser curve gastric ulcer often into branches of left gastric artery[29] and a posterior bulbar duodenal ulcer into gastroduodenal or pancreaticoduodenal arteries.[30] Due to abundant collateral circulation in the duodenum, cannulation of the superior mesen- teric artery is occasionally required to exclude collateral supply from inferior pancrea- ticoduodenal artery.[31] In a series by Loffroy and colleagues,[32] angiography showed contrast extravasation or false aneurysm at the bleeding site in 25 of 33 patients. Since ulcer bleeding is intermittent, blind therapy is sometimes based on endoscopic local- ization of bleeding site. Eriksson and colleagues[33] reported the technique of clip placement during endoscopy, which facilitates the localization of the bleeder. Various agents including coils, glue, microspheres, and gelatin particles can be used alone or in combination to occlude feeding vessels after their selective cannulations. Compli- cations including gastric and duodenal infarction, hepatic infarction, and late duodenal stenosis have been reported in early series.[34,35] Special precaution and technique are required, especially when using glue, due to the risk of ischemia when the glue regur- gitates to undesired vessels.[36] Case series reporting the efficacy of angiographic embolization usually comprises patients with a high operative risk, with previous failed endoscopic therapy or with recurrent bleeding after surgery. The reported technical

Table 2
Results of angiographic embolization in management of massive peptic ulcer bleeding

Study	Patient No.	Patient Characteristics	Techniques and Agents	Radiologic Success	Lasting Hemostasis	Complications of TAE	Mortality
Larssen and colleagues 2008[37]	36	Failed endoscopic treatment or rebleed, 2 prophylactic	Coils, microcoils, gelfoam	92%	72%	3% no clinical consequence	19%
Loffroy and colleagues 2008[32]	35	High operative risk patients	Coils, microcoils, gelatin powder, cyanoacrylate glue, microspheres	94%	77%	6% major complication (groin), 8% minimal complication	21%
Holme and colleagues 2006[38]	40	13 had previous surgery, only include hemodynamically stable patients	Superselective with microcoils (12) or sandwich technique with coils (28)	83%	50%	0	25%
Toyoda and colleagues 2005[30]	11	Severe comorbidities or malignancy	Coils, microcoils, or gelfoam embolized gastroduodenal, anterior and posterior superior pancreaticoduodenal arteries in 10	91%	91%	No major complication	27%
Ljungdahl and colleagues 2002[39]	18	5 had previous surgery	Coils, microcoils, or gelfoam	100%	83%	2 patients (11%)	5%
Walsh and colleagues 1999[40]	50	High operative risk patients	Coils, microcoils, polyvinyl alcohol, gelfoam	92%	46%	4% major leading to death	40%

success rate ranged from 90% to 100%, whereas clinical success rate is lower and ranged from 50% to 83% (**Table 2**). In these series, those who failed embolization or rebleed after embolization were treated with repeat endoscopy, surgery, or repeat embolization. An overall mortality of 5% to 40% was reported.

ANGIOGRAPHIC EMBOLIZATION VERSUS SURGERY

To date, there has been no controlled trial that compared angiographic embolization to surgery as a salvage procedure for failed endoscopic therapy. Two retrospective comparisons showed at least similar efficacy in terms of rate of rebleeding, morbidity, and mortality. Ripoll and colleagues[41] retrospectively analyzed the outcome of 70 patients with refractory peptic ulcer bleeding. About 31 patients underwent angiographic embolization, and 39 patients were managed with surgery. Although patients receiving angiographic embolization were 10 years older and more had heart disease, the incidence of recurrent bleeding (29% vs 23%) and mortality was similar (26% vs 21%). Another retrospective comparison study by Eriksson and colleagues[42] included 40 patients who underwent angiographic embolization and 51 patients who underwent surgery after failed endoscopic therapy. The angiographic embolization group was older with more comorbidity. The 30-day mortality was lower in the angiographic embolization group (3% vs 14%). These results are promising, and we are eagerly awaiting results of randomized, controlled trials to prove the benefits of angiographic embolization.

SUMMARY

Massive bleeding from a peptic ulcer remains a challenge. A multidisciplinary team of skilled endoscopists, intensive care specialists, experienced upper gastrointestinal surgeons, and intervention radiologists all have a role to play. Endoscopy is the first-line treatment. Even with larger ulcers, endoscopic hemostasis can be achieved in the majority of cases. Surgery is clearly indicated in patients in whom arterial bleeding cannot be controlled at endoscopy. Angiographic embolization is an alternate option, particularly in those unfit for surgery. In selected patients judged to belong to the high-risk group—ulcers 2 cm or greater in size located at the lesser curve and posterior bulbar duodenal, shock on presentation, and elderly with comorbid illnesses—a more aggressive postendoscopy management is warranted. The optimal course of action is unclear. Most would be expectant and offer medical therapy in the form of acid suppression. Surgical series suggest that early elective surgery may improve outcome. Angiography allows the bleeding artery to be characterized, and coil embolization of larger arteries may further add to endoscopic hemostasis. The role of early elective surgery or angiographic embolization in selected high-risk patients to forestall recurrent bleeding remains controversial. Prospective studies are needed to compare different management strategies in these high-risk ulcers.

REFERENCES

1. Read RC, Huebl HC, Thal AP. Randomized study of massive bleeding from peptic ulceration. Ann Surg 1965;165:561–77.
2. Gardner B, Baronofsky ID. Massive bleeding in duodenal ulcer with special reference to the significance of the presence of crater. Bull N Y Acad Med 1959;35:554–70.

3. Rockall TA, Logan RF, Devlin HB, et al. Incidence of and mortality from acute upper gastrointestinal haemorrhage in the United Kingdom. BMJ 1995;311: 222–6.
4. Rudolph SJ, Landsverk BK, Freeman ML. Endotracheal intubation for airway protection during endoscopy for severe upper GI hemorrhage. Gastrointest Endosc 2003;57:58–61.
5. Sacks HS, Chalmers TC, Blum AL, et al. Endoscopic hemostasis. An effective therapy for bleeding peptic ulcers. JAMA 1990;264(4):494–9.
6. Cook DJ, Guyatt GH, Salena BJ, et al. Endoscopic therapy for acute nonvariceal upper gastrointestinal hemorrhage: a meta analysis. Gastroenterology 1992; 102(1):139–48.
7. Kahi CJ, Jensen DM, Sung JJ, et al. Endoscopic therapy versus medical therapy for bleeding peptic ulcer with adherent clot: a meta-analysis. Gastroenterology 2005;129:855–62.
8. Vergara M, Calvet X, Gisbert JP. Epinephrine injection versus epinephrine injection and a second endoscopic method in high risk bleeding ulcers. Cochrane Database Syst Rev 2007;(2):CD005584.
9. Sung JJ, Tsoi KK, Lai LH, et al. Endoscopic clipping versus injection and thermocoagulation in the treatment of non-variceal upper gastrointestinal bleeding: a meta-analysis. Gut 2007;56:1364–73.
10. Lin HJ, Perng CL, Sun IC, et al. Endoscopic haemoclip versus heater probe thermocoagulation plus hypertonic saline-epinephrine injection for peptic ulcer bleeding. Dig Liver Dis 2003;35(12):898–902.
11. Swain CP, Storey DW, Bown SG, et al. Nature of the bleeding vessel in recurrently bleeding gastric ulcers. Gastroenterology 1986;90:595–608.
12. Osborn GR. The pathology of gastric arteries, with special reference to fatal haemorrhage from peptic ulcer. Br J Surg 1954;41:585–94.
13. Swain CP, Lai KC, Kalabakas A, et al. A comparison of size and pathology of vessel and ulcer in patients dying from bleeding gastric and duodenal ulcers [Abstract]. Gastroenterology 1993;104(Suppl):A202.
14. Johnston JH, Jensen DM, Auth D. Experimental comparison of endoscopic yttrium-aluminum-garnet laser, electrosurgery, and heater probe for canine gut arterial coagulation. Importance of compression and avoidance of erosion. Gastroenterology 1987;92:1101–8.
15. Elmunzer BJ, Young SD, Inadomi JM, et al. Systematic review of the predictors of recurrent hemorrhage after endoscopic hemostatic therapy for bleeding peptic ulcers. Am J Gastroenterol 2008;103:2625–32.
16. Kubba AK, Choudari C, Rajgopal C, et al. The outcome of urgent surgery for major peptic ulcer haemorrhage following failed endoscopic therapy. Eur J Gastroenterol Hepatol 1996;8:1175–8.
17. Robson AJ, Richards JM, Ohly N, et al. The effect of surgical subspecialization on outcomes in peptic ulcer disease complicated by perforation and bleeding. World J Surg 2008;32(7):1456–61.
18. Morris DL, Hawker PC, Brearley S, et al. Optimal timing of operation for bleeding peptic ulcer: prospective randomized trial. Br Med J 1984;228:1277–80.
19. Saperas E, Pique JM, Perez AR, et al. Conservative management of bleeding duodenal ulcer without a visible vessel: prospective randomized trial. Br J Surg 1987;74(9):784–6.
20. Lau JWY, Sung JJY, Lam Y, et al. Endoscopic retreatment compared with surgery in patients with recurrent bleeding after initial endoscopic control of bleeding ulcers. N Engl J Med 1999;340(10):751–6.

21. Imhof M, Ohmann C, Röher HD, et al. Endoscopic versus operative treatment in high-risk ulcer bleeding patients - results of a randomised study. Langenbecks Arch Surg 2003;387(9–10):327–36.

22. Imhof M, Schröders C, Ohmann C, et al. Impact of early operation on the mortality from bleeding peptic ulcer–ten years' experience. Dig Surg 1998; 15(4):308–14.

23. Bender JS, Bouwman DL, Weaver DW. Bleeding gastroduodenal ulcers: improved outcome from a unified surgical approach. Am Surg 1994;60(5):313–5.

24. Mueller X, Rothenbuehler JM, Amert A, et al. Outcome of peptic ulcer hemorrhage treated according to a defined approach. World J Surg 1994;18(3): 406–9.

25. Poxon VA, Keighley MR, Dykes PW, et al. Comparison of minimal and conventional surgery in patients with bleeding peptic ulcer: a multicentre trial. Br J Surg 1991;78(11):1344–5.

26. Millat B, Hay JM, Valleur P, et al. Emergency surgical treatment for bleeding duodenal ulcer: oversewing plus vagotomy versus gastric resection, a controlled randomized trial. World J Surg 1993;17(5):568–73.

27. Goldman ML, Land WC, Bradley EL, et al. Transcatheter therapeutic embolization in the management of massive upper gastrointestinal bleeding. Radiology 1976; 120(3):513–21.

28. Matolo NM, Link DP. Selective embolization for control of gastrointestinal hemorrhage. Am J Surg 1979;138(6):840–4.

29. Kelemouridis V, Athanasoulis C, Waltman A. Gastric bleeding sites: an angiographic study. Radiology 1983;149(3):643–8.

30. Toyoda H, Nakano S, Takeda I, et al. Transcatheter arterial embolization for massive bleeding from duodenal ulcers not controlled by endoscopic hemostasis. Endoscopy 1995;27(4):304–7.

31. Bell SD, Lau KY, Sniderman KW. Synchronous embolization of the gastroduodenal artery and the inferior pancreaticoduodenal artery in patients with massive duodenal hemorrhage. J Vasc Interv Radiol 1995;6(4):531–6.

32. Loffroy R, Guiu B, Cercueil JP, et al. Refractory bleeding from gastroduodenal ulcers: arterial embolization in high-operative-risk patients. J Clin Gastroenterol 2008;42(4):361–7.

33. Eriksson LG, Sundbom M, Gustavsson S, et al. Endoscopic marking with a metallic clip facilitates transcatheter arterial embolization in upper peptic ulcer bleeding. J Vasc Interv Radiol 2006;17(6):959–64.

34. Lang EK. Transcatheter embolization in management of hemorrhage from duodenal ulcer: long-term results and complications. Radiology 1992;182(3): 703–7.

35. Brown KT, Friedman WN, Marks RA, et al. Gastric and hepatic infarction following embolization of the left gastric artery: case report. Radiology 1989; 172(3):731–2.

36. Lee CW, Liu KL, Wang HP, et al. Transcatheter arterial embolization of acute upper gastrointestinal tract bleeding with N-butyl-2-cyanoacrylate. J Vasc Interv Radiol 2007;18(2):209–16.

37. Larssen L, Mogen T, Bjørnbeth BA, et al. Transcatheter arterial embolization in the management of bleeding duodenal ulcers: a 5.5-year retrospective study of treatment and outcome. Scand J Gastroenterol 2008;43(2):217–22.

38. Holme JB, Nielsen DT, Funch-Jensen P, et al. Transcatheter arterial embolization in patients with bleeding duodenal ulcer: an alternative to surgery. Acta Radiol 2006;47(3):244–7.

39. Ljungdahl M, Eriksson LG, Nyman R, et al. Arterial embolization in management of massive bleeding from gastric and duodenal ulcers. Eur J Surg 2002;168(7): 384–90.

40. Walsh RM, Anain P, Geisinger M, et al. Role of angiography and embolization for massive gastroduodenal hemorrhage. J Gastrointest Surg 1999;3(1):61–5.

41. Ripoll C, Bañares R, Beceiro I, et al. Comparison of transcatheter arterial embolization and surgery for treatment of bleeding peptic ulcer after endoscopic treatment failure. J Vasc Interv Radiol 2004;15(5):447–50.

42. Eriksson LG, Ljungdahl M, Sundbom M, et al. Transcatheter arterial embolization versus surgery in the treatment of upper gastrointestinal bleeding after therapeutic endoscopy failure. J Vasc Interv Radiol 2008;19(10):1413–8.

Stress-Induced Ulcer Bleeding in Critically Ill Patients

Tauseef Ali, MD, Richard F. Harty, MD*

KEYWORDS

- Stress ulcers • Intensive care unit • Critically ill patients
- Gastric mucosal damage • Gastrointestinal bleeding

Stress is defined as a response to severe demands on the human body resulting in the disruption of homeostasis through physical and psychological stimuli.[1] It has long been recognized that severe physiologic stress can cause gastric mucosal damage. More than 150 years ago, Curling described duodenal ulcer bleeding in patients with extensive burn injuries.[2] The syndrome of stress-related mucosal damage (SRMD) of the gastrointestinal (GI) tract was first described in 1971 by Lucas and colleagues[3] who used the term *stress-related erosive syndrome*. Since then, numerous terms have been used to describe stress-related mucosal damage in critically ill patients, including *stress ulcers, stress erosions, stress gastritis, hemorrhagic gastritis, erosive gastritis,* and *stress-related mucosal disease.*[4]

EPIDEMIOLOGY

Acute GI bleeding in critically ill patients has been described in the medical literature since the 1800s. Determining the true frequency of clinically important bleeding is complicated by variability in the definitions of end points, difficulty in measuring the end points, and the heterogeneity of the patient populations.[5] The reported incidence of stress-related mucosal damage varies from 6% to 100% in critically ill patients.[4] Endoscopic studies generally indicate that approximately 75% to 100% of critically ill patients have gross gastric lesions visible when endoscopy is performed within the first 1 to 3 days of illness.[3,6,7] The prevalence of stress-related mucosal damage ranges from 15% to 50% if occult bleeding (defined as a drop in hemoglobin level or positive stool occult blood test) is used as an end point.[8,9] Clinically overt bleeding

Financial disclosure: The authors have no relationship with a commercial company that has a direct financial interest in the subject matter or materials discussed in their article.

Section of Digestive Diseases and Nutrition, Department of Internal Medicine, University of Oklahoma Health Sciences Center, 1360 WP, 920 SL Young Boulevard, Oklahoma City, OK 73104, USA

* Corresponding author.

E-mail address: richard-harty@ouhsc.edu (R.F. Harty).

(hematemesis or nasogastric lavage positive for bright red blood) occurs in about 5% to 25% of critically ill patients who do not receive prophylactic therapy.[9–11] However, clinically overt bleeding does not predict impending clinically significant bleeding (defined as bleeding associated with hypotension, tachycardia, and a drop in hemoglobin level necessitating transfusion). Approximately 20% of clinically evident bleeding is reported to be clinically significant.[12] The incidence of clinically significant GI bleeding has been estimated to be approximately 3% to 4%.[4]

In a prospective study of more than 2000 patients, Cook and colleagues[13] reported an incidence of clinically significant bleeding of 1.5% in critically ill patients. Clinically important or significant bleeding was defined as overt bleeding complicated by one of the following within 24 hours after the onset of bleeding (in the absence of other causes): (1) a spontaneous decrease of more than 20 mm Hg in the systolic blood pressure; (2) an increase in heart rate of more than 20 beats per minute; or (3) a decrease in systolic blood pressure, measured on sitting up, of more than 10 mm Hg; or (4) a decrease in hemoglobin level of more than 2 g/dL and the need for subsequent transfusion, after which the hemoglobin did not increase by a value defined as the number of units transfused minus 2 g/dL. The mortality rate was 48.5% in the group with bleeding and 9.1% in the group without bleeding ($P<.001$).[13] Another recent prospective study examined the attributable mortality and length of intensive care unit (ICU) stay in relation to clinically important GI bleeding in more than 1500 patients.[14] Using the matched cohort method, the relative risk (RR; the ratio of the probability of the event occurring in the exposed group versus a nonexposed group) of mortality attributable to clinically significant GI bleeding was significant (RR 2.9, 95% confidence interval [CI] 1.6 to 5.5). The mortality attributable to bleeding was also statistically significant using the model-based matched cohort method (RR 1.8, 95% CI 1.1 to 2.9). The study also tested the risk of mortality attributable to bleeding over time, using the unadjusted regression method. Patients who bled earlier in their ICU stay had a lower risk of dying than patients who bled later ($P = .02$); the RR of mortality associated with clinically important bleeding was 0.4 (95% CI 0.06 to 2.0) at 2 weeks, 1.6 (95% CI 0.6 to 4.0) at 3 weeks, and 7.4 (95% CI 1.7 to 32.2) at 4 weeks.[14] After adjusting for age, APACHE II score, admitting diagnosis, ventilation status, and 6 Multiple Organ Dysfunction Score (MODS) domains, the ICU stay attributable to bleeding by the regression method was 6.2 days (95% CI 1.0 to 11.4 days).[14]

To summarize, the reported incidence of clinically significant bleeding is approximately 1.5% to 4% with the relative risk of mortality at two to four. The attributable length of ICU stay associated with clinically significant bleeding is approximated to five to seven days. However, the incidence of bleeding from stress-related mucosal damage seems to be decreasing secondary to therapeutic advancement and prevention of mucosal hypoperfusion.[15]

PATHOGENESIS

The gastric mucosa maintains structural integrity and function despite continuous exposure to noxious factors, including 0.1 mol/L HCl and pepsin, which are capable of digesting tissue.[16] An early hypothesis proposed by Hunter in 1772 and supported by Virchow in 1853 was that continuous circulation of alkaline blood through the mucosa neutralizes acid.[17,18] Subsequent work demonstrated that a large number of mucosal defense mechanisms prevent mucosal damage and maintain mucosal integrity. Vane discovered that the major mechanism by which aspirin and other nonsteroidal antiinflammatory drugs (NSAIDs) produce gastric damage involves inhibition of prostaglandin (PG) synthesis.[19] The concept of cytoprotection developed in the late 1970s and early 1980s by Robert and colleagues[20,21] sparked tremendous interest in gastric mucosal defense mechanisms. Gastric mucosal injury may occur if noxious factors "overwhelm" an intact mucosal defense or the mucosal defensive mechanisms are impaired.

Gastric Mucosal Defense Mechanisms

Defense mechanisms permit the gastric mucosa to withstand frequent exposure to damaging factors.[22,23] These include local mechanisms such as the mucus-bicarbonate-phospholipid barrier, continuous cell renewal from mucosal progenitor cells, alkaline tide, and mucosal microcirculation.[16] These concepts have been recently reviewed and illustrated by Laine and colleagues.[16] **Fig. 1** depicts the key components of gastric mucosal defense. Various peptides, including gastrin 17, cholecystokinin, thyrotropin-releasing hormone, bombesin, corticotropin-releasing factor (CRF), epidermal growth factor (EGF), peptide YY, neurokinin A analogs, and intragastric peptone, exert gastroprotection, which is abolished by afferent nerve denervation,

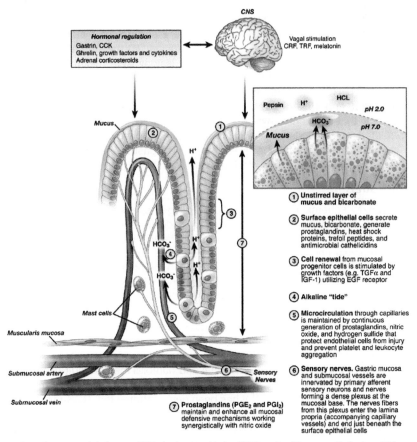

Fig. 1. Gastric mucosal defense. CCK, cholecystokinin; IGF, insulin-like growth factor; PGI$_2$, prostacyclin; TGF, transforming growth factor; TRF, thyrotropin-releasing factor. (*From* Laine L, Takeuchi K, Tarnawski A. Gastric mucosal defense and cytoprotection: bench to bedside. Gastroenterology 2008;135:42; with permission.)

blockade of calcitonin gene-related peptide receptors, and inhibition of NO synthase.[16]

Ischemia and Reperfusion Injury

Stress-related gastric mucosal injury seems to be related to local ischemia, although progression to significant mucosal injury also requires acid.[16] Critically ill patients developing acute gastric mucosal lesions show a significant decrease in gastric mucosal blood volume compared with controls.[24] Studies in the rat model revealed a significant correlation between blood pressure during hypotension and gastric mucosal blood flow. Mucosal blood flows measured by the hydrogen gas clearance technique in the corpus, antrum, and duodenum of rats all showed a significant linear correlation with mean blood pressure. Blood flow to the mucosa in the stomach and duodenum decreased progressively as systemic blood pressure fell. Significant gastric mucosal lesions occurred only after mean blood pressure and, hence, mucosal blood flow was reduced to less than 40% of baseline values.[25] A rat model of hemorrhagic shock and retransfusion-induced gastric injury revealed that histologic mucosal damage occurred even without acid, although it increased with intragastric instillation of acid in a dose-dependent fashion.[26] In addition, reperfusion after ischemia increased histologic injury compared with ischemia alone, although increasing the duration of ischemia (from 20 to 30 minutes) increased gastric histologic lesions to the same extent as a similar period of retransfusion (10 minutes after 20 minutes ischemia). In the absence of acid, gross gastric lesions were minimal, involving 4% of the body and 3% of the antrum surface area. However, intragastric instillation of acid (0.1 mol/L HCl) markedly increased the gross lesions in a dose-dependent fashion to 53% and 45% of the body and antral surface areas, respectively. These studies imply that splanchnic hypoperfusion in the presence of gastric acid leads to stress-related mucosal damage and suppression of gastric acid would minimize such injuries. This forms the basis for the use of gastric antisecretory agents as prophylactic agents for stress-related mucosal injuries.

Oxidative Stress

Under hypoxic-ischemic conditions, reactive oxygen species (ROS), such as superoxide anions, hydrogen peroxide, and hydroxyl radicals, are rapidly and continuously produced. Oxidative stress resulting from hypoxia and ischemia to the gastric and duodenal mucosa has proved to be an important element in the development and progression of epithelial necrosis and mucosal ulceration.[27,28] Overproduction of ROS results in oxidative damage, including lipid peroxidation, protein oxidation, and DNA damage, which can lead to cell death. Furthermore, ROS are known to act as second messengers to activate diverse redox-sensitive signaling transduction cascades, including mitogen-activated protein kinases (MAPKs) and downstream transcription factors such as NF-κB and AP-1. These signaling pathways and transcription factors regulate the expression of numerous pro-inflammatory genes and, thereby, lead to the elaboration of chemical and humoral mediators of tissue inflammation and injury.[29,30] The p38 MAPK is considered important in determining cellular adaptive responses and cell fate.[31] It has been demonstrated that ROS-mediated p38 activation plays an essential role in the pathogenesis of stress-induced gastric inflammatory damage in the rat model of cold immobilization stress.[32] These results suggest that local ROS generation could be an initiating or triggering event in the early phase of stress-induced gastric mucosal injury.[27] The clinically relevant translation of this area of research is the importance of restoring and maintaining systemic and regional circulation and tissue oxygenation in critically ill patients.

The Cyclooxygenase-2 Pathway

Whereas cyclooxygenase-2 (COX-2) has no essential role in the maintenance of gastric mucosal integrity under basal conditions, COX-2 is rapidly induced in a pro-ulcerogenic setting and contributes to mucosal defense by minimizing injury.[33] Ischemia/reperfusion has been shown to increase COX-2 messenger RNA levels in the rat gastric mucosa. It has also been discovered that hypoxia increases expression of the COX-2 gene in human vascular endothelial cells in culture, independent of other stimuli.[34] Therefore, COX-2 expression is assumed to be up-regulated as one of the protective mechanisms when the stomach is exposed to stress, and contributes to mucosal defense by minimizing injury. Therefore, it is reasonable to speculate that COX-2 may prevent gastric mucosal ulcers in mild stress by a phenomenon of adaptive cytoprotection, but may not be able to prevent stress-related mucosal damage in severe stress because of the intensity of the insult and activation of various other pro-ulcerogenic mechanisms. It is understandable why NSAID exposure in the critically ill patient may have profound adverse effects on sustaining the COX-2 defense mechanism.

Endogenous Nitric Oxide and Endothelin-1

Gastric microcirculatory disturbances are involved in the pathogenesis of stress ulcers; however, the vasomodulators causing this vascular instability are not fully understood. Reduced local mucosal nitric oxide (NO; a vasodilator) generation and increased endothelin-1 (a potent vasoconstrictor) levels seem to be involved in events associated with compromise of mucosal blood flow observed in SRMD.[35] In addition, NO plays an important role in the regulation of epithelial cell functions in the GI tract. Gene expression of inducible NO synthase (iNOS) is markedly up-regulated following ischemia/reperfusion and is accompanied by a significant increase in the mucosal NO content. Endogenous NO plays a dual role in ischemia/reperfusion-induced gastric injury; constitutive NO synthase/NO is protective, whereas inducible NO synthase/NO can be pro-ulcerogenic during ischemia/reperfusion.[36] The constitutive NO synthase/NO acts to maintain mucosal integrity through modulating various functions such as mucus secretion, bicarbonate secretion, and mucosal blood flow. In contrast, the inflamed mucosa is associated with recruitment of various inflammatory cells as well as up-regulation of iNOS, cytokines, and adhesion molecules. Under stress conditions, NO produced by iNOS reacts with O_2^- produced by neutrophils to form peroxynitrites. These NO-derived reactive compounds contribute to the nitrosative and oxidative stress burden of vulnerable tissue such as the mucosa of the stomach and duodenum. Thus, the duality of NO function is dependent on the vascular and metabolic integrity of the mucosal and submucosal tissues and the presence or absence of inflammation.[36] Similarly, endothelin-1 levels in plasma and injured mucosa of critically ill patients have been found to be elevated, suggesting endogenous ET-1 may play an important role in the local pathogenesis of stress ulcers.[37]

Mucosal Blood Flow

Critically ill patients may experience a decrease in gastric mucosal blood flow through systemic hypotension and splanchnic hypoperfusion.[38] In rats, gastric lesions began to appear when blood pressure fell to 33% of baseline during hemorrhagic shock. At blood pressure 80% below baseline, 26.8% of the total corpus area developed lesions. Normotensive critically ill septic patients on mechanical ventilation were reported to have a 50% to 60% reduction in gastric mucosal blood flow, measured by reflectance spectrophotometry, compared with controls.[39] **Fig. 2** illustrates the

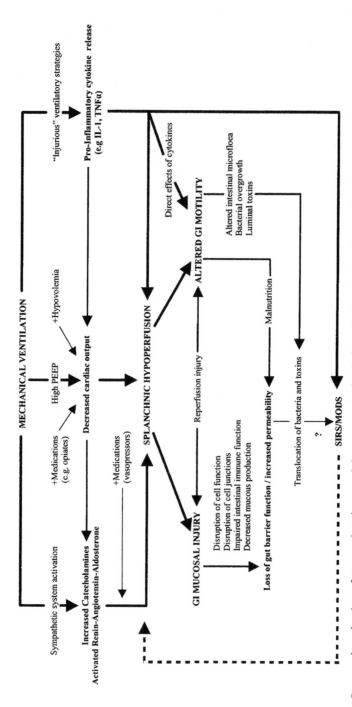

Fig. 2. Proposed mechanism of stress-related mucosal damage on mechanical ventilation. PEEP, positive end-expiratory pressure; SIRS, systemic inflammatory response syndrome; TNF-α, tumor necrosis factor-alpha. (*From* Mutlu GM, Mutlu EA, Factor P. GI complications in patients receiving mechanical ventilation. Chest 2001;119:1224; with permission.)

consequences of mechanical ventilation in critically ill patients. Splanchnic hypoperfusion in mechanically ventilated patients is caused by decreased cardiac output, release of pro-inflammatory cytokines, and sympathetic system activation. Mechanical ventilation as a risk factor for stress-related mucosal damage is discussed further in next section.

In summary, the etiology and pathophysiology of SRMD is multifactorial and, although several steps in this process have been elucidated, there are additional questions that require further investigation. Ischemia and reperfusion are believed to cause disruption of the mucosal defenses, resulting in mucosal injury and ulceration. The major causative factors of SRMD that have been recognized to date include reduced mucosal blood flow, ischemia, and reperfusion injury. The integrity of the gastric mucosa is maintained by several factors, including the microcirculation and the mucus-bicarbonate gel layer. Maintenance of these functional and structural elements provides nutrient and oxygen delivery to the epithelial cells, neutralization of hydrogen ions to prevent acid back diffusion, and dissipation of reactive substances and other toxic cellular byproducts. Thus, stress-related mucosal damage develops if these elements of protection are either compromised or breached. Tissue PG levels have been shown to be decreased, which in turn impairs mucus replenishment and microcirculation responsiveness. Elevated levels of nitric oxide synthase have also been shown to contribute to reperfusion injury and necrotic cell death, and tissue inflammation response.[40]

RISK FACTORS FOR STRESS-INDUCED ULCER BLEEDING

The frequency of clinically significant stress-related mucosal bleeding in critically ill patients is related to certain risk factors. A prospective multicenter cohort study evaluated potential risk factors for stress ulceration in patients admitted to ICUs.[13] Of 2252 patients, 33 (1.5%) had clinically important bleeding. Two strong independent risk factors for bleeding were identified: respiratory failure (odds ratio [OR] 15.6) and coagulopathy (OR 4.3). Of 847 patients who had one or both of these risk factors, 31 (3.7%) had clinically important bleeding. Of 1405 patients without these risk factors, 2 (0.1%) had clinically important bleeding.

In another multicenter cohort study involving medical and surgical ICUs in six tertiary care Department of Veterans Affairs Medical Centers, patients were evaluated prospectively for the development of acute upper GI hemorrhage while in the ICU.[41] Seventy-six (9%) patients had overt upper GI bleeding and a mortality rate of 49%, compared with a 15% mortality rate in patients who did not bleed (P<.001). By logistic regression analysis, the following factors were associated with an increased risk of bleeding: acute hepatic failure, prolonged duration of nasogastric tube placement, alcoholism, renal failure, and an increased serum concentration of anti–Helicobacter pylori (H pylori) immunoglobulin A.[41] The various risk factors identified from these two studies[13,41] are listed in **Table 1**.

These studies suggest that prophylaxis therapies for bleeding can be safely withheld in critically ill patients who do not have major risk factors. Restricting the use of prophylactic medicinal interventions to patients who have risk factors has not been shown to increase morbidity or mortality in critically ill patients and is more cost-effective.[12,42,43]

PROPHYLAXIS OF STRESS-ULCER BLEEDING

The incidence of significant stress-related bleeding has decreased dramatically in the past several decades as a result of advances in nursing care, monitoring, and support

Table 1		
Risk factors for stress-induced ulcer bleeding		
Risk Factors	**Odds Ratio**	**References**
Respiratory failure	15.6	[13]
Acute hepatic failure	6.67	[41]
Coagulopathy	4.3	[13]
Hypotension	3.7	[13]
Chronic renal failure	3.03	[41]
Prolonged duration of NG tube placement	2.59	[41]
History of alcohol abuse	2.23	[41]
Sepsis	2.0	[13]
Helicobacter pylori IgA >1	1.92	[41]

of critically ill patients, including optimization of hemodynamic status, tissue oxygenation, and treatment of sepsis.[5,20] The concept of cytoprotection came from earlier animal experiments showing that pretreatment of rats with intragastric prostaglandin E_2 (PGE_2) 15 to 30 minutes before intragastric instillation of 100% alcohol or boiling water completely prevented severe gastric mucosal necrosis.[20] Subsequent studies confirmed the cytoprotective effects of PGs in humans.[16] Since the first demonstration of cytoprotection by PGs, other agents have been developed to prevent gastric mucosal damage. A review of these agents is presented, divided into two categories: (1) current practices of prophylactic therapy for stress-ulcer bleeding in critically ill ICU patients; and (2) alternative approaches to prevention of stress-ulcer bleeding.

Current Practices of Prophylactic Therapy

Gastric antisecretory agents have been shown to substantially reduce the incidence of clinically important bleeding events secondary to stress ulceration in high-risk critically ill patients.[5,12] In 1999 therapeutic guidelines for stress-ulcer prophylaxis was reported by the American Society of Health-System Pharmacists (ASHP).[5] Earlier studies identified histamine-2 receptor antagonists (H_2RA) as efficacious therapy for stress-ulcer prophylaxis.[5] However, despite H_2RAs proven efficacy, the armamentarium of possible therapies has expanded to include proton pump inhibitors (PPIs). Superior gastric acid suppression and a favorable adverse effect profile with PPI therapy have been suggested as the reason for its selection over other agents. Earlier surveys indicated that H_2RAs were chosen as initial therapy in 67% to 77% of cases, and 3% of respondents chose a PPI, namely, omeprazole.[44,45] A survey of 500 intensivists published in 2004 assessed the current practice of stress-ulcer prophylaxis. The results indicated that 64% used H_2RAs by intermittent infusion and 23% used PPIs.[46] Based on our literature review, these survey data have not been updated. Our estimate is that PPI therapy has exceeded H_2RA therapy for SRMD prophylaxis.

Histamine₂-receptor antagonists

A variety of H_2RAs can be used for stress-ulcer prophylaxis in the ICU. The available H_2RAs are not equally potent on a dose (milligram) basis in blocking the actions of histamine on parietal cells. Cimetidine is the least potent, ranitidine and nizatidine are more potent, and famotidine is the most potent. However, cimetidine is the only H_2RA with US Food and Drug Administration (FDA) approval for the prevention of upper GI bleeding in the ICU.[39]

Cimetidine has a well-established safety profile. Drug interactions occur more frequently with cimetidine than with other H$_2$RAs. Other side effects include thrombocytopenia[47] and neurologic sides effects, especially in elderly patients and patients with hepatic or renal dysfunction.[48] Ranitidine has 5 to 12 times greater antisecretory potency than cimetidine.[39] Famotidine is the most potent H$_2$RA available in the United States. It is 8 to 10 times more potent than ranitidine.[39] A lower volume of intravenously administrated drug (10 mL/d) is required with famotidine compared with cimetidine and ranitidine (60–80 mL/d). This characteristic may be particularly useful in patients with congestive heart failure or those requiring fluid restriction.[39] Drug interactions seem to be minimal with famotidine. In controlled trials of famotidine, no drug interactions were observed with agents metabolized by the cytochrome P450 (CYP) enzyme system, including warfarin, theophylline, phenytoin, and diazepam.[49]

Continuous infusion of H$_2$RAs is superior to intermittent bolus administration in maintaining gastric pH at levels >4.[50–52] The enteral route has also been studied and in one study, enteral administration of ranitidine every 12 hours led to effective absorption of the drug from the upper GI tract of ICU patients. Serum concentrations of ranitidine for 150-mg and 300-mg enteral doses remained within, or exceeded, the therapeutic range in more than 90% of ICU patients with clinically important criteria of stress.[53]

Development of tolerance to H$_2$RAs is a major concern and has been reported to develop within 42 hours after intravenous administration by repeated bolus and continuous infusion.[54] A critical review of the efficacy of H$_2$RAs in the prevention of stress ulcers, performed 10 years ago, indicated wide fluctuation in the results and no clear consensus was provided.[5]

Proton pump inhibitors

PPIs are the most potent antisecretory agents available and act by irreversibly blocking the H$^+$ K$^+$–ATPase pump (the proton pump) in gastric parietal cells. Prospective randomized trials have proved the efficacy of PPIs in stress-ulcer prophylaxis.[55]

Omeprazole was the first PPI approved in the United States for oral administration. In prospective studies, omeprazole suspension administered by nasogastric tube prevented clinically significant GI bleeding and maintained gastric pH at favorable levels.[56,57] In one prospective open-label study, simplified omeprazole suspension prevented clinically significant upper GI bleeding and maintained a gastric pH of greater than 5.5 in 75 patients on mechanical ventilation with at least one additional risk factor for stress-related mucosal damage.[56] In another trial on 60 trauma patients on mechanical ventilation, omeprazole suspension prevented clinically significant GI bleeding, maintained excellent control of gastric pH, produced no toxicity, and was the least costly medication alternative.[57] Esomeprazole is the S-isomer of omeprazole available in an oral and parenteral formulation. In contrast with omeprazole, no significant drug interactions between esomeprazole and phenytoin, warfarin, quinidine, clarithromycin, or amoxicillin have been demonstrated in clinical studies.[58] Administration of intravenous esomeprazole has been found to be an effective and safe approach for prophylaxis of stress ulcers in a study of 48 patients subjected to mechanical ventilation over 48 hours.[59] Lansoprazole is available in oral form only in the United States. Nasogastric lansoprazole (30 mg daily) has been shown to be effective in suppressing gastric acid secretion in critically ill patients.[60] To compare the pharmacodynamic response between enteral and intravenous lansoprazole in ICU patients requiring stress-ulcer prophylaxis therapy, patients on mechanical ventilation were randomized to receive 72 hours of daily enteral (lansoprazole oral disintegrating tablet [LODT] 30 mg mixed in 10 mL of water through a nasal gastric tube) or intravenous (30 mg over 30 minutes) lansoprazole therapy. LODT bioavailability was 76%. LODT maintained gastric pH above four longer than intravenous lansoprazole at 24 hours (7.4 vs 5.9 hours; $P = .039$) and 72 hours (10.4 and 8.9 hours; $P = .046$) and resulted in a greater average pH over the first 24 hours (3.67 vs 2.89; $P = .03$). The study concluded that despite a lower bioavailability, enteral lansoprazole suppresses acid in ICU patients to a greater extent than intravenous lansoprazole.[61] Among the PPIs, pantoprazole has the lowest pH of activation and the highest stability under moderately acidic conditions.[62] This feature, in addition to its high potency and the availability of an intravenous form, makes it well suited for the prophylaxis of stress ulcer in the ICU.[39] A recent multicenter, randomized, open-label, dose-ranging pilot study involving 200 ICU patients was conducted to assess the effectiveness of intermittent intravenous pantoprazole for control of gastric acid. Intravenous pantoprazole (40 mg every 24 hours, 40 mg every 12 hours, 80 mg every 24 hours, 80 mg every 12 hours, 80 mg every 8 hours) or continuously infused cimetidine (300 mg bolus; 50 mg/h) in patients at risk for upper GI bleeding were studied. The primary end point was the percent time that gastric pH was maintained at or greater than four. Of all the pantoprazole treatments, 80 mg every 12 hours and 80 mg every 8 hours showed the greatest effects on the percent time that pH was 4.0 or greater, regardless of day. On day 2 of treatment, 40 mg every 12 hours and 80 mg every 12 hours were similar in percent time that pH was 4.0 or greater. This suggested that patients might obtain adequate control of gastric pH with an initial treatment using an 80-mg dosing regimen (80 mg every 24 hours, every 12 hours, or every 8 hours) followed by 40 mg every 12 hours.[52] An interesting finding of this study was the improved control of gastric pH by the five different dosing regimens of intermittent intravenous pantoprazole compared with continuous infusion of cimetidine (300 mg bolus followed by 50 mg/h infusion) in patients fed enterally. In contrast to pantoprazole, patients treated with cimetidine had a decreased percent time pH was 4.0 or greater after initiation of enteral feeding; this decrease occurred within 8 hours of switching to enteral.[52]

All delayed-released PPIs are acid labile and must be protected from acid degradation within the stomach. The enteric coating on delayed-release PPIs protects them from acid degradation but impairs absorption. Immediate-release (IR) omeprazole powder for oral suspension, which consists of pure, uncoated omeprazole with 20 mEq of sodium bicarbonate, is constituted with 15 to 30 mL of water. The T_{max} for the precommercial formulation of IR omeprazole is achieved in approximately 25 minutes, compared with 127 minutes for the delayed-release formulation of omeprazole.[63] IR omeprazole is the only PPI that has received FDA approval for stress-ulcer prophylaxis. A large, multicenter, prospective double-blind trial demonstrated the efficacy of IR omeprazole in preventing GI bleeding in critically ill patients.[64]

Intragastric pH studies have demonstrated that, whereas a pH of more than four may be adequate to prevent stress ulceration, a pH of greater than six may be necessary to maintain clotting in patients at risk of rebleeding from peptic ulcer. Studies comparing the ability of intravenous administration of H_2RAs and PPIs to raise and maintain intragastric pH suggest that, although both can raise the pH to more than four, PPIs are much more likely to maintain a pH of more than six. Unlike H_2RAs, PPIs can elevate and maintain intragastric pH at more than six, which is relevant for patients in the ICU at risk for rebleeding from peptic ulcers after hemostasis.[11]

The first comparison of a PPI with another drug for the prevention of bleeding in critically ill was published by Levy and colleagues.[55] This study found a significantly lower rate of stress-induced GI bleeding when using omeprazole compared with ranitidine (6% vs 31%). However, the number of patients in this study (n = 67) was too low to yield conclusive results with sufficient power. In addition, the ranitidine group had a higher rate of risk factors and the bleeding rate in this group was unexplainably high and much higher than in other trials; therefore, the validity of the results is questionable.[65] Comparisons between clinical and pharmacologic features of H_2RAs and PPIs are provided in **Table 2**.

Alternative Therapies

Misoprostol

Misoprostol is a synthetic PGE_1 analog with gastric cytoprotective and antisecretory properties when administered at a high dose.[16] Few studies have evaluated PG analogs for the prophylaxis of stress-related bleeding in the ICU. One prospective double-blind, double-placebo study compared the effectiveness of antacid titration with fixed doses of a synthetic PGE_1 analog (misoprostol) for preventing stress gastritis and bleeding. No statistically significant differences were identified between the two treatment groups concerning upper GI tract lesions or serious adverse effects. The rate of diarrhea was considerably higher than that reported with other prophylactic agents for stress ulcers.[66] The low rate of misoprostol use in United Stated may be due to GI side effects, such as diarrhea and abdominal discomfort, and the need for multiple daily doses.

Sucralfate

Sucralfate consists of a core of sucrose molecules surrounded by aluminum hydroxide sulfate salts. It coats the gastric mucosa and forms a thin protective layer between the mucosa and the gastric acid in the lumen.[39] Another cytoprotective mechanism of action may be the stimulation of mucosal defenses that trigger the release of PGE_2.[67] In a metaanalysis of stress-ulcer prophylaxis,[68] the efficacy of sucralfate was compared with H_2RAs in nine studies and with antacids in 8 studies. Sucralfate was significantly more effective than H_2RAs (typical OR 0.532, 95% CI 0.303 to 0.933) and equally as effective as antacids (typical OR 0.868, 95% CI 0.452 to 1.667). The occurrence of pneumonia in those patients who were administered sucralfate was compared with the patients who were given H_2RAs in five studies, and with those patients who were given antacids in four studies. Pneumonia was a significantly more frequent occurrence under prophylaxis with H_2RAs (typical OR 0.498, 95% CI 0.316 to 0.783) and with antacids (typical OR 0.402, 95% CI 0.235 to 0.687). Due to the availability of more potent acid-suppression therapy, sucralfate has never gained popularity for stress-ulcer prophylaxis in the United States.

Table 2
Comparison between H_2RAs and PPIs for stress-ulcer prophylaxis

	H_2 Blockers	Proton Pump Inhibitors
FDA approved medications for stress-ulcer prophylaxis	Cimetidine	IR omeprazole
Potency to reduce gastric acid secretion	++	++++
Common side effects	+++	++
Risk of pneumonia	++	++++
Drug interactions	+++	+
Tachyplaxis	+	None
Cost-effectiveness	++++	++
Therapeutic effectiveness	++	++++

Antacids

Antacids containing aluminum and magnesium hydroxide heal ulcers by neutralizing gastric acid and inactivating the proteolytic activity of pepsin. In a randomized trial of 100 critically ill patients at risk of developing GI bleeding, one group (51 patients) received antacid prophylaxis, and the other (49 patients) received no prophylaxis.[69] Hourly antacid titration kept the pH of the gastric contents above 3.5. Two of the 51 patients who received antacid prophylaxis had GI bleeding whereas 12 of the 49 control patients bled ($P<.005$). Analysis of all the patients showed that an increasing prevalence of respiratory failure, sepsis, peritonitis, jaundice, renal failure, and hypotension was correlated with a greater frequency of bleeding.[69] These data indicate that the occurrence of acute GI bleeding in critically ill patients can be reduced by antacid titration. However, frequent dosing of antacids is labor intensive and more potent acid-suppression therapy is available. Moreover, antacids are associated with electrolyte abnormalities and changes in bowel motility. Preparations containing magnesium create a predisposition to diarrhea and cannot be given to patients with renal insufficiency. On the other hand, use of preparations containing aluminum/calcium leads to constipation.[39] Currently, antacids are not used as stress-ulcer prophylaxis therapy due to the availability of more potent medications and frequently associated side effects.

Helicobacter pylori *eradication*

The role of *H pylori* in the pathogenesis of stress-related mucosal damage is controversial. In a prospective observational study, all patients admitted consecutively to seven ICUs during a 1-year period were monitored for signs of clinically relevant upper GI bleeding. *H pylori* infection was more frequent in patients who bled than in matched controls (36% vs 16%; $P = .04$).[70] Another prospective study included serologic analysis of samples from all consecutive patients over a 1-year period who showed significant upper GI bleeding (defined as hematemesis, melena, or grossly bloody nasogastric aspirate) after cardiac surgery.[71] Patients with no evidence of GI hemorrhage after cardiac surgery were chosen as controls. *H pylori* was not found to be a risk factor for upper GI bleeding, although patients who required prolonged mechanical ventilation were at high risk.[71] Antibiotic treatment of *H pylori* infection in the ICU setting can be associated with unwanted consequences such as selection for resistant organisms, acquisition of methicillin-resistant *Staphylococcus aureus*, promotion of ventilator-associated pneumonia, and induction of *Clostridium difficile* colitis.[39] The use of antibiotics for eradication of *H pylori* in the acute setting is not recommended until further evidence proves that the benefit of early treatment outweighs the risks.[72,73] At the present time, the role of *H pylori* infection on the development of SRMD is uncertain.

Enteral feeding

Early enteral nutrition has been proven effective in preventing stress ulceration of the upper GI tract in critically ill patients, especially in burn patients.[74] Intragastric administration of enteral nutrition has variable effects on gastric pH, enhances regional distribution of GI blood flow, and may lower intramucosal pH.[75] All substrates (carbohydrate, lipid, amino acid), when administered into the stomach, reduce the occurrence of mucosal erosions but do not entirely prevent their development. Limited retrospective data suggest that enteral nutrition support may be effective for preventing GI hemorrhage, but the results of prospective studies are confounded by poor study design.[75] Definitive recommendations regarding the role of enteral nutrition for stress-ulcer prophylaxis are not possible due to the lack of prospective, randomized studies. Therefore, the use of enteral nutrition as the only therapeutic agent for stress-ulcer prophylaxis should be discouraged until definitive data are available. Initiation and discontinuation of pharmacologic stress-ulcer prophylaxis should be independent of enteral nutrition. Care should be taken when choosing prophylactic drug therapies to be administered with continuous enteral nutrition. Gastric feeding has been shown to reduce the effectiveness of sucralfate, whereas coadministration of enteral nutrition and ranitidine for the prophylaxis of stress ulcers has been associated with reduced bleeding rates.[39]

Adverse Effects Associated with Stress-Ulcer Prophylaxis

Risks of infection

Gastric juice of normal adults usually contains less than 10^3 microorganisms per milliliter that are predominantly anaerobes.[76] Gastric acidity constitutes a major defense mechanism against ingested pathogens and loss of normal stomach acidity has been associated with bacterial overgrowth of the upper GI tract.[77] Acid suppressive agents such as PPIs and H_2RAs increase gastric pH and PPIs have also been shown to affect leukocyte function.[78] These factors contribute to the reported associations between acid-suppression therapy and increased risk of respiratory tract[79] and enteric infections in critically ill patients. With regard to enteric infections in this clinical setting, PPI therapy has been reported to be a risk factor for hospital-acquired *Clostridium difficile*–associated diarrhea (CDAD).[80]

Pneumonia

Increased respiratory tract infections, such as pneumonia, have always been a concern in ventilator-dependent patients on acid-suppression therapy. In earlier studies comparing sucralfate with H_2 blockers, fewer respiratory tract infections were associated with sucralfate therapy.[81,82] Subsequent studies confirmed the association of acid suppression with pneumonia, especially in critically ill patients. A meta-analysis performed by Messori and colleagues[83] showed ranitidine to be ineffective in the prevention of GI bleeding in patients in intensive care and may increase the risk of pneumonia. However, these findings are based on small numbers of patients, and firm conclusions cannot be made. In 2004, a large nested case-control analysis of more than 300,000 individuals was reported.[79] The incidence rates of pneumonia in non–acid-suppressive drug users and acid-suppressive drug users were 0.6 and 2.45 per 100 person-years, respectively. The adjusted relative risk for pneumonia among persons currently using PPIs was 1.89.[79] Hence, the judicious use of acid suppression is warranted. Stress-ulcer prophylaxis should be used only in patients who have compelling risk factors and unnecessary use of acid-suppressive therapy must be avoided.

Clostridium difficile *infection*

Recent data suggest that the rates and severity of nosocomial *C difficile* infection are increasing.[84] The hypothesis that reduction in gastric acid might be relevant to *C difficile* acquisition is biologically plausible. The spores of clostridial organisms are resistant to acid, whereas vegetative cells of the bacteria are highly susceptible to a low pH environment. It has been demonstrated in a hamster model that 75% of ingested spores transformed into the vegetative state within an hour of ingestion.[85] Accordingly, in patients receiving acid-suppression therapy, it is feasible that vegetative cells derived from spores could survive in an intragastric milieu of elevated pH. In a large community-based case-control study, adjusted OR of *C difficile*–associated disease was found to be 2.9 with current use of PPIs.[86] A recent systematic review concluded that there was an increased risk of antisecretory therapy in patients infected with

C difficile (pooled OR 1.94, 95% CI 1.37 to 2.75) The association was greater for PPI use (OR 1.96, 95% CI 1.28 to 3.00) compared with H_2RA use (OR 1.40, 95% CI 0.85 to 2.29).[87] Therefore, judicious use of acid-suppression therapy for stress-ulcer prevention in critically ill patients is warranted.

Other enteric infections

The "gastric bactericidal barrier" is believed to reflect mainly low intragastric pH, because other constituents of the gastric juice seem to contribute little to the barrier function.[88] Indeed, the concept of a "gastric bactericidal barrier" was introduced many decades ago. In 1934, Hurst stated that "the Services would have saved much invaliding if men with achlorhydria were not sent to the tropics" on the basis of observations that dysentery and similar infections were over-represented in people with impaired gastric acid secretion.[89] A prolonged gastric acid inhibitor–induced hypochlorhydria has been suggested as a risk factor for severe GI infections.[90,91] Recently, pediatric population data showed increased risk of acute gastroenteritis (OR 3.58, 95% CI 1.87 to 6.86) and pneumonia (OR 6.39, 95% CI 1.38 to 29.70) in subjects using acid-suppressive drugs.[92] A systematic review conducted by Leonard and colleagues[87] showed an increased risk of taking acid suppression in those with enteric infections (OR 2.55, 95% CI 1.53 to 4.26). The association was greater for PPI use (OR 3.33, 95% CI 1.84 to 6.02) compared with H_2RA use (OR 2.03, 95% CI 1.05 to 3.92). Heretofore, this has not been a problem with extensive with H_2RAs and PPIs in an acute setting if acid-suppression therapy is used for a short period of time. The increased risk of enteric infections may apply to long-term users of acid-suppression therapy. This also implies that therapy for acid suppression must be discontinued once patients recover from critical illness and are no longer at increased risk for stress-ulcer mucosal damage.

Discontinuation of Prophylaxis

There are wide variations in prescribing practices for stress-ulcer prophylaxis. Many clinicians continue stress-ulcer prophylaxis until patients begin an oral diet or are transferred from the ICU.[44] However, in a recent survey 39% of institutions reported that approximately 50% of patients who received stress-ulcer prophylaxis in the ICU were continuing treatment, mostly intravenous agents, after being discharged to non-ICU settings.[45] Most experts consider the risk of clinically important bleeding outside the ICU to be too low to justify continued prophylaxis.[40] Treatment algorithms or protocols for stress ulcer based on prescribing patterns, hospital formulary restrictions, and cost analysis should be considered for each institution to guide critical care physicians on the proper use of stress-ulcer therapies.[44] Introduction by pharmacists of a treatment algorithm for stress-ulcer prophylaxis in ICUs has been shown to allow a reduction of inappropriate prescriptions and, thus, a reduction in the cost of drugs.[42] Adherence to published guidelines for stress-ulcer prophylaxis will prevent unwanted side effects of medications and will also be cost-effective.

Management of Active Stress-Ulcer Bleeding

Stress-related mucosal damage can lead to either diffuse superficial mucosal erosions or discrete stress ulcers, which are focal lesions and may penetrate into the submucosa. Focal stress ulcers are most often located in the gastric body and fundus but may also be present in the duodenum.[40] In critically ill patients GI bleeding may become clinically evident, with a bloody or coffee ground gastric aspirate, hematemesis or melena. Unexplained hypotension or a decrease in hemoglobin level greater than 2 g/dL should also prompt evaluation for bleeding due to stress-related mucosal damage necessitating appropriate management as outlined earlier.

Medical Therapy

Because hypoperfusion seems to be an important factor in the development of SRMD, high-risk patients should be aggressively monitored and treated.[40] Gastrotoxic agents such as NSAIDs or aspirin should be avoided.[40] Measures should be taken to improve hemodynamic parameters to restrict the use of vasopressors if possible, because use of these agents can worsen ischemia of the GI tract. Vasopressors do increase blood pressure, but at the expense of mesenteric perfusion.[93] Early enteral nutrition should be considered. Packed red blood cell transfusion may be required to maintain hemoglobin at an adequate level. Acid-suppression therapy should be initiated. Although studies specifically addressing the choice of therapy for stress-related bleeding are lacking, PPIs are the preferred agents as they have been shown to be more potent agents and reduce the risk of rebleeding, and the need for surgical intervention in non-variceal GI bleeding.[94]

Interventional Therapy

More aggressive therapies are indicated if prophylactic therapy fails and clinically significant stress-related GI bleeding persists. Esophagogastroduodenoscopy (EGD) is the principal diagnostic procedure. EGD can accurately identify the site of bleeding, provides prognostic information about rebleeding risk, and offers therapeutic potential. The precise role of endoscopic therapy in the management of clinically significant stress-related bleeding is difficult to define due, in part, to the diffuse nature of mucosal lesions, which do not lend themselves readily to endoscopic hemostasis.[95] Isolated bleeding sites may be treated by endoscopic or angiographic techniques, although little has been published regarding the efficacy of these modalities in the treatment of stress-related GI bleeding.[95] Several different types of endoscopic treatment described for peptic ulcers, including thermal coagulation, injection therapy, hemostatic clips, argon plasma coagulation, and combination therapy can be applied for a discrete bleeding site of a stress-related ulcer. No prospective comparative trials of endoscopy with and without therapeutic interventions have been performed for stress-related ulcers. Although a clean-based peptic ulcer has 3% to 5% rebleeding rate,[96] stress-related ulcers almost never rebleed once the risk factors are ameliorated. However, data supporting this assertion are lacking. Diagnostic EGD is a safe and simple procedure with a morbidity of 1% and mortality of less than 0.1%.[97] Angiographic and surgical interventions can be considered if the lesions are not amenable to endoscopic therapy.

FUTURE THERAPEUTIC INTERVENTIONS

Newer interventions are needed for monitoring, prevention, and treatment of stress ulcers. Preliminary in vitro data suggest that delivery of the amino acid glutamine to the gastric mucosa might attenuate pro-inflammatory cytokine expression and increase heat shock protein, which protects cells from stress.[98] The beneficial role of growth factors, such as EGF and transforming growth factor alpha formulations, on stress-ulcer bleeding is under investigation.[99] Endothelin-1 (ET-1) has been shown to be involved in the pathogenesis of stress ulceration with elevated plasma and mucosal ET-1 levels found in critically ill patients with stress-ulcer bleeding.[37] ET-1 antagonists could have a potential role in the future in the management of stress ulceration and bleeding. New techniques for detecting and treating hypoperfusion in ICU patients are also needed. A device inserted in a nasogastric tube that could continuously measure local blood flow would help detect gut ischemia.[40] Although these new techniques are conceptually intriguing, their advancement to therapies or diagnostic modalities for stress-related ulcer bleeding has not occurred. This may be due, in part, to the low prevalence of SRMD and the widespread use of potent antisecretory therapies.

SUMMARY

Increased knowledge of risk factors and improved ICU care has decreased the incidence of stress-related bleeding. Not all critically ill patients need prophylaxis for SRMD and withholding such prophylaxis in suitable low-risk candidates is a reasonable and cost-effective approach. Mechanical ventilation for more than 48 hours and coagulopathy are the main risk factors for stress-induced upper GI bleeding. Although intravenous H_2RAs can prevent clinically important bleeding, their benefits seem to be limited by the rapid development of tolerance. The availability of intravenous formulations of PPIs makes it possible to critically compare their prophylactic efficacy and safety to different classes of acid-suppressive agents, such as H_2RAs, in critically ill patients. The appropriate dose of PPI and the role of newer PPI formulations need to be further defined along with proposed guidelines for the use of intravenous and oral/enteral formulations of PPIs in patients at risk for stress-related mucosal damage.[100]

REFERENCES

1. Selye H. A syndrome produced by diverse nocuous agents. 1936. J Neuropsychiatry Clin Neurosci 1998;10(2):230–1.
2. Curling TB. On acute ulceration of the duodenum in cases of burn. Med Chir Trans (Lond) 1842;25:260–81.
3. Lucas CE, Sugawa C, Riddle J, et al. Natural history and surgical dilemma of "stress" gastric bleeding. Arch Surg 1971;102:266–73.
4. Choung RS, Talley NJ. Epidemiology and clinical presentation of stress-related peptic damage and chronic peptic ulcer. Curr Mol Med 2008;8:253–7.
5. ASHP therapeutic guidelines on stress ulcer prophylaxis. ASHP commission on therapeutics and approved by the ASHP board of directors on 1998. Am J Health Syst Pharm 1999;56:347–79.
6. Peura DA, Johnson LF. Cimetidine for prevention and treatment of gastroduodenal mucosal lesions in patients in an intensive care unit. Ann Intern Med 1985;103:173–7.
7. Czaja AJ, McAlhany JC, Pruitt BA Jr. Acute gastroduodenal disease after thermal injury. An endoscopic evaluation of incidence and natural history. N Engl J Med 1974;291:925–9.
8. Duerksen DR. Stress-related mucosal disease in critically ill patients. Best Pract Res Clin Gastroenterol 2003;17:327–44.
9. Shuman RB, Schuster DP, Zuckerman GR. Prophylactic therapy for stress ulcer bleeding: a reappraisal. Ann Intern Med 1987;106:562–7.
10. Mutlu GM, Mutlu EA, Factor P. GI complications in patients receiving mechanical ventilation. Chest 2001;119:1222–41.
11. Fennerty MB. Pathophysiology of the upper gastrointestinal tract in the critically ill patient: rationale for the therapeutic benefits of acid suppression. Crit Care Med 2002;30:S351–5.

12. Cook DJ, Reeve BK, Guyatt GH, et al. Stress ulcer prophylaxis in critically ill patients. Resolving discordant meta-analyses. JAMA 1996;275:308–14.
13. Cook DJ, Fuller HD, Guyatt GH, et al. Risk factors for gastrointestinal bleeding in critically ill patients. Canadian Critical Care Trials Group. N Engl J Med 1994; 330:377–81.
14. Cook DJ, Griffith LE, Walter SD, et al. The attributable mortality and length of intensive care unit stay of clinically important gastrointestinal bleeding in critically ill patients. Crit Care 2001;5:368–75.
15. Allen ME, Kopp BJ, Erstad BL. Stress ulcer prophylaxis in the postoperative period. Am J Health Syst Pharm 2004;61:588–96.
16. Laine L, Takeuchi K, Tarnawski A. Gastric mucosal defense and cytoprotection: bench to bedside. Gastroenterology 2008;135:41–60.
17. Hunter J. Digestion of the stomach after death. Philos Trans R Soc Lond B Biol Sci 1772;62:447–54.
18. Virchow R. Historisches, kritisches und positives zur lehre der unterleibsaffektionen. Arch Anat Pathol 1853;5:281–375.
19. Vane JR. Inhibition of prostaglandin synthesis as a mechanism of action for aspirin-like drugs. Nat New Biol 1971;231:232–5.
20. Robert A, Nezamis JE, Lancaster C, et al. Cytoprotection by prostaglandins in rats. Prevention of gastric necrosis produced by alcohol, HCl, NaOH, hypertonic NaCl, and thermal injury. Gastroenterology 1979;77:433–43.
21. Robert A, Nezamis JE, Lancaster C, et al. Mild irritants prevent gastric necrosis through "adaptive cytoprotection" mediated by prostaglandins. Am J Phys 1983; 245:G113–21.
22. Dong MH, Kaunitz JD. Gastroduodenal mucosal defense. Curr Opin Gastroenterol 2006;22:599–606.
23. Ham M, Kaunitz JD. Gastroduodenal defense. Curr Opin Gastroenterol 2007;23: 607–16.
24. Kamada T, Sato N, Kawano S, et al. Gastric mucosal hemodynamics after thermal or head injury. A clinical application of reflectance spectrophotometry. Gastroenterology 1982;83:535–40.
25. Leung FW, Itoh M, Hirabayashi K, et al. Role of blood flow in gastric and duodenal mucosal injury in the rat. Gastroenterology 1985;88:281–9.
26. Yasue N, Guth PH. Role of exogenous acid and retransfusion in hemorrhagic shock-induced gastric lesions in the rat. Gastroenterology 1988;94:1135–43.
27. Das D, Bandyopadhyay D, Bhattacharjee M, et al. Hydroxyl radical is the major causative factor in stress-induced gastric ulceration. Free Radic Biol Med 1997; 23:8–18.
28. Shian WM, Sasaki I, Kamiyama Y, et al. The role of lipid peroxidation on gastric mucosal lesions induced by water-immersion-restraint stress in rats. Surg Today 2000;30:49–53.
29. Sun Y, Oberley LW. Redox regulation of transcriptional activators. Free Radic Biol Med 1996;21:335–48.
30. Droge W. Free radicals in the physiological control of cell function. Physiol Rev 2002;82:47–95.
31. Branger J, van den Blink B, Weijer S, et al. Anti-inflammatory effects of a p38 mitogen-activated protein kinase inhibitor during human endotoxemia. J Immunol 2002;168:4070–7.
32. Jia YT, Wei W, Ma B, et al. Activation of p38 MAPK by reactive oxygen species is essential in a rat model of stress-induced gastric mucosal injury. J Immunol 2007;179:7808–19.

33. Maricic N, Ehrlich K, Gretzer B, et al. Selective cyclo-oxygenase-2 inhibitors aggravate ischaemia-reperfusion injury in the rat stomach. Br J Pharmacol 1999;128:1659–66.
34. Schmedtje JF Jr, Ji YS, Liu WL, et al. Hypoxia induces cyclooxygenase-2 via the NF-kappaB p65 transcription factor in human vascular endothelial cells. J Biol Chem 1997;272:601–8.
35. Wada K, Kamisaki Y, Ohkura T, et al. Direct measurement of nitric oxide release in gastric mucosa during ischemia-reperfusion in rats. Am J Phys 1998;274:G465–71.
36. Kobata A, Kotani T, Komatsu Y, et al. Dual action of nitric oxide in the pathogenesis of ischemia/reperfusion-induced mucosal injury in mouse stomach. Digestion 2007;75:188–97.
37. Michida T, Kawano S, Masuda E, et al. Endothelin-1 in the gastric mucosa in stress ulcers of critically ill patients. Am J Gastroenterol 1997;92:1177–81.
38. Maynard N, Bihari D, Beale R, et al. Assessment of splanchnic oxygenation by gastric tonometry in patients with acute circulatory failure. JAMA 1993;270: 1203–10.
39. Spirt MJ. Stress-related mucosal disease: risk factors and prophylactic therapy. Clin Ther 2004;26:197–213.
40. Spirt MJ, Stanley S. Update on stress ulcer prophylaxis in critically ill patients. Crit Care Nurse 2006;26:18–20, 22–8.
41. Ellison RT, Perez-Perez G, Welsh CH, et al. Risk factors for upper gastrointestinal bleeding in intensive care unit patients: role of Helicobacter pylori. Federal Hyperimmune Immunoglobulin Therapy Study Group. Crit Care Med 1996;24: 1974–81.
42. Coursol CJ, Sanzari SE. Impact of stress ulcer prophylaxis algorithm study. Ann Pharmacother 2005;39:810–6.
43. Erstad BL, Camamo JM, Miller MJ, et al. Impacting cost and appropriateness of stress ulcer prophylaxis at a university medical center. Crit Care Med 1997;25: 1678–84.
44. Lam NP, Le PD, Crawford SY, et al. National survey of stress ulcer prophylaxis. Crit Care Med 1999;27:98–103.
45. Barletta JF, Erstad BL, Fortune JB. Stress ulcer prophylaxis in trauma patients. Crit Care 2002;6:526–30.
46. Daley RJ, Rebuck JA, Welage LS, et al. Prevention of stress ulceration: current trends in critical care. Crit Care Med 2004;32:2008–13.
47. Wade EE, Rebuck JA, Healey MA, et al. H(2) antagonist-induced thrombocytopenia: is this a real phenomenon? Intensive Care Med 2002;28:459–65.
48. Epstein CM. Histamine H2 antagonists and the nervous system. Am Fam Physician 1985;32:109–12.
49. Humphries TJ, Merritt GJ. Review article: drug interactions with agents used to treat acid-related diseases. Aliment Pharmacol Ther 1999;3:18–26.
50. Siepler JK, Trudeau W, Petty DE. Use of continuous infusion of histamine 2-receptor antagonists in critically ill patients. DICP 1989;23:S40–3.
51. Ostro MJ, Russell JA, Soldin SJ, et al. Control of gastric pH with cimetidine: boluses versus primed infusions. Gastroenterology 1985;89:532–7.
52. Somberg L, Morris J Jr, Fantus R, et al. Intermittent intravenous pantoprazole and continuous cimetidine infusion: effect on gastric pH control in critically ill patients at risk of developing stress-related mucosal disease. J Trauma 2008;64:1202–10.
53. Pemberton LB, Schaefer N, Goehring L, et al. Oral ranitidine as prophylaxis for gastric stress ulcers in intensive care unit patients: serum concentrations and cost comparisons. Crit Care Med 1993;21:339–42.

54. Mathot RA, Geus WP. Pharmacodynamic modeling of the acid inhibitory effect of ranitidine in patients in an intensive care unit during prolonged dosing: characterization of tolerance. Clin Pharmacol Ther 1999;66:140–51.
55. Levy MJ, Seelig CB, Robinson NJ, et al. Comparison of omeprazole and ranitidine for stress ulcer prophylaxis. Dig Dis Sci 1997;42:1255–9.
56. Phillips JO, Metzler MH, Palmieri MT, et al. A prospective study of simplified omeprazole suspension for the prophylaxis of stress-related mucosal damage. Crit Care Med 1996;24:1793–800.
57. Lasky MR, Metzler MH, Phillips JO. A prospective study of omeprazole suspension to prevent clinically significant gastrointestinal bleeding from stress ulcers in mechanically ventilated trauma patients. J Trauma 1998;44:527–33.
58. Andersson T, Hassan-Alin M, Hasselgren G, et al. Drug interaction studies with esomeprazole, the (S)-isomer of omeprazole. Clin Pharm 2001;40:523–37.
59. Stefanov C, Batashki I, Dimitrov D, et al [Efficiency and safety of the intravenous application of esomeprazole (Nexium—Astra Zeneca) in high risk patients subjected to mechanical ventilation]. Khirurgiia 2007;3:25–8 [Bulgarian].
60. Tsai WL, Poon SK, Yu HK, et al. Nasogastric lansoprazole is effective in suppressing gastric acid secretion in critically ill patients. Aliment Pharmacol Ther 2000;14:123–7.
61. Olsen KM, Devlin JW. Comparison of the enteral and intravenous lansoprazole pharmacodynamic responses in critically ill patients. Aliment Pharmacol Ther 2008;3:326–33.
62. Huber R, Kohl B, Sachs G, et al. Review article: the continuing development of proton pump inhibitors with particular reference to pantoprazole. Aliment Pharmacol Ther 1995;9:363–78.
63. Harty RF, Ancha HB. Stress ulcer bleeding. Curr Treat Options Gastroenterol 2006;9:157–66.
64. Conrad SA, Gabrielli A, Margolis B, et al. Randomized, double-blind comparison of immediate-release omeprazole oral suspension versus intravenous cimetidine for the prevention of upper gastrointestinal bleeding in critically ill patients. Crit Care Med 2005;33:760–5.
65. Klebl FH, Scholmerich J. Therapy insight: prophylaxis of stress-induced gastrointestinal bleeding in critically ill patients. Nat Clin Pract Gastroenterol Hepatol 2007;4:562–70.
66. Zinner MJ, Rypins EB, Martin LR, et al. Misoprostol versus antacid titration for preventing stress ulcers in postoperative surgical ICU patients. Ann Surg 1989;210:590–5.
67. Szabo S, Hollander D. Pathways of gastrointestinal protection and repair: mechanisms of action of sucralfate. Am J Med 1989;86:23–31.
68. Tryba M. Sucralfate versus antacids or H2-antagonists for stress ulcer prophylaxis: a meta-analysis on efficacy and pneumonia rate. Crit Care Med 1991; 19:942–9.
69. Hastings PR, Skillman JJ, Bushnell LS, et al. Antacid titration in the prevention of acute gastrointestinal bleeding: a controlled, randomized trial in 100 critically ill patients. N Engl J Med 1978;298:1041–5.
70. Maury E, Tankovic J, Ebel A, et al. An observational study of upper gastrointestinal bleeding in intensive care units: is *Helicobacter pylori* the culprit? Crit Care Med 2005;33:1513–8.
71. Halm U, Halm F, Thein D, et al. *Helicobacter pylori* infection: a risk factor for upper gastrointestinal bleeding after cardiac surgery? Crit Care Med 2000;28: 110–3.

72. van der Voort PH, van der Hulst RW, Zandstra DF, et al. Prevalence of *Helicobacter pylori* infection in stress-induced gastric mucosal injury. Intensive Care Med 2001;27:68–73.

73. Schilling D, Haisch G, Sloot N, et al. Low seroprevalence of *Helicobacter pylori* infection in patients with stress ulcer bleeding–a prospective evaluation of patients on a cardiosurgical intensive care unit. Intensive Care Med 2000;26: 1832–6.

74. Yan R, Sun Y, Sun R [Early enteral feeding and supplement of glutamine prevent occurrence of stress ulcer following severe thermal injury]. Zhonghua Zheng Xing Shao Shang Wai Ke Za Zhi 1995;11:189–92 [Chinese].

75. MacLaren R, Jarvis CL, Fish DN. Use of enteral nutrition for stress ulcer prophylaxis. Ann Pharmacother 2001;35:1614–23.

76. O'May GA, Reynolds N, Macfarlane GT. Effect of pH on an in vitro model of gastric microbiota in enteral nutrition patients. Appl Environ Microbiol 2005;71: 4777–83.

77. Thorens J, Froehlich F, Schwizer W, et al. Bacterial overgrowth during treatment with omeprazole compared with cimetidine: a prospective randomised double blind study. Gut 1996;39:54–9.

78. Zedtwitz-Liebenstein K, Wenisch C, Patruta S, et al. Omeprazole treatment diminishes intra- and extracellular neutrophil reactive oxygen production and bactericidal activity. Crit Care Med 2002;30:1118–22.

79. Laheij RJ, Sturkenboom MC, Hassing RJ, et al. Risk of community-acquired pneumonia and use of gastric acid-suppressive drugs. JAMA 2004;292: 1955–60.

80. Cunningham R, Dale B, Undy B, et al. Proton pump inhibitors as a risk factor for *Clostridium difficile* diarrhoea. J Hosp Infect 2003;54:243–5.

81. Tryba M. Risk of acute stress bleeding and nosocomial pneumonia in ventilated intensive care unit patients: sucralfate versus antacids. Am J Med 1987;83: 117–24.

82. Driks MR, Craven DE, Celli BR, et al. Nosocomial pneumonia in intubated patients given sucralfate as compared with antacids or histamine type 2 blockers. The role of gastric colonization. N Engl J Med 1987;317:1376–82.

83. Messori A, Trippoli S, Vaiani M, et al. Bleeding and pneumonia in intensive care patients given ranitidine and sucralfate for prevention of stress ulcer: meta-analysis of randomised controlled trials. BMJ 2000;321:1103–6.

84. Pepin J, Valiquette L, Alary ME, et al. *Clostridium difficile*-associated diarrhea in a region of Quebec from 1991 to 2003: a changing pattern of disease severity. CMAJ 2004;171:466–72.

85. Wilson KH, Sheagren JN, Freter R. Population dynamics of ingested *Clostridium difficile* in the gastrointestinal tract of the Syrian hamster. J Infect Dis 1985;151: 355–61.

86. Dial S, Delaney JA, Barkun AN, et al. Use of gastric acid-suppressive agents and the risk of community-acquired *Clostridium difficile*-associated disease. JAMA 2005;294:2989–95.

87. Leonard J, Marshall JK, Moayyedi P. Systematic review of the risk of enteric infection in patients taking acid suppression. Am J Gastroenterol 2007;102: 2047–56.

88. Martinsen TC, Bergh K, Waldum HL. Gastric juice: a barrier against infectious diseases. Basic Clin Pharmacol Toxicol 2005;96:94–102.

89. Hurst AF. The clinical importance of achlorhydria. BMJ 1934;2:665–9.

90. Neal KR, Briji SO, Slack RC, et al. Recent treatment with H2 antagonists and antibiotics and gastric surgery as risk factors for Salmonella infection. BMJ 1994;308:176.
91. Neal KR, Scott HM, Slack RC, et al. Omeprazole as a risk factor for campylobacter gastroenteritis: case-control study. BMJ 1996;312:414–5.
92. Canani RB, Cirillo P, Roggero P, et al. Therapy with gastric acidity inhibitors increases the risk of acute gastroenteritis and community-acquired pneumonia in children. Pediatrics 2006;117:e817–20.
93. Marik PE, Mohedin M. The contrasting effects of dopamine and norepinephrine on systemic and splanchnic oxygen utilization in hyperdynamic sepsis. JAMA 1994;272:1354–7.
94. Khuroo MS, Yattoo GN, Javid G, et al. A comparison of omeprazole and placebo for bleeding peptic ulcer. N Engl J Med 1997;336:1054–8.
95. Beejay U, Wolfe MM. Acute gastrointestinal bleeding in the intensive care unit. The gastroenterologist's perspective. Gastroenterol Clin North Am 2000;29: 309–36.
96. Katschinski B, Logan R, Davies J, et al. Prognostic factors in upper gastrointestinal bleeding. Dig Dis Sci 1994;39:706–12.
97. Kovacs TO. Management of upper gastrointestinal bleeding. Curr Gastroenterol Rep 2008;10:535–42.
98. Wischmeyer PE, Riehm J, Singleton KD, et al. Glutamine attenuates tumor necrosis factor-alpha release and enhances heat shock protein 72 in human peripheral blood mononuclear cells. Nutrition 2003;19:1–6.
99. Akbulut KG, Gonul B, Turkyilmaz A, et al. The role of epidermal growth factor formulation on stress ulcer healing of the gastric mucosa. Surg Today 2002; 32:880–3.
100. Woofter A, Goodgame R. Grand rounds in gastroenterology from Baylor College of Medicine. Upper gastrointestinal bleeding in the ICU. MedGenMed 2006;8:43.

Refractory Peptic Ulcer Disease

Lena Napolitano, MD, FACS, FCCP, FCCM

KEYWORDS

- Peptic ulcer disease • *Helicobacter pylori* • Gastrin
- Zollinger-Ellison syndrome • Hypersecretion

Although the incidence of peptic ulcer disease (PUD) in Western countries has declined over the past 100 years, about 1 in 10 Americans are still affected.[1] As the prevalence of PUD increased with advancing age, it is expected that this common disease will continue to have a significant global impact on health care delivery, health economics, and the quality of life of patients.[2]

PUD is the main cause for upper gastrointestinal (UGI) hemorrhage, and *Helicobacter pylori* infection is the main etiologic factor for PUD. Medical regimens to identify and eradicate the organism and the widespread use of proton pump inhibitor (PPI) therapy to suppress gastric acid secretion have resulted in successful medical management of PUD in the vast majority of patients.[3–5] As a result, successful medical management of PUD has largely supplanted the need for gastric surgery by general surgeons.[6]

Surgery of PUD is now limited to treatment of more emergent complications of the disease (hemorrhage, perforation, gastric outlet obstruction), refractory disease and intractability (related to bleeding or gastrointestinal [GI] complications), or rare causes of ulcer disease, such as gastrinoma and the Zollinger-Ellison syndrome (ZES). Indications for elective peptic ulcer surgery include the following: resection of ulcers suspicious for malignancy, failure to heal despite maximal medical therapy, intolerance or noncompliance with medical therapy, and relapse while on maximal medical therapy.

In this article diagnostic and treatment issues related to refractory PUD are reviewed.[7] It is most important to ensure that appropriate standard therapy for PUD is provided with subsequent confirmation of eradication of *H pylori* infection, because this is the best method for prevention of refractory PUD. If refractory PUD does occur, it is important to have a systematic approach for diagnosis and treatment. Refractory PUD manifests as either *hemorrhagic complications* (persistent or recurrent bleeding) or *GI complications* (perforation, stricture, obstruction). Treatment strategies for hemorrhagic complications include endoscopic therapy, surgery, and transcatheter

Department of Surgery, University of Michigan Health System, University of Michigan School of Medicine, Room 1C421, University Hospital, 1500 East Medical Drive, Ann Arbor, MI 48109-0033, USA
E-mail address: lenan@umich.edu

Gastroenterol Clin N Am 38 (2009) 267–288
doi:10.1016/j.gtc.2009.03.011
0889-8553/09/$ – see front matter © 2009 Elsevier Inc. All rights reserved.

angiographic embolization. Treatment strategies for GI complications include endoscopic dilation for stricture and surgery for perforation and obstruction. Potential etiologies of persistent or worsening PUD must be considered in these cases and include the following: patient risk factors and noncompliance, persistent *H pylori* infection, and non–*H pylori*–related infection, related to underlying idiopathic gastric hypersecretion or ZES and gastrinoma. An appropriate and meticulous diagnostic work-up for refractory PUD is mandatory.

STANDARD THERAPY FOR PEPTIC ULCER DISEASE

The widespread use of effective antisecretory therapies, including PPIs, and the recognition and successful eradication of *H pylori* infection have made peptic ulcer a disease that can be cured by medical management in most cases.[8] Surgical intervention had once been the dominant form of definitive therapy, but it is now reserved for emergent, life-threatening complications of PUD, such as bleeding, perforation, and obstruction.[9] Intractability, failure to comply with or tolerate medical therapy, and rare cases of gastrinoma or ZES are indications for elective surgery for PUD.

H pylori is associated with 95% of duodenal ulcers and 70% of gastric ulcers, and eradication of *H pylori* reduces the relapse rate of ulcers. The 2004 Cochrane evidence-based review of 53 randomized controlled trials of short- and long-term treatment of PUD in *H pylori*-positive adults examined the effect of this treatment. Patients received at least 1 week of *H pylori* eradication therapy compared with ulcer-healing drug, placebo, or no treatment. In duodenal ulcer healing, *H pylori* eradication therapy was superior to ulcer-healing drug (34 trials, 3910 patients, relative risk [RR] of ulcer persistence, 0.66; 95% confidence interval [CI], 0.58–0.76) and no treatment (two trials, 207 patients, RR, 0.37; 95% CI, 0.26–0.53). In gastric ulcer healing, no significant differences were detected between eradication therapy and ulcer-healing drug (13 trials, 1469 patients, RR, 1.32; 95% CI, 0.92–1.90). This confirmed that a 1- to 2-week course of *H pylori* eradication therapy is an effective treatment for *H pylori*-positive PUD.[10]

There is now a worldwide consensus that the first-line treatment of *H pylori* infection should be triple therapy with a PPI twice daily plus clarithromycin 500 mg twice daily and either amoxicillin 1 g twice daily or metronidazole 500 mg twice daily for 7 to 14 days.[11] Treatment with PPIs twice daily is superior to treatment once daily.[12] Bismuth-containing quadruple therapy, if available, is also a first choice treatment option.[13] Successful eradication with first-line treatments varies from 70% to 95%, and 10- and 14-day treatments are generally 7% to 9% more effective than the most commonly used 7-day regimens.[14] Rescue treatment should be based on antimicrobial susceptibility.

Eradication of *H pylori* infection should be confirmed after the completion of therapy and noninvasive testing with the urea breath test is the preferred choice, 4 to 8 weeks after the completion of therapy (**Table 1**).[15] If the ulcer recurs after the eradication therapy, a more careful search for reinfection or eradication failure should be performed by testing for the presence of active infection (by histologic examination and culture, together with an antibiotic-sensitivity test). The diagnosis of *H pylori* infection in patients with a bleeding PUD is limited by the decreased sensitivity of standard invasive tests; usually, both the rapid urease test and histologic testing should be performed during endoscopy and then combined with the urea breath test. Infection should be considered as present when any test is positive, whereas the invasive tests and the urea breath test should be negative to establish the absence of *H pylori* infection.

		Table 1

Table 1
Helicobacter pylori testing, particularly to confirm eradication after treatment
for peptic ulcer disease

Diagnostic Test	Specific Issues	Can Be Used to Confirm Eradication
Serologic ELISA	Useful only for initial testing Sensitivity 85% Specificity 79%	No
Urea breath test	Sensitivity 95%–100% Specificity 91%–98% Expensive	yes (PPI therapy should be stopped for 2 weeks before test for eradication)
Stool antigen test	Inconvenient but accurate Sensitivity 91%–98% Specificity 94%–99%	Yes
Urine-based ELISA and rapid urine test	Sensitivity 70%–96% Specificity 77%–85%	No
Endoscopic biopsy	*Culture* Sensitivity 70%–80% Specificity 100% *Histology* Sensitivity >95% Specificity 100% *Rapid urease (CLO) test* Sensitivity 93%–97% Specificity 100%	Yes

Abbreviation: CLO, *Campylobacter*-like organism.
Data from University of Michigan Health System. Peptic ulcer disease. Available at: http://www. cme.med.umich.edu/pdf/guideline/PUD05.pdf. Accessed January 12, 2009.

Furthermore, it is well accepted that in patients with uncomplicated PUD, *H pylori* eradication therapy need not be followed by antisecretory treatment. A 5-year prospective controlled study randomized 82 patients with *H pylori*-associated bleeding peptic ulcers to 1 of 4 16-week maintenance treatment groups after successful *H pylori* eradication with a 1-week PPI-based triple therapy and an additional 43-week treatment with 20 mg of omeprazole daily for ulcer healing. The four experimental groups were as follows: group A received 15 mL of an antacid suspension four times daily; group B received 300 mg of colloidal bismuth subcitrate four times daily, group C received 20 mg of famotidine twice daily; and group D, the control group, received placebo twice daily. Follow-up included a urea breath test labeled with carbon 13, biopsy-based tests, and repeated endoscopic examination. During a mean follow-up of 56 months, there was no peptic ulcer recurrence among the three treatment groups, and all the patients remained free of *H pylori* infection during the study period. This study documented that in patients with bleeding peptic ulcers, antiulcer maintenance treatment was not necessary to prevent ulcer recurrence after successful *H pylori* eradication and ulcer healing. Besides, the 1-week PPI-based triple therapy had the efficacy to ensure long-term eradication of *H pylori* in a region of high prevalence.[16]

REFRACTORY PEPTIC ULCER DISEASE

Refractory PUD is defined as a disease that fails to heal after 8 to 12 weeks of therapy or one that is associated with complications. It is most challenging to evaluate and treat patients with complicated and/or refractory PUD. A recent analysis regarding admission rates for PUD in the United Kingdom during 1972 to 2000 determined that emergency admission rates as a whole changed little, a decline in the young being offset by an increase in the elderly. Hemorrhage was the most common reason (approximately 115 per million population for duodenal ulcer and 87 for gastric ulcer) throughout (compared with perforation [80 and 21] and pain [90 and 68]).[17]

Refractory Peptic Ulcer Disease and Bleeding

Acute UGI bleeding related to refractory PUD remains a challenging clinical problem owing to significant patient morbidity and mortality. PUD accounts for 28% to 59% of all episodes of UGI bleeding.[18] The mortality rate associated with bleeding duodenal ulcer disease is about 10%. The first priority in treatment of bleeding due to refractory PUD is the initiation of resuscitation, critical care support, and PPI therapy (**Fig. 1**). A systematic review of the clinical efficacy of PPI in acute UGI bleeding concluded that PPI treatment compared with placebo or histamine-2 receptor antagonists (H2RAs) reduces mortality following PUD bleeding among patients with high-risk endoscopic findings, and reduces hemorrhage recurrence rates and surgical intervention.[19] PPI treatment initiated before endoscopy in UGI bleeding significantly reduced the proportion of patients with stigmata of recent hemorrhage (SRH) at index endoscopy but did not reduce mortality, rebleeding, or the need for surgery in this analysis. More recently, the initiation of PPI bolus followed by continuous infusion after endoscopic therapy in patients with bleeding ulcers significantly improved outcome compared with placebo/no therapy (RR, 0.40, 95% CI, 0.28–0.59; number needed to treat [NNT], 12, 95% CI, 10–18), but not compared with H2RA.[20] The strategy of giving PPI before and after endoscopy, with endoscopic hemostatic therapy for those with major SRH, is the most cost-effective. Treatment of H pylori infection was found to be more effective than antisecretory therapy in preventing recurrent bleeding from PUD.[21] Further large randomized controlled trials are needed to address areas, such as PPI administration before endoscopic diagnosis, different doses and administration of PPIs, as well as the primary and secondary prevention of UGI bleeding.

Endoscopy is the preferred first-line management of refractory bleeding due to PUD.[22] Current endoscopic modalities, both thermal and nonthermal, offer a wide range of choices in high-risk PUD bleeding (active arterial bleeding or nonbleeding

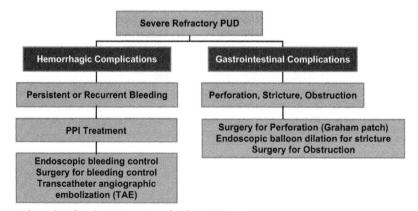

Fig. 1. Algorithm for the treatment of refractory PUD.

visible vessel). Combinations of injection (epinephrine) along with thermal therapy or endoclips are recommended for better clinical outcomes. A recent review concluded that all endoscopic treatments are superior to pharmacotherapy alone in peptic ulcer bleeding. Optimal endoscopic therapies include thermal therapy or clips, either alone or in combination with other methods, but epinephrine injection should not be used alone.[19,23] The role of endotherapy for adherent clots is controversial. A second-look endoscopy may be beneficial in high-risk patients.

Primary endoscopic hemostasis is successful in more than 90% of patients, but in 15% to 25% of the patients, either the bleeding cannot be controlled endoscopically or there is recurrence of bleeding, requiring alternative treatment. The combination of endoscopic intervention for hemostasis and PPI therapy is necessary to achieve hemostasis of active bleeding related to PUD.[24] Continued bleeding after attempted endoscopic control may warrant surgical intervention. A multidisciplinary team approach should be part of all treatment protocols for the ideal management of refractory UGI hemorrhage related to PUD, and early surgical consultation is required.

An emerging strategy for bleeding control in refractory PUD is angiographic embolization (see **Fig. 1**). In patients who are poor surgical candidates because of their high operative risk, percutaneous transcatheter angiographic arterial embolization (TAE) is a therapeutic option. A recent study evaluated the efficacy and medium-term outcomes of TAE to control massive bleeding from gastroduodenal ulcers after failed endoscopic treatment in high-operative-risk patients. This was a retrospective study of 35 consecutive emergency embolization procedures in hemodynamically unstable patients (24 men, 11 women, mean age 71±11.6 y) referred from 1999 to 2006 for selective angiography after failed endoscopic treatment. Mean follow-up was 27 months. Endovascular treatment was feasible in 33 patients and consistently stopped the bleeding. "Sandwich" coiling of the gastroduodenal artery was performed in 11 patients and superselective occlusion of the terminal-feeding artery with glue, coils, or gelatin particles in 22 patients. Early rebleeding occurred in six patients and was managed successfully using endoscopy (n = 2), reembolization (n = 1), or surgery (n = 3). No major complications related to TAE occurred. Seven patients died within 30 days of TAE and three died later during the follow-up, but none of the deaths were due to rebleeding. No late bleeding recurrences were reported. These investigators concluded that selective TAE is safe and effective for controlling life-threatening bleeding from gastroduodenal ulcers, usually obviating the need for emergency surgery in critically ill patients, whose immediate survival depends on their underlying conditions.[25]

Previous reports also evaluated the efficacy and safety of TAE. In a 6-year review of 40 consecutive patients with bleeding/rebleeding after endoscopic therapy and/or surgery for duodenal ulcer, superselective angiographic catheterization and coil embolization were performed by the same interventional radiologist. Lasting hemostasis was achieved in 26 of 40 patients (65%). Transfusion requirement was reduced from median 14 (range, 3–35) units of blood before TAE to two (range, 0–53) units after TAE. Ten patients died, half of them because of continuous bleeding. No adverse effects as a result of TAE were observed.[26]

A recent retrospective review identified all patients admitted to Ullevål University Hospital with hematemesis and/or melena and endoscopically verified duodenal ulcer from June 2000 to 2005. The indication for TAE was endoscopically unmanageable bleeding/rebleeding or rebleeding after surgery. Technical success was defined as acute hemostasis. Clinical success was defined as technical success without rebleeding within 30 days. A total of 278 patients (mean age, 73 years) were included in the study. Primary endoscopic hemostasis failed in 13 patients (5%) and 53 patients

(20%) experienced rebleeding. An attempt was made to treat 36 patients with TAE. Technical success in the TAE group was 92% and clinical success was 72%. In total, 10 patients underwent surgery, three because of rebleeding after TAE. The 30-day mortality was 10% for all patients, 19% in the TAE group, and 20% in the surgical group. High technical and clinical success was obtained with TAE in patients with bleeding duodenal ulcer after failure of endoscopic treatment in this cohort study.[27]

A retrospective review of the outcome of TAE and surgery as salvage therapy of UGI bleeding after failed endoscopic treatment was recently performed in 658 patients referred for diagnostic/therapeutic emergency endoscopy and diagnosed with UGI bleeding (January 1998–December 2005).[28] Of these 658 patients, 91 (14%) had repeat bleeding or continued to bleed. Forty of those 91 patients were treated with TAE and 51 were underwent surgery. Patients treated with TAE were older (mean age, 76 years; age range, 40–94 years) and had slightly more comorbidities compared with patients who underwent surgery (mean age, 71 years; age range, 45–89 years). The 30-day mortality rate in patients treated with TAE was 1 of 40 (3%) compared with 7 of 51 (14%) in patients who underwent surgery ($P<.07$). Most repeat bleeding could be effectively treated with TAE, both in the surgical and TAE groups. The results of this study suggest that, after failure of therapeutic endoscopy for UGI bleeding, TAE should be the treatment of choice before surgery and that TAE can also be used to effectively control bleeding after failed surgery or TAE. There was a clear trend to lower 30-day mortality with the use of TAE instead of surgery.

The data from these cohort studies document that TAE is an effective and safe treatment in a significant proportion of patients with bleeding/rebleeding duodenal ulcers after therapeutic endoscopy and/or surgery and may serve as an alternative to surgery in high-risk patients (**Fig. 2**).

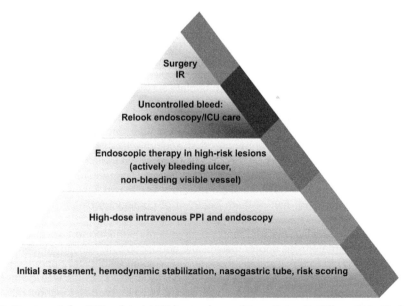

Fig. 2. Treatment for PUD-related UGI hemorrhage. (*From* Peter S, Wilcox CM. Modern endoscopic therapy of peptic ulcer bleeding. Dig Dis 2008;26:291–9; with permission.)

Refractory Peptic Ulcer Disease and Gastrointestinal Complications

GI complications related to refractory PUD include perforation (duodenal or gastric perforation) and obstruction, either partial or complete gastric outlet obstruction related to stenosis and stricture at the ulcer site. These GI complications can be challenging to treat and frequently require surgical intervention.

Perforation related to Peptic Ulcer Disease

Perforation occurs in approximately 2% to 10% of patients with PUD.[29] It usually involves the anterior wall of the duodenum (60%), although it may also occur in antral (20%) and lesser-curve (20%) gastric ulcers. Recent data strongly implicate *H pylori* infection as the cause of perforated duodenal ulcer, with reported *H pylori* infection rates of 70% to 92% in these patients.[30–34] A randomized study in 129 patients with duodenal ulcer perforation documented that 104 (81%) were infected with *H pylori*, diagnosed by esophagogastroduodenoscopy and biopsy at the time of laparotomy. Postoperatively, patients were randomized to receive *H pylori* treatment or PPI therapy for 4 weeks. Repeat endoscopy at 1 year confirmed that the incidence of recurrent ulceration was significantly lower in the *H pylori* treatment group (5%) compared with the PPI therapy group (38%). Based on these findings, surgical treatment for perforated duodenal ulcer is simple patch closure with postoperative *H pylori* treatment, including PPI therapy and antimicrobial agents, and documentation of eradication. Some patients with complicated perforated ulcer, either with destruction of proximal duodenum and penetration into adjacent organs, giant perforations measuring more than 20 mm in diameter or with severe duodenal stenosis, may require resectional surgery.[35,36]

Perforated duodenal ulcer with perforation free into the peritoneal cavity is associated with peritonitis and warrants emergency surgical intervention. Both conventional laparotomy and laparoscopic techniques for suture closure with omental patch are acceptable surgical options for treatment in these patients.[37–39] A randomized clinical trial (n = 130) did identify that laparoscopic repair of perforated PUD was associated with a shorter operating time, less postoperative pain, reduced pulmonary complications, shorter postoperative hospital stay, and earlier return to normal daily activities compared with the conventional open surgery, but surgeon's laparoscopic experience and severity of illness of the patient must be considered in this decision making.[40] A Cochrane Systematic Review concluded that laparoscopic surgery results are not clinically different from those of open surgery in patients with perforated PUD.[41] Another systematic review concluded that laparoscopic repair seemed better than open surgery for low-risk patients, and that limited knowledge about its benefits and risks compared with open surgery suggests that the open approach may be more appropriate in high-risk studies.[42] A more recent small prospective cohort study (n = 33) suggested that laparoscopic repair should be considered for all patients provided the necessary expertise is available.[43] Specific factors have been identified that qualify as criteria for open laparotomy, including shock, delayed presentation— for more than 24 hours, confounding medical conditions, age more than 70 years, poor laparoscopic expertise, and American Society of Anesthesiologists score III to IV.[44] However, additional studies are warranted in this area.

Obstruction related to Peptic Ulcer Disease

In patients presenting with gastric outlet obstruction, PUD is the underlying cause in up to 8% of patients. Many of them, however, have refractory PUD related to recurrent or persistent duodenal or pyloric channel ulcers that evolve into pyloric stenosis and obstruction as a result of acute and chronic inflammation, spasm, edema, scarring, and fibrosis. Initial management includes nasogastric decompression, antisecretory therapy, and eradication of *H pylori*.[45] Endoscopic evaluation is necessary to determine the site, cause, and degree of obstruction and to evaluate for carcinoma as an etiology of the obstruction, because malignancy is the most common cause of gastric outlet obstruction in this era of antisecretory therapy.[46]

Treatment of gastric outlet obstruction related to refractory PUD includes endoscopic pyloric balloon dilation and surgery. Endoscopic balloon dilation has been used for treatment of gastric outlet obstruction with variable results.[47] Several large studies have demonstrated high rates of success for the relief of symptoms from pyloric stenosis using balloon dilation, which increases the diameter of the stenotic pylorus on average from 6 to 16 mm.[48] Patients who require more than two dilations are at a high risk of endoscopic failure and the need for surgical intervention. Because many patients with benign pyloric stenosis have underlying ulcer disease, *H pylori* infection is a common finding. Eradication of this infection at the time of balloon dilation will ensure higher long-term success rates.[49] Endoscopic balloon dilation should therefore be the first-line therapy in appropriate patients with benign pyloric stenosis related to PUD.

Obstruction necessitates operation in about 2000 patients per year in the United States.[50] Surgical procedures that are considered in gastric outlet obstruction related to refractory PUD include vagotomy and pyloroplasty, antrectomy, and gastroenterostomy. Minimally invasive laparoscopic techniques (truncal vagotomy, gastrojejunostomy) have been developed for some of these surgical procedures that are associated with reduced postoperative recovery time.[51,52] The largest series of laparoscopic procedures for the management of refractory PUD included 263 patients who were treated for either refractory PUD or obstruction due to PUD. Laparoscopic posterior truncal vagotomy with anterior proximal gastric vagotomy for refractory disease and laparoscopic bilateral truncal vagotomy with stapled gastrojejunostomy for obstructive disease have become the standard surgical management at this institution.[53]

DIAGNOSTIC EVALUATION OF PATIENTS WITH REFRACTORY PEPTIC ULCER DISEASE

The diagnostic evaluation of patients with refractory PUD can be challenging. Potential etiologies of persistent or worsening PUD include the following: patient risk factors and noncompliance, persistent *H pylori* infection, and non–*H pylori*–related infection, related to underlying idiopathic gastric hypersecretion, or ZES and gastrinoma (**Fig. 3**). The evaluation of the etiology of the severe PUD in any patient may require multiple

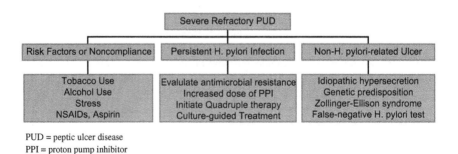

PUD = peptic ulcer disease
PPI = proton pump inhibitor
H. pylori = Helicobacter pylori

Fig. 3. Algorithm for the diagnostic work-up of refractory PUD.

diagnostic studies. Diagnostic endoscopy in UGI series can evaluate gastric emptying. Laboratory diagnostic studies including fasting gastrin level, neuroendocrine markers, and octreotide scan may be performed for the evaluation of gastrinoma or ZES as a cause of intractable PUD. Pancreatic polypeptide and chromogranin level A are additional diagnostic laboratory studies that may be helpful. Therapy for refractory PUD involves treatment of the underlying cause. Recent data and studies regarding each of these potential etiologies of refractory PUD are reviewed in the following sections.

Patient Risk Factors and Noncompliance

Although curative treatment of H pylori infection markedly reduces the relapse of peptic ulcers, the details of the ulcers that do recur has not been well characterized until recently. A multicenter study involving 4940 PUD patients who were H pylori negative after successful eradication treatment were followed for up to 48 months. The crude peptic ulcer recurrence rate was 3.02% (149/4940). The annual recurrence rates of gastric, duodenal, and gastroduodenal ulcer were 2.3%, 1.6%, and 1.6%, respectively. Exclusion of patients who took nonsteroidal anti-inflammatory drugs (NSAIDs) led annual recurrence rates to 1.9%, 1.5%, and 1.3%, respectively. The recurrence rate was significantly higher in gastric ulcer. Recurrence rates of patients who smoked, consumed alcohol, and used NSAIDs were significantly higher in those with gastric ulcer recurrence compared with duodenal ulcer recurrence, and relapsed ulcers recurred at the same or adjacent sites as the previous ulcers.[54]

Persistent or recurrent PUD may occur because of specific patient risk factors or noncompliance with medical therapies. Patient risk factors for PUD include smoking or alcohol use, stress, and the use of NSAIDs.[55] A population-based prospective cohort study (Danish adults, n = 2416) confirmed that the main risk factors for PUD were H pylori infection (OR, 4.3, 95% CI, 2.2–8.3), tobacco smoking (OR, 3.8, CI, 1.7–9.8), and stress due to the use of minor tranquilizers (OR, 3.0, CI, 1.4–6.6). In patients with documented H pylori, tobacco and alcohol use both increased the risk of PUD, whereas moderate leisure time physical activity protected against PUD in Danish adults.[56]

Multiple studies support a causal relationship between smoking and peptic ulcers in men and women. A Centers for Disease Control and Prevention study (the First National Health and Nutrition Examination Survey Epidemiologic Follow-up Study) used data from a nationally representative prospective study of adults in the United States, to evaluate the impact of smoking on the incidence of peptic ulcers in women (n = 2851) who had not been diagnosed as having a peptic ulcer before the baseline interview.[57] Among these women, 140 (4.9%) developed PUD. During 12.5 years of follow-up, the estimated cumulative incidence of ulcers was 10.0% for current smokers, 6.4% for former smokers, and 5.4% for never smokers. After adjusting for age, education, regular aspirin use, coffee consumption, and use of alcohol, current smokers were 1.8 times more likely to develop ulcers than never smokers (95% CI, 1.2–2.6); the risk of peptic ulcer increased as the amount smoked increased.

Because tobacco and alcohol use are independent risk factors for PUD, and interfere with patient compliance and rate of ulcer healing, cessation should be considered in patients with refractory or severe PUD.[58]

NSAIDs are widely used for their anti-inflammatory, analgesic, and antipyretic effects, and low-dose aspirin (also an NSAID) is used for cardiovascular prophylaxis. The main concern limiting the use of these drugs is their GI toxicity. GI side effects include the following: ulcers (found at endoscopy in 15%–30% of patients using NSAIDs regularly); complications, such as upper GI bleeding (annual incidence of

1.0%–1.5%); and the development of upper GI symptoms, such as dyspepsia (occurring in up to 60% of patients taking NSAIDs). H2RAs are not effective at preventing NSAID-induced gastric ulcers when used at standard doses, although they can decrease upper GI symptoms. Misoprostol effectively decreases NSAID-induced ulcers and GI complications but is used infrequently in the United States—perhaps because of issues of compliance (multiple daily doses) and side effects (eg, diarrhea, dyspepsia). Once-daily PPI therapy also decreases the development of NSAID-associated ulcers and recurrent NSAID-related ulcer complications; it also decreases upper GI symptoms in NSAID users. In patients using aspirin, the addition of a cyclo-oxygenase-2-specific inhibitor seems to significantly increase GI risk to the level of a nonselective NSAID; aspirin plus a nonselective NSAID seems to increase GI risk still higher. Patients taking low-dose aspirin who have risk factors for GI complications (including concomitant nonselective NSAID therapy) should therefore receive medical co-therapy, such as a PPI.[59]

Clinical trials have reproducibly demonstrated that the healing of NSAID-associated gastric and duodenal ulcers is accelerated with the use of acid suppressive agents, such as H2RAs and PPIs, even with the continued use of the NSAIDs. The risk of developing gastroduodenal ulcers or ulcer complications with the continued and long-term use of NSAIDs is now well recognized as an important problem commonly encountered in daily clinical practice. Clinical trials have shown that co-prescription of misoprostol, high-dose H2RAs or PPIs can effectively prevent or reduce the rate of gastroduodenal mucosal damage associated with the use of nonselective NSAIDs. Approaching the problem in a different way, cyclooxygenase-2-selective inhibitors circumvent the problem; based on their mechanism of action, these agents are less ulcerogenic in UGI tract as compared with nonselective NSAIDs.[60]

Multiple studies have examined whether PPI prophylaxis could prevent ulcer relapse in patients with NSAID-related peptic ulcers. In one study, patients who presented with PUD and infected with H pylori while receiving NSAIDs were recruited. Patients with healed ulcers and H pylori eradication were given naproxen 750 mg daily and randomly assigned to receive lansoprazole 30 mg daily or no treatment for 8 weeks. At the end of the 8-week treatment period, significantly fewer patients (1/22, 4.5%, 95% CI, 0–23) in the lansoprazole group compared with the group that received H pylori eradication alone (9/21, 42.9%, 95% CI, 22–66) developed recurrence of symptomatic and complicated ulcers (log rank test, $P = .0025$). Lansoprazole significantly reduced the cumulative relapse of symptomatic and complicated ulcers in patients requiring NSAIDs after eradication of H pylori.[61] This and other studies confirmed that PPI treatment is more effective than H pylori eradication in preventing ulcer recurrence in long term NSAID users.

Although a tremendous amount of research supports the use of preventative therapies and interventions to reduce and/or avoid NSAID- or aspirin-associated ulcers and ulcer complications in the UGI tract, these strategies are often not applied sufficiently, not optimally dosed, and/or associated with poor patient compliance. This reinforces the need for continued clinician and patient education to improve the outcomes of care.

Persistent H pylori Infection

H pylori is the primary cause of PUD.[62] H pylori infection is curable with regimens of multiple antimicrobial agents, but antimicrobial resistance is a leading cause of treatment failure.[63] Current treatment for H pylori infections generally includes two or more antimicrobial agents (eg, amoxicillin, clarithromycin, metronidazole), but treatment fails in 10% to 20% of all cases, often because of drug resistance. The eradiation rates of *H pylori* with standard treatments are decreasing worldwide (**Fig. 4**).[64,65] The choice of antibiotic treatment for refractory *H pylori* infections should be based on in vitro susceptibility data, and physicians should consider local resistance patterns when treating these infections empirically.[66]

The efficacy of a culture-guided treatment approach for the eradication of persistent *H pylori* infection was analyzed in 94 consecutive patients in whom *H pylori* infection persisted after two eradication attempts. Susceptibility analysis was performed for amoxicillin, clarithromycin, metronidazole, tetracycline, and levofloxacin. Patients were then treated with a culture-guided, third-line regimen: 89 patients with a 1-week quadruple regimen, including omeprazole, bismuth, doxycycline, and amoxicillin and five patients with a 1-week triple regimen containing omeprazole, amoxicillin, and levofloxacin or clarithromycin. Ninety-four subjects (100%) were resistant to metronidazole, 89 (95%) to clarithromycin, 29 (31%) to levofloxacin, and five (5%) to tetracycline. No resistance to amoxicillin was found in any patient. Overall, *H pylori* eradication was obtained in 90% of subjects. The quadruple regimen was effective in 81 patients (92% by per protocol and 91% by intention-to-treat [ITT] analysis). Four patients (80%, both per protocol and ITT analysis) were *H pylori* negative after the triple regimen. This study confirmed that the culture-guided, third-line therapeutic approach is effective for the eradication of *H pylori*. Furthermore, the 1-week doxycycline- and amoxicillin-based quadruple regimen is a good third-line 'rescue' treatment option.[67]

The *H pylori* Antimicrobial Resistance Monitoring Program is a prospective, multicenter United States network that tracks national incidence rates of *H pylori* antimicrobial resistance. Of 347 clinical *H pylori* isolates collected from December 1998 to 2002, 101 (29.1%) were resistant to 1 antimicrobial agent and 17 (5%) were resistant to two or more antimicrobial agents. Eighty-seven (25.1%) isolates were resistant to metronidazole, 45 (12.9%) to clarithromycin, and three (0.9%) to amoxicillin. On multivariate analysis, black race was the only significant risk factor (*P*<.01, hazard ratio, 2.04) for infection with a resistant *H pylori* strain.[68]

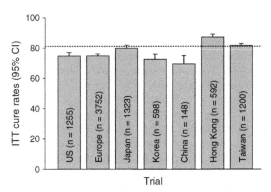

Fig. 4. Results of recent comparative studies on more than 100 patients tested for the combined effect of a PPI plus amoxicillin and clarithromycin. The dotted line signifies the threshold for an acceptable result. The results are shown as mean cure rates (ITT) and upper limits of 95% CIs. The number of patients in the studies and the country where the study was performed are shown within each column. (*From* Graham DY, Lu H, Yamaoka Y. A report card to grade *Helicobacter pylori* therapy. Helicobacter 2007;12(4):275–8; with permission from Blackwell Publishers Ltd.)

Owing to rising drug-resistant *H pylori* infections, currently recommended PPI-based triple therapies are losing their efficacy, and regimens efficacious in the presence of drug resistance are needed. A recent meta-analysis examined the efficacy, safety, and adherence of first-line quadruple *H pylori* therapies in adults. Quadruple therapy containing a gastric acid inhibitor, bismuth, metronidazole, and tetracycline was enhanced when omeprazole was included, treatment duration lasted 10 to 14 days, and when therapy took place in the Netherlands, Hong Kong, and Australia. Treatment efficacy decreased as the prevalence of metronidazole resistance increased. Even in areas with a high prevalence of metronidazole resistance, this quadruple regimen eradicated more than 85% of *H pylori* infections when it contained omeprazole and was given for 10 to 14 days. Furthermore, in the presence of clarithromycin resistance, this quadruple regimen eradicated 90% to 100% of *H pylori* infections, whereas the currently recommended triple therapy containing clarithromycin, amoxicillin, and a PPI eradicated only 25% to 61% (*P*<.001). Adherence and adverse events for quadruple therapy were similar to currently recommended triple therapies. This study questions whether quadruple therapy with a PPI, a bismuth compound, metronidazole and tetracycline should be recommended as first-line anti-*H pylori* therapy.[69]

In patients who present with persistent or worsening PUD, it is important to assess for active *H pylori* infection, and to determine whether antimicrobial resistance is present.[70,71] Bacteriologic methods are necessary for detection of the putative antimicrobial resistance of *H pylori*. The main cause for failure of *H pylori* eradication therapy is resistance to clarithromycin, which is due to point mutations. In these patients with resistant isolates, the provision of alternative therapeutic regimens for the successful eradication of *H pylori* infection is mandatory.

High-dose PPI/amoxicillin therapy can also be used as an alternative strategy for retreatment of *H pylori* after failure to eradicate the infection. High-dose dual therapy with rabeprazole (10 mg four times a day) and amoxicillin (500 mg four times a day) for 2 weeks was a useful treatment strategy after failure of eradication of *H pylori* by the usual triple PPI/amoxicillin/clarithromycin therapy.[72] *H pylori* infections are difficult to cure and successful treatment generally requires the administration of several antibacterial agents simultaneously. Duration of therapy is also important and depends on whether resistance is present; 14 days is often best. With few exceptions, worldwide increasing macrolide resistance now undermines the effectiveness of the legacy triple therapy (PPI, clarithromycin, and amoxicillin) and, in many areas, cure rates have declined to unacceptable levels. The development of sequential therapy was one response to this problem. Sequential therapy has repeatedly been shown in head-to-head studies to be superior to legacy triple therapy. Sequential therapy, as originally described, is the sequential administration of a dual therapy (PPI plus amoxicillin) followed by a Bazzoli-type triple therapy (PPI plus clarithromycin and tinidazole) and has been shown to be especially useful where there is clarithromycin resistance. However, the cure rates of the original sequential treatment can probably be further improved by changes in dose, duration, or administration, such as by continuing the amoxicillin into the triple therapy arm. The sequential approach may also be more complicated than necessary, based on the fact that the same four drugs have also been given concomitantly (at least nine publications with >700 patients) as a quadruple therapy with excellent success.[73]

The future development of new anti-*H pylori* therapies presents enormous challenges to clinical pharmacologists, not only in the identification of novel targets but also in ensuring adequate drug delivery to the unique gastric mucus niche of *H pylori*.[74] It is now recognized that *H pylori* infects about half of the world's population and is a major cause of diseases in the UGI tract. Based on results of clinical studies, the World Health Organization has assigned *H pylori* as a class I carcinogen. The prevention of the initial infection by a suitable vaccination might be the new therapeutic strategy for the future.[75] Several lines of evidence from experimental animal models of infection have clearly demonstrated the feasibility of a prophylactic and therapeutic vaccine against *H pylori*.[76] However, comparatively few clinical studies have been performed to evaluate whether the positive results obtained in animals can be reproduced in humans. These studies are also needed for deciphering those aspects of the effector immune responses that correlate with protection against *H pylori* infection and disease.[77] The recent report of a phase I study of an intramuscular *H pylori* vaccine in noninfected volunteers documented satisfactory safety and immunogenicity, produced antigen-specific T-cell memory, and warrants further clinical study.[78]

Non–H pylori–*Related Ulcer*

The proportion of ulcers that are not associated with *H pylori* infection is increasing, especially in the United States and Australia.[79] The increase in this type of ulcer warrants an analysis of the diagnostic and treatment approaches to *H pylori*-negative ulcers. Review of the medical literature documents show that up to 52% of duodenal ulcers and 47% of gastric ulcers are not caused by *H pylori* infection. The cause of *H pylori*-negative ulceration seems to be multifactorial. Contributing factors include covert NSAID use, false-negative *H pylori* tests, genetic predisposition, and in rare cases, Crohn's disease or ZES.[80] *H pylori*-negative ulcers tend to be associated with hypersecretion and can have serious clinical sequelae.

H pylori-negative ulcers are often refractory to treatment, and may have an aggressive clinical course, possibly because they lack the beneficial effect of *H pylori* infection on antisecretory therapy. PPIs appear to effectively treat both *H pylori*-positive and *H pylori*-negative ulcers.[81] Furthermore, the recent availability of intravenous PPIs has simplified therapy in patients who cannot receive enteral therapy, such as in patients with partial gastric outlet obstruction, and when there is a question or concern for adequate absorption of enteral PPIs.

Recent studies document that NSAID/aspirin use is the most common cause of *H pylori*-negative duodenal ulcer disease.[82,83] The priority, therefore, is cessation of NSAID/aspirin use if possible in these patients with refractory PUD. In patients with hypersecretion as the etiology of the non–*H pylori*–related ulcer, the potential etiologies include idiopathic gastric hypersecretion or ZES and/or gastrinoma. The most frequent conditions of hypergastrinemia in humans are the ZES with autonomous gastrin hypersecretion by the tumor cell and reactive hypergastrinemia in type A autoimmune chronic atrophic gastritis with achlorhydria causing unrestrained gastrin release from the gastrin-producing antral G cells. Both entities differ with respect to the pH in the gastric fluid, which is less than two in patients with ZES and neutral in patients with type A gastritis. Other conditions with moderate hypergastrinemia are treatment with PPIs, gastric outlet obstruction, previous vagotomy, chronic renal failure, or short bowel syndrome.[84]

The diagnostic evaluation in these patients, however, is difficult, because most of these patients have hypergastrinemia due to chronic treatment with acid suppressive therapy and medical regimens for eradication of *H pylori*. PPIs are potent acid suppressants which, at normal doses, can result in hypergastrinemia. In fact, there is a significant inverse correlation between the fasting serum gastrin concentration and gastric acid profile in patients with gastroesophageal reflux and PUD. An elevated fasting serum gastrin concentration while on PPI therapy suggests that gastric acid secretion is adequately suppressed.[85] Additionally, gastric outlet obstruction may be a contributing etiology of elevated serum gastrin.

Therefore, the use of PPIs could delay or mask the diagnosis of gastrinoma.[86] In patients receiving PPI therapy, an attempt should be made to eliminate PPI therapy as a possible cause of hypergastrinemia. It is critical to determine the etiology of the refractory PUD and hypergastrinemia in these patients. A short course of high-dose H2RA therapy can be initiated with PPI discontinuation and before repeat gastrin measurements. However, this strategy is not recommended in the treatment of acute PUD, because it has been well established that ulcer-healing rates are superior with PPI therapy.[87]

Because PPIs have been released and come into widespread use, the diagnosis of gastrinoma has been masked and will probably be delayed, with the result that patients with gastrinoma will be diagnosed at more advanced stages in the course of the disease.[88] Physicians must therefore maintain a high index of suspicion for this disease and not mask a potential malignancy with prolonged control of acid-related symptoms without taking steps to diagnose gastrinoma.

Furthermore, differentiation of idiopathic gastric hypersecretion versus gastrinoma or ZES can be difficult, and frequently requires multiple diagnostic studies. This work-up is necessary, however, because the medical and surgical therapy of these patients differs. Patients with "idiopathic" ulcers are characterized by postprandial hypersecretion of acid and hypergastrinemia with accelerated gastric emptying. Any patient with intractable or recurrent PUD requires diagnostic evaluation for the ZES or gastrinoma.

ZES is characterized by severe PUD due to gastric acid hypersecretion that results from gastrin-secreting tumors (gastrinomas) of the GI tract. Gastrin stimulates the parietal cell to secrete acid directly and indirectly by releasing histamine from enterochromaffin-like cells, and induces hyperplasia of parietal and enterochromaffin-like cells. ZES should be suspected in patients with severe erosive or ulcerative esophagitis, multiple peptic ulcers, peptic ulcers in unusual locations, refractory peptic ulcers, complicated peptic ulcers, peptic ulcers associated with diarrhea, and a family history of multiple endocrine neoplasia type 1 (MEN-1) or any of the endocrinopathies associated with MEN-1. In about 75% of patients the tumors are sporadic, and 25% of patients have MEN-1. Patients with ZES have two problems that require treatment—the hypersecretion of gastric acid and the gastrinoma itself. Although most gastrinomas grow slowly, 60% to 90% are malignant and 25% show rapid growth.

The clinical signs and symptoms of patients presenting with ZES can be myriad. The classic triad of abdominal pain, weight loss, and diarrhea in the presence of ulcer disease suggests gastrinoma and should prompt investigation. A prospective evaluation of the initial presenting symptoms in 261 patients with ZES was performed over a 25-year period at the National Institutes of Health (NIH). A mean delay to diagnosis of 5.2±0.4 years occurred in all patients. Abdominal pain and diarrhea were the most common symptoms, present in 75% and 73% of patients, respectively. Heartburn and weight loss, which were reported uncommonly in early series, were present in 44% and 17% of patients, respectively. GI bleeding was the initial presentation in a quarter of the patients. Patients rarely presented with only one symptom (11%); pain and diarrhea was the most frequent combination, occurring in 55% of patients. An important presenting sign that should suggest ZES is prominent gastric body folds, which were noted on endoscopy in 94% of patients; however, esophageal stricture and duodenal or pyloric scarring, reported in numerous case reports, were noted in only 4% to 10%. A correct diagnosis of ZES was made by the referring physician initially in only 3% of the patients. The most common misdiagnoses made were idiopathic PUD (71%), idiopathic gastroesophageal reflux disease (7%), and chronic idiopathic diarrhea (7%). The introduction of successful antisecretory therapy has probably led to patients presenting with less severe symptoms and fewer complications.[89]

Despite numerous publications and widespread awareness of ZES, delay in diagnosis persists. Analysis of reported series indicates several features that should lead the physician to suspect ZES and shorten the delay in diagnosis including the following: (1) the combination of abdominal pain, diarrhea, and weight loss; (2) recurrent or refractory ulcers; (3) prominent gastric rugal folds (secondary to the trophic effect of gastrin) seen on endoscopy (94% in NIH series), and (4) GI symptoms with or without ulcers occurring in an MEN-1 patient. It is recommended that patients in these groups have a fasting serum gastrin determination off PPIs for a minimum of 72 hours and possibly up to 7 days.

An algorithm for the diagnosis and localization of gastrinoma is helpful (**Fig. 5**).[80] The initial diagnostic test for ZES should be a fasting serum gastrin level when antisecretory medications are discontinued. Patients with ZES have significantly increased serum gastrin concentrations, frequently between 150 and 1000 pg/mL and higher. Fasting gastrin levels tend to be higher in patients with extensive disease. If the gastrin level is elevated, gastric acidity should be assessed through pH or gastric analysis. It should be noted that hypochlorhydria causes feedback stimulation of antral gastrin secretion. In suspected cases of ZES with mild hypergastrinemia, the secretin stimulation test may be useful.

An elevation of fasting gastrin is not diagnostic of ZES; provocative testing is necessary. The most commonly used tests are secretin, calcium, and meal stimulation. The release of gastrin from gastrinoma tissue is sensitive to alterations in the serum

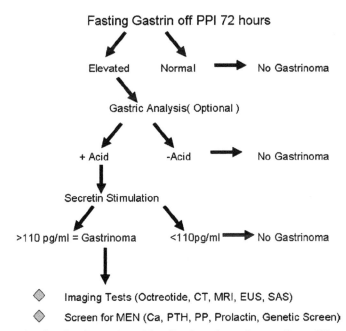

Fig. 5. Algorithm for the diagnosis and localization of gastrinoma. (*From* Ellison EC. Zollinger-Ellison syndrome: a personal perspective. Am Surg 2008;74:563–71; with permission.)

calcium level, and the calcium infusion test is recommended in ZES when the results of the secretin stimulation test are equivocal or if secretin is not available.[90]

Serologic markers helpful in reaching a diagnosis of gastrinoma are also available, as serum chromogranin A has been shown to be a general marker for neuroendocrine tumors. It is elevated in gastrinoma, and the elevation has been reported to correlate with tumor volume.[91] It is less sensitive and specific than fasting serum gastrin for the diagnosis of ZES, but can be a confirmatory test. Chromogranin A is considered the most accurate marker in the diagnosis of gastro-entero-pancreatic (GEP) endocrine tumors. Pancreatic polypeptide has also been proposed to play this role, but then not used because of its low sensitivity. The combined assessment of pancreatic poly-peptide and Chromogranin A leads to a significant increase in sensitivity in the diag-nosis of GEP tumors.[92]

Imaging for gastrinoma localization can be accomplished using computed tomog-raphy or magnetic resonance imaging, but perhaps the best modality with highest sensitivity and specificity for localization is by means of somatostatin-receptor scintig-raphy with 111-In-pentetreotide and spectroscopy.[93] Somatostatin-receptor scintig-raphy, which images the entire body at one time, is more sensitive for detecting gastrinomas than any conventional imaging study.[93] Since this test became available, all liver metastases detected at exploration have been detected by the test, and it is therefore the initial localization study of choice. This study, however, has limited sensi-tivity for detection of the primary gastrinoma. Somatostatin-receptor scintigraphy is superior to computed tomography and ultrasonography for determining the extent of the disease in patients with gastrinomas. However, the problem of detecting primary tumors in these patients is not solved by somatostatin-receptor scintig-raphy.[94] Endoscopic ultrasound may have a similar sensitivity for identifying primary tumors. A combination of somatostatin-receptor scintigraphy and endoscopic ultra-sound detects more than 90% of gastrinomas.

Initial treatment for ZES should be oral high-dose PPIs. Maintenance per os panto-prazole therapy at a dose of 80 to 240 mg/d in divided doses was both effective and generally well tolerated for patients with ZES and idiopathic hypersecretion in a recent study.[95] If parenteral therapy is needed, intermittent bolus injection of pantoprazole is recommended.[96] The dose and duration of therapy depends on the response of the patient, based on symptoms and documented ulcer healing.

The role of surgery in patients with the ZES is controversial.[97] Because the use of PPIs, the number of acid-reducing procedures has decreased substantially. Total gastrectomy and antisecretory surgery is rarely required. In patients without metas-tasis and without MEN-1, surgical cure is possible in 30%. It has been suggested that patients with gastrinomas larger than 2.5 cm, irrespective of whether they have MEN-1, should undergo surgical resection in an effort to decrease the risk for metas-tasis.[98] A recent study examined the outcomes of 151 ZES patients who underwent surgical intervention. Of these patients, 123 had sporadic gastrinomas and 28 had MEN-1 with an imaged tumor of at least 3 cm in diameter. Among the patients with sporadic gastrinomas, 34% were free of disease at 10 years, as compared with none of the patients with MEN-1. The overall 10-year survival rate was 94%. This study concluded that all patients with the ZES who do not have MEN-1 or metastatic disease should be offered surgical exploration for possible cure.[99] The role of surgery in the ZES MEN-1 patients may be determined by imaging: (1) image-negative patients should be observed and not undergo surgery given the low cure rates; and (2) image-positive patients with no distant metastases (liver, bone) should undergo explo-ration for surgical resection because resection has been shown to improve survival, independent of a biochemical cure.[80]

SURGERY FOR REFRACTORY PUD

Surgery is indicated in patients who are intolerant of medications or do not comply with medication regimes, and those at high risk for complications (eg, transplant recipients, patients dependent on steroids or NSAIDs, those with giant gastric or duodenal ulcer, and those with ulcers that fail to heal with adequate medical treatment). Surgery should also be considered for patients who have a relapse during maintenance treatment or who have had multiple courses of medications. Surgical options for duodenal ulcers include truncal vagotomy and drainage (pyloroplasty or gastrojejunostomy), selective vagotomy (preserving the hepatic and celiac branches of the vagus) and drainage, highly selective vagotomy (division of only the gastric branches of the vagus, preserving Latarjet's nerve to the pylorus), or partial gastrectomy. Surgery for gastric ulcers usually involves a partial gastrectomy. Procedures other than highly selective vagotomy may be complicated by postprocedure dumping and diarrhea.[53,100,101]

SUMMARY

Refractory PUD is a diagnostic and therapeutic challenge. Optimal management of severe or refractory PUD requires a multidisciplinary team approach, using primary care providers, gastroenterologists, and general surgeons. Medical management has become the cornerstone of therapy. Identification and eradication of H pylori infection combined with acid reduction regimens can heal ulceration and also prevent recurrence. Severe, intractable or recurrent PUD and associated complications mandates a careful and methodical evaluation and management strategy to determine the potential etiologies and necessary treatment (medical or surgical) required.

REFERENCES

1. Sonnenberg A, Everhart JE. The prevalence of self-reported peptic ulcer in the United States. Am J Public Health 1996;86:200–5.
2. Ramakrishnan K, Salinas RC. Peptic ulcer disease. Am Fam Physician 2007; 76(7):1005–12.
3. Soll AH. Consensus conference. Medical treatment of peptic ulcer disease. Practice guidelines. Practice Parameters Committee of the American College of Gastroenterology. JAMA 1996;275:622–9.
4. Walsh JH, Peterson WL. The treatment of Helicobacter pylori infection in the management of peptic ulcer disease. N Engl J Med 1995;333:984–91.
5. Hopkins RJ, Girardi LS, Turney EA. Relationship between H. pylori eradication and reduced duodenal and gastric ulcer recurrence: a review. Gastroenterology 1996;110:1244–52.
6. Yuan Y, Padol IT, Hunt RH. Peptic ulcer disease today. Nat Clin Pract Gastroenterol Hepatol 2006;3(2):80–9.
7. Guzzo JL, Duncan M, Bass BL, et al. Severe and refractory peptic ulcer disease: the diagnostic dilemma: case report and comprehensive review. Dig Dis Sci 2005;50(11):1999–2008.
8. Verma S, Giaffer MH. Helicobacter pylori eradication ameliorates symptoms and improves quality of life in patients on long-term acid suppression. A large prospective study in primary care. Dig Dis Sci 2002;47(7):1567–74.
9. Bardhan KD, Nayyar AK, Royston C. History in our lifetime: the changing nature of refractory duodenal ulcer in the era of histamine H2 receptor antagonists. Dig Liver Dis 2003;35(8):529–36.

10. Ford A, Delaney B, Forman D, et al. Eradication therapy for peptic ulcer disease in *Helicobacter pylori* positive patients. Cochrane Database Syst Rev 2004;(4):CD003840.

11. Malfertheiner P, Megraud F, O'Morain C, et al. European Helicobacter pylori Study Group (EHPSG). Current concepts in the management of *Helicobacter pylori* infection—the Maastricht 2-2000 consensus report. Aliment Pharmacol Ther 2002;16:167–80.

12. Vallve M, Vergara M, Gisbert JP, et al. Single versus double dose of a proton pump inhibitor in triple therapy for *Helicobacter pylori* eradication: a meta-analysis. Aliment Pharmacol Ther 2002;16:1149–56.

13. Malfertheiner P, Megraud F, O'Morain C, et al. Current concepts in the management of *Helicobacter pylori* infection: the Maastricht III consensus report. Gut 2007;56(6):772–81.

14. Calvet X, Garcia N, Lopez T, et al. A meta-analysis of short versus long therapy with a proton pump inhibitor, clarithromycin and either metronidazole or amoxicillin for treating *Helicobacter pylori* infection. Aliment Pharmacol Ther 2000;14: 603–9.

15. Bilardi C, Biagini R, Dulbecco P, et al. Stool antigen assay (HpSA) is less reliable than urea breath test for post-treatment diagnosis of *Helicobacter pylori* infection. Aliment Pharmacol Ther 2002;16:1733–8.

16. Liu CC, Lee CL, Chan CC, et al. Maintenance treatment is not necessary after *Helicobacter pylori* eradication and healing of bleeding peptic ulcer: a 5-year prospective, randomized, controlled study. Arch Intern Med 2003;163(17):2020–4.

17. Bardhan KD, Williamson M, Royston C, et al. Admission rates for peptic ulcer in the Trent Region, UK, 1972–2000. Changing pattern, a changing disease? Dig Liver Dis 2004;36(9):577–88.

18. Van Leerdam ME. Epidemiology of acute upper gastrointestinal bleeding. Best Pract Res Clin Gastroenterol 2008;22:209–24.

19. Leontiadis GI, Sreedharan A, Dorward S, et al. Systematic review of the clinical effectiveness and cost-effectiveness of proton pump inhibitors in acute upper gastrointestinal bleeding. Health Technol Assess 2007;11(51). iii–iv, 1–164.

20. Laine L, McQuaid KR. Endoscopic therapy for bleeding ulcers: an evidence-based approach based on meta-analyses of randomized controlled trials. Clin Gastroenterol Hepatol 2009;7(1):33–47.

21. Gisbert JP, Khorrami S, Carballo F, et al. *H. pylori* eradication therapy vs. antisecretory non-eradication therapy (with or without long-term maintenance antisecretory therapy) for the prevention of recurrent bleeding from peptic ulcer. Cochrane Database Syst Rev 2004;(2):CD004062.

22. Peter S, Wilcox CM. Modern endoscopic therapy of peptic ulcer bleeding. Dig Dis 2008;26:291–9.

23. Barkun AN, Martel M, Toubouti Y, et al. Endoscopic hemostasis in peptic ulcer bleeding for patients with high-risk lesions: a series of meta-analyses. Gastrointest Endosc 2009;69:786–99.

24. Tajima A, Koizumi K, Suzuki K, et al. Proton pump inhibitors and recurrent bleeding in peptic ulcer disease. J Gastroenterol Hepatol 2008;23(Suppl 2):S237–41.

25. Loffroy R, Guiu B, Cercueil JP, et al. Refractory bleeding from gastroduodenal ulcers: arterial embolization in high operative risk patients. J Clin Gastroenterol 2008;42(4):361–7.

26. Holme JB, Nielsen DT, Funch-Jensen P, et al. Transcatheter arterial embolization in patients with bleeding duodenal ulcer: an alternative to surgery. Acta Radiol 2006;47(3):244–7.

27. Larssen L, Moger T, Bjornbeth BA, et al. Transcatheter arterial embolization in the management of bleeding duodenal ulcers: a 5.5 year retrospective study of treatment and outcome. Scand J Gastroenterol 2008;43(2):217–22.

28. Eriksson LG, Ljungdahl M, Sundbom M, et al. Transcatheter arterial embolization versus surgery in the treatment of upper gastrointestinal bleeding after therapeutic endoscopy failure. J Vasc Interv Radiol 2008;19(10): 1413–8.

29. Behrman SW. Management of complicated peptic ulcer disease. Arch Surg 2005;140:201–8.

30. Ng EK, Chung SC, Sung JJ, et al. High prevalence of Helicobacter pylori infection in duodenal ulcer perforations not caused by non-steroidal anti-inflammatory drugs. Br J Surg 1996;83:1779–81.

31. Matsukura N, Onda M, Tokunaga A, et al. Role of Helicobacter pylori infection in perforation of peptic ulcer: an age and gender-matched case-control study. J Clin Gastroenterol 1997;25:S235–9.

32. Sebastian M, Chandran VP, Elashaal YI, et al. Helicobacter pylori infection in perforated peptic ulcer disease. Br J Surg 1995;82:360–2.

33. Tokunaga Y, Hata K, Ryo J, et al. Density of Helicobacter pylori infection in patients with peptic ulcer perforation. J Am Coll Surg 1998;186:659–63.

34. Gisbert JP, Pajares JM. Helicobacter pylori infection and perforated peptic ulcer prevalence of the infection and role of antimicrobial treatment. Helicobacter 2003;8(3):159–67.

35. Kujath P, Schwandner O, Bruch HP. Morbidity and mortality of perforated peptic gastroduodenal ulcer following emergency surgery. Langenbecks Arch Surg 2002;387(7–8):298–302.

36. Tsugawa K, Koyanagi N, Hashizume M, et al. The therapeutic strategies in performing emergency surgery for gastroduodenal ulcer perforation in 130 patients over 70 years of age. Hepatogastroenterology 2001;48(37):156–62.

37. Lunevicius R, Morkevicius M. Comparison of laparoscopic versus open repair for perforated duodenal ulcers. Surg Endosc 2005;19(12):1565–71.

38. Song KY, Kim TH, Kim SN, et al. Laparoscopic repair of perforated duodenal ulcers: the simple 'one-stitch' suture with omental patch technique. Surg Endosc 2008;22(7):1632–5.

39. Lam PW, Lam MC, Hui EK, et al. Laparoscopic repair of perforated duodenal ulcers: the "three-stitch" Graham patch technique. Surg Endosc 2005;19(12): 1627–30.

40. Siu WT, Leong HT, Law BK, et al. Laparoscopic repair for perforated peptic ulcer: a randomized controlled trial. Ann Surg 2002;235(3):313–9.

41. Sanabria AE, Morales CH, Villegas MI. Laparoscopic repair for perforated peptic ulcer disease. Cochrane Database Syst Rev 2005;(4):CD004778.

42. Lunevicius R, Morkevicius M. Systematic review comparing laparoscopic and open repair for perforated peptic ulcer. Br J Surg 2005;92(10):1195–207.

43. Bhogal RH, Athwal R, Durkin D, et al. Comparison between open and laparoscopic repair of perforated peptic ulcer disease. World J Surg 2008;32(11): 2371–4.

44. Lunevicius R, Morkevicius M. Management strategies, early results, benefits and risk factors of laparoscopic repair of perforated peptic ulcer. World J Surg 2005; 29(10):1299–310.

45. Gisbert JP, Pajares JM. Review article: Helicobacter pylori infection and gastric outlet obstruction—prevalence of the infection and role of antimicrobial treatment. Aliment Pharmacol Ther 2002;16(7):1203–8.

46. Shone DN, Nikoomanesh P, Smith-Meek MM, et al. Malignancy is the most common cause of gastric outlet obstruction in the era of H2 blockers. Am J Gastroenterol 1995;90:1769–70.

47. Kochhar R, Sethy PK, Nagi B, et al. Endoscopic balloon dilation of benign gastric outlet obstruction. J Gastroenterol Hepatol 2004;19(4):418–22.

48. Yusuf TE, Brugge WR. Endoscopic therapy of benign pyloric stenosis and gastric outlet obstruction. Curr Opin Gastroenterol 2006;22(5):570–3.

49. Cherian PT, Cherian S, Singh P. Long-term followup of patients with gastric outlet obstruction related to peptic ulcer disease treated with endoscopic balloon dilatation and drug therapy. Gastrointest Endosc 2007;66(3):491–7.

50. Gibson JB, Behrman SW, Fabian TC, et al. Gastric outlet obstruction resulting from peptic ulcer disease requiring surgical intervention is infrequently associated with Helicobacter pylori infection. J Am Coll Surg 2000;191:32–7.

51. Yang PJ, Yang CY, Lin TH, et al. A novel surgical technique: gasless laparoscopy-assisted gastrojejunostomy. Hepatogastroenterology 2008;55(86–87): 1948–50.

52. Abdel-Salam WN, Katri KM, Bessa SS, et al. Laparoscopic-assisted truncal vagotomy and gastrojejunostomy: trial of simplification. J Laparoendosc Adv Surg Tech A 2009, in press.

53. Palanivelu C, Jani K, Rajan PS, et al. Laparoscopic management of acid peptic disease. Surg Laparosc Endosc Percutan Tech 2006;16(5):312–6.

54. Miwa H, Sakaki N, Sugano K, et al. Recurrent peptic ulcers in patients following successful Helicobacter pylori eradication: a multicenter study of 4940 patients. Helicobacter 2004;9(1):9–16.

55. Lanas AI, Remacha B, Esteva F, et al. Risk factors associated with refractory peptic ulcers. Gastroenterology 1995;109:1124.

56. Rosenstock S, Jorgensen T, Bonnevie O, et al. Risk factors for peptic ulcer disease: a population based prospective cohort study comprising 2416 Danish adults. Gut 2003;52(2):186–93.

57. Anda RF, Williamson DF, Escobedo LG, et al. Smoking and the risk of peptic ulcer disease among women in the United States. Arch Intern Med 1990; 150(7):1437–41.

58. Reynolds JC, Schoen RE, Maislin G, et al. Risk factors for delayed healing of duodenal ulcers treated with famotidine and ranitidine. Am J Gastroenterol 1994;89(4):571–80.

59. Laine L. Proton pump inhibitor co-therapy with nonsteroidal anti-inflammatory drugs-nice or necessary? Rev Gastroenterol Disord 2004;4(Suppl 4): S33–41.

60. Goldstein JL. Challenges in managing NSAID-associated gastrointestinal tract injury. Digestion 2004;69(Suppl 1):25–33.

61. Lai KC, Lam SK, Chu KM, et al. Lansoprazole reduces ulcer relapse after eradication of Helicobacter pylori in nonsteroidal anti-inflammatory drug users— a randomized trial. Aliment Pharmacol Ther 2003;18(8):829–36.

62. Goddard AF, Logan RP. Diagnostic methods for Helicobacter pylori detection and eradication. Br J Clin Pharmacol 2003;56(3):273–83.

63. Howden CW, Hunt RH. Guidelines for the management of Helicobacter pylori infection. Ad Hoc Committee on Practice Parameters of the American College of Gastroenterology. Am J Gastroenterol 1998;93(12):2330–8.

64. Kadayifci A, Buyukhatipoglu H, Cemil Savas M, et al. Eradication of H. pylori with triple therapy: an epidemiologic analysis of trends in Turkey over 10 years. Clin Ther 2006;28(11):1960–6.

65. Graham DY, Lu H, Yamaoka Y. A report card to grade *Helicobacter pylori* therapy. Helicobacter 2007;12(4):275–8.
66. Branca G, Spanu T, Cammarota G, et al. High levels of dual resistance to clarithromycin and metronidazole and in vitro activity of levofloxacin against *Helicobacter pylori* isolates from patients after failure of therapy. Int J Antimicrob Agents 2004;24(5):433–8.
67. Cammarota G, Martino A, Pirozzi G, et al. High efficacy of 1-week doxycycline- and amoxicillin-based quadruple regimen in a culture-guided, third-line treatment approach for *Helicobacter pylori* infection. Aliment Pharmacol Ther 2004; 19(7):789–95.
68. Duck WM, Sobel J, Pruckler JM, et al. Antimicrobial resistance incidence and risk factors among *Helicobacter pylori*-infected persons, United States. Emerg Infect Dis 2004;10(6):1088–94.
69. Fischbach LA, Zanten SV, Dickason J. Meta-analysis: the efficacy, adverse events, and adherence related to first-line anti-*Helicobacter pylori* quadruple therapies. Aliment Pharmacol Ther 2004;20(10):1071–82.
70. Gerrits MM, van Vliet AH, Kuipers EJ, et al. *Helicobacter pylori* and antimicrobial resistance: molecular mechanisms and clinical implications. Lancet Infect Dis 2006;6(11):699–709.
71. Megraud F, Lehours P. *Helicobacter pylori* detection and antimicrobial susceptibility testing. Clin Microbiol Rev 2007;20(2):280–322.
72. Furuta T, Shirai N, Xiao F, et al. High-dose rabeprazole/amoxicillin therapy as the second-line regimen after failure to eradicate *H. pylori* by triple therapy with the usual doses of a proton pump inhibitor, clarithromycin and amoxicillin. Hepatogastroenterology 2003;50(54):2274–8.
73. Graham DY, Lu H, Yamaoka Y. Therapy for *Helicobacter pylori* infection can be improved: sequential therapy and beyond. Drugs 2008;68(6):725–36.
74. Jodlowski TZ, Lam S, Ashby DR Jr. Emerging therapies for the treatment of *Helicobacter pylori* infections. Ann Pharmacother 2008;42(11):1621–39.
75. Selgrad M, Malfertheiner P. New strategies for *Helicobacter pylori* eradication. Curr Opin Pharmacol 2008;8(5):593–7.
76. Kabir S. The current status of *Helicobacter pylori* vaccines: a review. Helicobacter 2007;12(2):89–102.
77. Ruggiero P, Peppoloni S, Rappuoli R, et al. The quest for a vaccine against *Helicobacter pylori*: how to move from mouse to man? Microbes Infect 2003;5(8):749–56.
78. Malfertheiner P, Schultze V, Rosenkranz B, et al. Safety and immunogenicity of an intramuscular *Helicobacter pylori* vaccine in noninfected volunteers: a phase I study. Gastroenterology 2008;135(3):787–95.
79. Freston JW. *Helicobacter pylori*-negative peptic ulcers: frequency and implications for management. J Gastroenterol 2000;35(Suppl 12):29–32.
80. Ellison EC, Johnson JA. The Zollinger-Ellison syndrome: a comprehensive review of historical, scientific and clinical considerations. Curr Probl Surg 2009;46(1):13–106.
81. Freston JW. Review article: role of proton pump inhibitors in non-*H. pylori*-related ulcers. Aliment Pharmacol Ther 2001;15(Suppl 2):2–5.
82. Chen TS, Chang FY. Clinical characteristics of *Helicobacter pylori*-negative duodenal ulcer disease. Hepatogastroenterology 2008;55(86–87):1615–8.
83. Gisbert JP, Blanco M, Mateos JM, et al. *H. pylori*-negative duodenal ulcer prevalence and causes in 774 patients. Dig Dis Sci 1999;44(11):2295–302.
84. Arnold R. Diagnosis and differential diagnosis of hypergastrinemia. Wien Klin Wochenschr 2007;119(19–20):562–9.

85. Bonapace ES, Fisher RS, Parkman HP. Does fasting serum gastrin predict gastric acid suppression in patients on proton-pump inhibitors? Dig Dis Sci 2000;45(1):34–9.

86. Ellison EC, Sparks J. Zollinger-Ellison syndrome in the era of effective acid suppression: are we unknowingly growing tumors? Am J Surg 2003;186(3): 245–8.

87. Kaneko E, Hoshihara Y, Sakaki N, et al. Peptic ulcer recurrence during maintenance therapy with H2-receptor antagonist following first-line therapy with proton pump inhibitor. J Gastroenterol 2000;35(11):824–31.

88. Corleto VD, Annibale B, Gibril F, et al. Does the widespread use of proton pump inhibitors mask, complicate and/or delay the diagnosis of Zollinger-Ellison syndrome? Aliment Pharmacol Ther 2001;15(10):1555–61.

89. Roy PK, Venzon DJ, Shojamanesh H, et al. Zollinger-Ellison syndrome. Clinical presentation in 261 patients. Medicine (Baltimore) 2000;79(6):379–411.

90. Wada M, Komoto I, Doi R, et al. Intravenous calcium injection test is a novel complementary procedure in differential diagnosis for gastrinoma. World J Surg 2002;26(10):1291–6.

91. Nobels FR, Kwekkeboom DJ, Coopmans W, et al. Chromogranin A as serum marker for neuroendocrine neoplasia: comparison with neuron-specific enolase and the alpha-subunit of glycoprotein hormones. J Clin Endocrinol Metab 1997; 82(8):2622–8.

92. Panzuto F, Severi C, Cannizzaro R, et al. Utility of combined use of plasma levels of chromogranin A and pancreatic polypeptide in the diagnosis of gastrointestinal and pancreatic endocrine tumors. J Endocrinol Invest 2004;27(1):6–11.

93. Gibril F, Reynolds JC, Doppman JL, et al. Somatostatin receptor scintigraphy: its sensitivity compared with that of other imaging methods in detecting primary and metastatic gastrinomas. A prospective study. Ann Intern Med 1996; 125(1):26–34.

94. Kisker O, Bartsch D, Weinel RJ, et al. The value of somatostatin-receptor scintigraphy in newly diagnosed endocrine gastroenteropancreatic tumors. J Am Coll Surg 1997;184(5):487–92.

95. Metz DC, Soffer E, Forsmark CE, et al. Maintenance oral pantoprazole therapy is effective for patients with Zollinger-Ellison syndrome and idiopathic hypersecretion. Am J Gastroenterol 2003;98(2):301–7.

96. Lew EA, Pisegna JR, Starr JA, et al. Intravenous pantoprazole rapidly controls gastric acid hypersecretion in patients with Zollinger-Ellison syndrome. Gastroenterology 2000;118(4):696–704.

97. Norton JA, Jensen RT. Resolved and unresolved controversies in the surgical management of patients with Zollinger-Ellison syndrome. Ann Surg 2004; 240(5):757–73.

98. Hung PD, Schubert ML, Mihas AA. Zollinger-Ellison syndrome. Curr Treat Options Gastroenterol 2003;6(2):163–70.

99. Norton JA, Fraker DL, Alexander HR, et al. Surgery to cure the Zollinger-Ellison syndrome. N Engl J Med 1999;341(9):635–44.

100. Millat B, Fingerhut A, Borie F. Surgical treatment of complicated duodenal ulcers: controlled trials. World J Surg 2000;24(3):299–306.

101. Kauffman GL Jr. Duodenal ulcer disease: treatment by surgery, antibiotics, or both. Adv Surg 2000;34:121–35.

Management of Patients with High Gastrointestinal Risk on Antiplatelet Therapy

Byron Cryer, MD[a,b,]*

KEYWORDS

- Antiplatelet therapy • Clopidogrel prasugrel • Thienopyridines
- Aspirin • Gastrointestinal bleeding • Risk • *Helicobacter pylori*

In treating cardiovascular disease, clinicians are commonly caught between competing considerations of cardiovascular benefit and gastrointestinal (GI) risks. Because platelets have an important role in the pathophysiology of coronary artery and coronary stent thrombosis, drugs that prevent platelet thrombosis have acquired a critical role in the prevention of atherothrombotic complications of vascular disease. In recent years, the use of antiplatelet therapies has been markedly increasing, primarily for the prevention of coronary artery and coronary stent occlusion.[1–4] Additionally, in the prevention of cerebrovascular occlusion, antiplatelet therapies are among the principal treatments.[5] As evidence accumulates regarding the benefits of antiplatelet therapies in the treatment of cardiovascular and cerebrovascular diseases, the use of these agents in clinical practice continues to increase even more.

Currently, two categories of oral antiplatelet therapies, aspirin and the thienopyridines (clopidogrel and prasugrel), are available or are under clinical development for the prevention of atherothrombotic complications in patients with the acute coronary syndrome or who are undergoing percutaneous coronary intervention (PCI).[6] Although the evidence is clear from several well-designed trials that antiplatelet therapies have clinical benefit, the increasing use of these agents in clinical practice is associated with increasing GI complications, such as ulceration and GI bleeding. Because of the increasing rates of ulcer and GI complications being encountered with these drugs, this article focuses on management strategies that may reduce the GI risks of patients who take antiplatelet therapy, especially those patients at highest risk for development of a GI event while using these antiplatelet agents.

[a] Department of Veterans Affairs Medical Center, Medical Service, Digestive Diseases (111B1), North Texas VA Medical Center, 4500 S Lancaster Road, Dallas, TX 75216, USA
[b] Department of Internal Medicine, University of Texas Southwestern Medical School, Dallas, TX, USA
* Corresponding author. Department of Veterans Affairs Medical Center, Medical Service, Digestive Diseases (111B1), North Texas VA Medical Center, 4500 S Lancaster Road, Dallas, TX 75216.
E-mail address: byron.cryer@utsouthwestern.edu

Gastroenterol Clin N Am 38 (2009) 289–303
doi:10.1016/j.gtc.2009.03.005
0889-8553/09/$ – see front matter. Published by Elsevier Inc.

gastro.theclinics.com

MECHANISMS OF GASTROINTESTINAL INJURY WITH ANTIPLATELET THERAPIES

Aspirin reduces platelet activity by inhibiting the cyclooxygenase (COX) enzymes. Although aspirin can inhibit COX-1 and COX-2 isoenzymes, the platelet primarily comprises COX-1. Aspirin permanently inhibits platelet COX-1 at relatively low dosages, resulting in inhibition of platelet activity.[7] COX-2–mediated effects of aspirin, primarily the analgesic and anti-inflammatory consequences, are inhibited at higher aspirin dosages. Aspirin irreversibly inhibits the metabolism of arachidonic acid to thromboxane A_2 (TXA$_2$), which is highly sensitive to aspirin's effects, causing complete suppression of platelet TXA$_2$ production with a few doses of aspirin.[7] This inhibition of TXA$_2$ decreases platelet aggregation, causes vasodilation, reduces the proliferation of vascular smooth muscle cells, and decreases atherogenicity.

In the GI mucosa, the principal metabolic products of COX enzymes are the prostaglandins, substances that protect against GI mucosal injury. In the presence of a COX inhibitor, such as aspirin or other nonsteroidal anti-inflammatory drugs (NSAIDs), GI COX is inhibited, which results in increased degrees of GI mucosal injury. At daily aspirin dosages that are much lower than that desired for optimal cardiovascular efficacy, such as with 10 mg aspirin per day, gastric COX is markedly inhibited, mucosal prostaglandins are reduced to 60% of baseline, and GI ulceration occurs.[8] Therefore, there is likely no dose of daily administered aspirin that is therapeutically efficacious without conferring gastric mucosal injury.

Clopidogrel is an effective antithrombotic, because it blocks platelet activation of adenosine diphosphate (ADP) by irreversibly binding to platelets' ADP receptor, thereby preventing the ADP-dependent activation of the GpIIb-IIIa complex, the primary platelet receptor for fibrinogen. In the CAPRIE trial, a randomized trial comparing clopidogrel and aspirin for the prevention of ischemic events, a randomized, prospective study of the efficacy of clopidogrel 75 mg and aspirin 325 mg daily for secondary prevention of thrombotic vascular events, clopidogrel was marginally more effective than aspirin and resulted in modestly lower GI bleeding than aspirin (0.5% vs 0.7%).[9] In short-term endoscopic evaluations of healthy volunteers, clopidogrel causes less gastroduodenal damage than aspirin 325 mg daily,[10] and, in observational trials of populations undergoing antiplatelet therapies, clopidogrel has a nonsignificant, slightly lower rate of GI bleeding than that with aspirin.[11] Despite this reduction, the GI risks of thienopyridines are not zero. In fact, the use of prasugrel in patients with acute coronary syndromes with scheduled PCI is associated with significantly reduced rates of cardiovascular ischemic events when compared with those with clopidogrel.[12] However, prasugrel's increased cardiovascular efficacy is somewhat offset by an increased risk of major GI bleeding, including fatal bleeding.[12] Furthermore, the use of thienopyridines in high GI risk patients can result in high rates of GI bleeding. In patients with a prior history of GI bleeding, recurrent GI bleeding after only 1 year of clopidogrel can be observed in as high as 9% of patients taking this agent.[13] These observations indicate that, although it may have previously been assumed that the thienopyridines were the GI-safe alternatives to aspirin, these agents in fact are associated with considerable GI risks as well.

The mechanism that underlies the GI injury of thienopyridines is currently unclear. However, it has been hypothesized that agents such as clopidogrel and prasugrel may cause their GI injury through an impairment of ulcer healing.[14] Platelet aggregation plays a critical role in ulcer healing through the release of various platelet-derived growth factors that promote angiogenesis, which is essential for ulcer healing. For example, thrombocytopenic animals have reduced ulcer angiogenesis and impaired gastric ulcer healing.[15] ADP receptor antagonists impair gastric ulcer healing by inhibiting platelet release of proangiogenic growth factors such as vascular endothelial growth factor (VEGF),[15] which promotes endothelial proliferation and accelerates ulcer healing. Interestingly, new chemotherapeutic agents comprising monoclonal antibodies directed at circulating VEGF have GI bleeding as a major clinical toxicity.[16] Impairment of platelet activity has also been suggested in endoscopic studies to contribute to the mechanism of clinical GI bleeding associated with clopidogrel.[17] Although clopidogrel and other agents that impair angiogenesis might not be primarily responsible for GI ulcer induction, their antiangiogenic effects may impair healing of background ulcers, which, when combined with their propensity to increase bleeding, may convert small, silent ulcers into large ulcers that bleed profoundly.

MAGNITUDE OF GASTROINTESTINAL ULCERATION COMPLICATIONS WITH ANTIPLATELET THERAPIES

Aspirin

Estimates of the incidence of GI complications with cardioprotective doses of aspirin come from several prospectively conducted studies of patients taking low-dose aspirin for primary or secondary prevention of cardiovascular events. Although the point estimate of the incidence of GI events with aspirin varies across the prospective trials, meta-analyses of these studies indicate that the relative risk (RR) of a GI event in a patient taking low-dose aspirin increases by 1.5- to 3.2-fold when compared with that of non–aspirin-taking individuals.[18,19] However, the absolute risk of aspirin's clinical risks on an individual basis are small and are estimated to range from one to five out of 1000 exposed patients.[20,21] On the other hand, when these data are viewed from a population perspective, the population impact of the GI adverse effects of low-dose aspirin is likely substantial when considering that it has been estimated that 50% of adults aged 20 to 80 years in the United States are candidates for low-dose aspirin.[21] Furthermore, the excess risk attributable to aspirin will vary in parallel to the underlying GI risk of a patient. In a patient with a combination of risk factors, such as age more than 70 years and past history of ulcer complication, the attributable risk is increased to more than 10 extra cases per 1000 person years.[22]

Clopidogrel

In the CAPRIE trial, clopidogrel had modestly lower rates of GI bleeding compared with those with aspirin (0.5% vs 0.7%, respectively),[9] Extrapolating from that trial, substituting clopidogrel for aspirin in 1000 patients would result in a reduction of two patients with GI bleeding. In patients at high risk for GI bleeding, rates of GI bleeding on clopidogrel will be considerably higher.[13] In clinical practice, however, clopidogrel is rarely given as a stand-alone antiplatelet therapy, and the dual antiplatelet strategy of clopidogrel plus aspirin is a much more commonly encountered combination. Thus, rates of GI events with dual antiplatelet therapy better reflect clopidogrel's actual GI effects in clinical practice.

Dual Antiplatelet Therapy

In patients who are at high risk for development of coronary occlusion, such as those with drug-eluting coronary stents, at least 1 year of dual antiplatelet therapy is currently recommended.[23] In clinical trials comparing the dual antiplatelet strategy of clopidogrel plus aspirin to aspirin therapy alone, the dual antiplatelet strategy is associated with an approximate 2-fold greater incidence of GI complications when compared with either agent alone[2,24,25] Observational studies indicate a seven-fold increase in upper GI bleeding with the combination therapy when compared with aspirin,[26] with GI risk increasing in patients who are at higher risk. Clearly, in certain patients dual antiplatelet therapy can be a strategy associated with considerable risks of GI bleeding. Therefore, identification of high-risk patients and, in such patients, incorporation of strategies to reduce their GI risk would be clinically prudent.

PATIENTS AT RISK FOR ULCERS AND GASTROINTESTINAL COMPLICATIONS WHILE ON ANTIPLATELET THERAPIES

Across all therapeutic categories, strategies aimed at reducing GI risks should ideally target patients most at risk for the development of complications. With the antiplatelet therapies, there has not been as much work done in the identification of patients at greatest risk of developing GI complications as with other categories of medications such as the NSAIDs. However, because of several large-scale clinical trials that have been conducted in the evaluation of efficacy of aspirin and the thienopyridines, there are sufficient emerging data to suggest which groups constitute the highest GI risk patients among those undergoing antiplatelet therapies (**Table 1**).[1–4,9,13,19,20,22]

Aspirin

Among aspirin-taking patients, analyses of large patient care databases in the United Kingdom and Spain indicate that patients taking aspirin with advancing age, a past history of uncomplicated ulcer, and a past history of complicated ulcer are all at increased risk for the development of an ulcer (**Fig. 1**).[22,27] The most significant risk factor for an aspirin-induced complication is a history of prior complicated ulcer disease, as 15% of patients with a prior history of bleeding ulcer who are taking aspirin at a dose of 100 mg/d will have a recurrent bleeding ulcer at 1 year.[28] Advancing age is also a risk factor. Although there does not appear to be a threshold age at which the risk dramatically increases, the risk increases linearly at the rate of approximately 1% per decade of advancing age.[27]

Helicobacter pylori (H pylori) infection is also a risk factor for the development of ulcers and of ulcer complications in patients taking low-dose aspirin. In endoscopic studies of aspirin users, H pylori-infected patients aged 60 years or older who received low-dose aspirin were more likely to develop duodenal ulcers than aspirin-taking patients without the infection.[29,30] In a case-control study of low-dose aspirin users, H pylori increased the risk of upper GI bleeding five-fold when compared with noninfected patients with upper GI bleeding.[31] It is clear that H pylori increases risk of ulcers related to low-dose aspirin. However, the data have not been as straightforward as to whether eradication of H pylori before starting aspirin will reduce future ulcer risk in patients with a history of ulcer. In a 6-month randomized trial of H pylori eradication

Table 1	
Demonstrated risk factors for ulcers on antiplatelet therapies[a]	
Aspirin	**Clopidogrel**
Prior ulcer complication	Prior ulcer complication
Prior ulcer disease	Combination of clopidogrel with NSAID
Advanced age	Combination of clopidogrel with aspirin
H pylori	Combination of clopidogrel with anticoagulant
Dose of cardioprotective aspirin	
Combination of aspirin with NSAID	
Combination of aspirin with anticoagulant	

[a] Risk factors were compiled from data presented in several studies; References.[1–4,9,13,19,20,22]

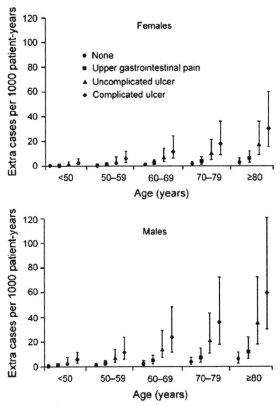

Fig. 1. Risk factors for development of gastroduodenal ulcers and ulcer complications in patients taking cardioprotective doses of low-dose aspirin. This meta-analysis, which used data derived from prospective trials of low-dose aspirin for primary and secondary prevention of cardiovascular events, assesses risk factors associated with the development of ulcer and ulcer complications. (*Reproduced from* Hernandez-Diaz S, Garcia Rodriguez L. Cardioprotective aspirin users and their excess risk of upper gastrointestinal complications. BMC Med 2006;4:22; with permission.)

that compared maintenance therapy with omeprazole in aspirin users with *H pylori* infection and a bleeding ulcer history, rates of recurrent ulcer bleeding were comparable among the two treatment groups, suggesting that *H pylori* eradication alone may reduce ulcer risk with low-dose aspirin to the level obtained with proton pump inhibitor (PPI) cotherapy.[32] In another prospective, randomized study, all low-dose aspirin users with *H pylori* infection and a history of ulcer bleeding were treated for *H pylori* before being randomized to a PPI or placebo. One year later, rates of recurrent bleeding were significantly nine times higher in those who had received eradication therapy alone, suggesting that treatment for *H pylori* alone in high-risk users of low-dose aspirin may be insufficient to reduce their subsequent bleeding risks.[28] However, in this study two-thirds of the patients with recurrent ulcer bleeding who had received *H pylori* treatment had persistent *H pylori* infection after treatment or were concomitantly taking NSAIDs. Thus, recurrent bleeding in patients in this study reflected failure to eliminate the *H pylori* infection rather than failure of effective eradication to reduce subsequent aspirin-related GI bleeding. In a more recent and larger prospective trial, patients with a prior history of bleeding ulcer who were infected with *H* pylori, but who also had confirmation of successful *H pylori* eradication before starting low-dose aspirin, had very low (~1%) rates of recurrent bleeding ulcers in up to 4 years of follow-up without concomitant PPI therapy.[20] Therefore, a reasonable conclusion from these studies regarding the contribution by *H pylori* to the risk of aspirin-related GI bleeding is that confirmed eradication of *H pylori* results in considerable reductions in risk of recurrent bleeding in high GI risk patients who take aspirin.

The dose of aspirin also appears to be related to GI ulcer risk, as a higher range of low-dose aspirin, between 100 and 325 mg/d, contributes to an increased risk of gastric or duodenal ulcer.[18,19] Although meta-analyses of the risk of aspirin dose and GI bleeding certainly suggest a trend in favor of lower doses of aspirin being associated with reduced GI risk, no study has been able to prove that 81 mg of aspirin daily is associated with statically fewer GI complications than 325 mg of aspirin per day. It has also been suggested that modifications to the formulation of aspirin might be associated with a lower GI bleeding risk. However, when enteric-coated and buffered aspirin formulations were compared with plain aspirin for their risks of major GI bleeding, GI risks were not lowered by the modified formulations of aspirin.[33,34]

Concurrent use of low-dose aspirin with an NSAID is also a risk factor for GI ulcer complications. Observational studies have noted that, compared with the risk of low-dose aspirin taken alone, when low-dose aspirin is combined with an NSAID, the RR of upper GI complications increases by two- to four-fold.[35,36] In certain clinical scenarios, patients achieve cardiovascular benefit from the addition of anticoagulants, such as heparin or coumadin, to low-dose aspirin. However, the addition of heparin or coumadin to low-dose aspirin may increase risks of major bleeding by 50% to two-fold, respectively.[37,38]

Clopidogrel

Similar to observations with low-dose aspirin, in patients taking clopidogrel as the sole antiplatelet therapy, a prior history of bleeding has been observed in several studies to be a risk factor that places these patients at substantial risk for GI complications on clopidogrel. In a retrospective cohort analysis of patients taking clopidogrel, 22% of patients with a prior history of GI bleeding had recurrent GI bleeding while taking clopidogrel, whereas no patients without a prior history of GI bleeding had bleeding while on this antiplatelet agent.[39] Prospectively conducted trials of patients with prior histories of ulcers have demonstrated rates of recurrent GI bleeding ranging from 9% to 13% of patients by 1 year.[13,40]

Concomitant use of clopidogrel with an NSAID has also been suggested by observational studies to increase the GI risks of clopidogrel. In one observational study, concurrent use of clopidogrel with an NSAID increased the RR of upper GI bleeding by 15.2 (95% confidence interval [CI], 4.1–56.5).[36] A substantial increase in GI bleeding risk is also conferred by the combined used of clopidogrel, anticoagulants, and aspirin.[41] Studies of clopidogrel have not yet reported the effects of advancing age or *H pylori* on clopidogrel's GI risks. However, since all other risk factors studied with clopidogrel have shown consistent similarity to GI risk factors with aspirin, for now it would be prudent to assume that these other as of yet unstudied GI risk factors with clopidogrel are similar to those seen with aspirin. Furthermore, any risk factor demonstrated in association with either of the individual antiplatelet therapies should be similarly assumed to be associated with GI risk with combination antiplatelet therapy.

STRATEGIES TO REDUCE GASTROINTESTINAL RISK OF ANTIPLATELET THERAPIES

Therapy for management of GI risks with antiplatelet agents needs to be tailored depending on whether one is attempting to treat an already established ulcer or GI bleed associated with antiplatelet therapies or attempting to prevent an ulcer or GI bleeding from developing in patients taking these medications.

Prevention of Ulcers and Gastrointestinal Bleeding in Patients Taking Antiplatelet Agents

As discussed in previous sections, although the RR of a GI bleed is increased 1.5- to 3.2-fold in patients undergoing antiplatelet therapies,[18,19] the absolute risk to any individual patient is relatively small. Thus, it is not likely cost efficient to treat all patients taking antiplatelet agents with strategies that will reduce their subsequent risks of a GI event. A more tailored approach that identifies those patients at greatest risk of developing GI bleeding on antiplatelet therapy is a more efficient approach to manage GI risk (**Table 1**). Recent guidelines have been published that suggest an approach for reducing GI risks in patients taking antiplatelet agents (**Fig. 2**).[42]

The initial step in reducing GI risk of antiplatelet therapies is to assess whether the patient has a continued requirement for antiplatelet therapy. Depending on the indication for aspirin and/or clopidogrel and the length of time on therapy, some patients may be able to have antiplatelet therapy withdrawn. For example, clopidogrel in combination with aspirin is recommended for specifically defined time periods for patients presenting with acute coronary syndrome and following PCI or coronary artery bypass grafting.[4] In patients who require continued treatment with antiplatelet therapies, the next step is to assess the presence of factors that may place the patient at greater GI risk. Because the majority of patients who chronically take antiplatelet agents will never develop clinically significant ulceration, the ideal candidates for cotherapy are those considered as at high risk for NSAID-induced ulcers (**Fig. 2 and Table 1**). Patients with multiple GI risk factors will certainly be the most compelling candidates for strategies to reduce their risk. All patients with a prior history of peptic ulcer or a history of ulcer complications should be tested for the presence of *H pylori* infection and those with the infection should be given therapies for the eradication of *H pylori* before starting antiplatelet therapy.[42,43]

After assessment and treatment of *H pylori* in patients with prior ulcer or GI bleeding histories, further reduction in GI risk in other high-risk patients who require antiplatelet agents is primarily accomplished by prescribing drugs that when coadministered with antiplatelet agents protect against mucosal ulceration. Although various cotherapies that have been considered are discussed in the following sections, PPIs are the risk reduction strategy most commonly recommended by guidelines (see **Fig. 2**).[42]

Prostaglandins

Prevention of upper GI injury with low-dose aspirin is dependent on the presence of GI mucosal prostaglandins.[8] In short-term studies of healthy volunteers, misoprostol, the synthetic prostaglandin E1 analogue, reduces gastric mucosal injury.[44] Studies using capsule endoscopy demonstrate that low-dose enteric-coated aspirin frequently damages the small intestine, and misoprostol significantly reduces small intestinal injury related to aspirin.[45] In patients taking low-dose aspirin plus an NSAID, misoprostol can effectively reduce the incidence of endoscopic ulcers.[46] The disadvantages to misoprostol are that it may cause dose-related diarrhea and is not effective in treating dyspepsia associated with aspirin.

Nitrates

Since a component of GI injury is felt to be related to a reduction in mucosal blood flow, compounds that maintain GI blood flow are conceptual targets as agents that might reduce GI injury due to antiplatelet therapies. As nitrates are vasodilators, their

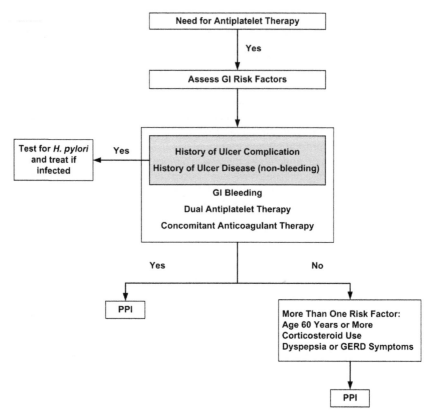

Fig. 2. Approach to reducing GI risks in patients taking antiplatelet therapies. Expert consensus guideline recommended by the American College of Cardiology Foundation, American College of Gastroenterology, and the American Heart Association. (*Reproduced from* Bhatt DL, Scheiman J, Abraham NS, et al; American College of Cardiology Foundation Task Force on Clinical Expert Consensus Documents. ACCF/ACG/AHA 2008 expert consensus document on reducing the gastrointestinal risks of antiplatelet therapy and NSAID use: a report of the American College of Cardiology Foundation Task Force on Clinical Expert Consensus Documents. J Am Coll Cardiol 2008;52(18):1502–17; with permission.)

efficacy in prevention of GI injury with antiplatelet agents has been evaluated in products in clinical development. Endoscopic trials indicate that a fixed-dose combination tablet of aspirin and nitric oxide (NO), NO-aspirin, causes fewer endoscopic lesions in the upper GI tract than aspirin.[47] In addition, an epidemiologic study reported that the use of nitrates is associated with risk reduction of ulcer bleeding in patients who take low-dose aspirin.[48] However, a subsequent case-control study by the same group revealed that nitrates did not effectively reduce the RR of hospitalizations for upper GI bleeding in patients taking low-dose aspirin (100–300 mg/d) or clopidogrel (**Fig. 3**).[49] Therefore, nitrates cannot be recommended with confidence as effective strategies to reduce the GI risks of antiplatelet therapies.

H_2-Receptor Antagonists

Very few studies have evaluated the efficacy of H_2-receptor antagonists (H_2RAs) in the prevention of GI injury with antiplatelet agents. A small retrospective cohort analysis demonstrated that after 1 year of clopidogrel, 22% of patients taking concomitant

Hospitalizations for Upper GI Bleeding

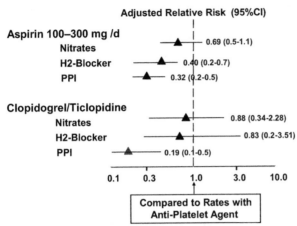

Adjusted Relative Risk (95%CI)

Aspirin 100–300 mg /d
Nitrates — 0.69 (0.5-1.1)
H2-Blocker — 0.40 (0.2-0.7)
PPI — 0.32 (0.2-0.5)

Clopidogrel/Ticlopidine
Nitrates — 0.88 (0.34-2.28)
H2-Blocker — 0.83 (0.2-3.51)
PPI — 0.19 (0.1-0.5)

0.1   0.3   1.0   3.0   10.0

Compared to Rates with
Anti-Platelet Agent

Fig. 3. Comparison of strategies for prevention of upper GI bleeding. The adjusted RRs (and 95% CI) of hospitalizations for upper GI bleeding in Spain are presented in this case-control study of 2777 cases of patients with upper GI bleeding and 5532 controls without bleeding. The RRs of upper GI bleeding with nitrates, H_2-receptor antagonists, and proton pump inhibitors (PPI) are shown compared with the bleeding rates associated with aspirin or clopidogrel/ticlopidine without cotherapy. Figure constructed using data presented in reference. (*Data from* Lanas A, Garcia-Rodriguez LA, Arroyo MT, et al. Effect of antisecretory drugs and nitrates on the risk of ulcer bleeding associated with nonsteroidal anti-inflammatory drugs, antiplatelet agents, and anticoagulants. Am J Gastroenterol 2007;102:507–15.)

H_2RAs had recurrent upper GI bleeding, whereas no patient taking clopidogrel plus a PPI had recurrent bleeding.[39] A recent case-control study revealed that, compared with patients undergoing antiplatelet therapy without protective cotherapy, H_2RAs can significantly reduce the risk of patients admitted to hospital with upper GI bleeding while taking low-dose aspirin (RR, 0.32; 95% CI, 0.2–0.5) but not in those taking clopidogrel (RR, 0.83; 95% CI, 0.2–3.5) (see **Fig. 3**).[49] Although this study did not assess the efficacy of H_2RAs in prevention of upper GI bleeding in patients undergoing dual antiplatelet therapies, it can be assumed that H_2RAs would not be effective in prevention of GI bleeding with clopidogrel plus aspirin, since this strategy was ineffective in preventing GI bleeding with clopidogrel alone.

Proton Pump Inhibitors

Use of PPIs (omeprazole, lansoprazole, rabeprazole, pantoprazole, and esomeprazole) as prophylaxis for GI injury due to antiplatelet therapies has become an attractive strategy for many clinicians. Support for this practice comes from several randomized, control trials and observational studies. In a randomized, control trial of low-dose aspirin in users with prior histories of bleeding ulcers, after eradication of *H pylori*, use of a PPI was associated with a statistically significant 89% reduction in recurrent ulcer bleeding at 1 year.[28] In a 6-month randomized trial of *H pylori* eradication compared with maintenance therapy with omeprazole in aspirin users with *H pylori* infection and a recent history of ulcer bleeding, rates of recurrent ulcer bleeding were comparable between the two treatment groups (0.9% and 1.9%, respectively).[32] In a more recent prospective study of *H pylori*-negative patients with histories of aspirin-induced upper GI bleeding, PPI administered along with low-dose aspirin was much more effective than clopidogrel alone in reducing rates of recurrent upper GI bleeding (0.7% and 8.6%, respectively; P = .001).[13] Finally, observational studies suggest that PPIs very effectively reduce upper GI bleeding risks associated with monotherapy with low-dose aspirin (RR, 0.32; 95% CI, 0.2–3.5) and with monotherapy with clopidogrel (RR, 0.19; 95% CI, 0.1–0.5).[49]

The sum of the above evidence from trials of differing design indicated that PPIs are very effective therapies in the prevention of GI injury with either aspirin or clopidogrel monotherapy. However, for the more commonly used dual-antiplatelet therapies, there are fewer data evaluating the effectiveness of PPIs. A recent prospectively placebo-controlled, endoscopic trial of the efficacy of various dosages of omeprazole as a strategy to reduce gastroduodenal erosions and ulcers indicated that omeprazole at doses of 20 and 40 mg significantly reduced short-term erosive GI injury by as much as 80% in patients taking clopidogrel and low-dose aspirin (**Fig. 4**).[50] The COGENT-1 (Clopidogrel and the Optimization of Gastrointestinal Events; NCT00557921) study was designed to evaluate GI events in patients with coronary artery disease taking low-dose aspirin randomized to a fixed-dose, single combination tablet of clopidogrel plus omeprazole 20 mg or to clopidogrel alone. This study, which had the recruitment goal of 8000 patients, was powered to evaluate clinically significant GI outcomes with the PPI/clopidogrel combination. Unfortunately, the study was prematurely terminated in January 2009 after enrolling only 2000 patients. Therefore, the only currently available data supporting PPIs as effective therapies to prevent GI injury from dual antiplatelet therapies are from a short-term endoscopic trial.[50]

Treatment of Ulcers and Gastrointestinal Bleeding in Patients Taking Antiplatelet Agents

Healing of bleeding ulcers formed as a consequence of antiplatelet therapy can be effectively accomplished, assuming that these agents can be discontinued. A clinical challenge that clinicians frequently encounter is when a patient who requires chronic antiplatelet therapy presents with GI bleeding, for example, a patient with recent percutaneous revascularization. In a clinical trial of patients chronically taking low-dose aspirin for cardiovascular indications who presented with bleeding gastric or duodenal ulcers, after initial withholding of aspirin, successful endoscopic treatment of bleeding ulcers, and treatment with PPIs, patients were randomized to low-dose aspirin or to placebo.[51] Rates of recurrent upper GI bleeding 1 month after endoscopic

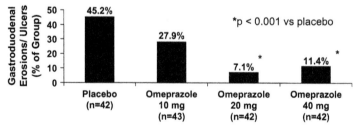

Fig. 4. Omeprazole for the prevention of endoscopic gastroduodenal mucosal injury with clopidogrel plus aspirin. *H. pylori*-negative healthy volunteers (n = 174) taking clopidogrel 75 mg daily plus aspirin 325 mg daily for 14 d were randomized to placebo or omeprazole 10 mg, 20 mg, or 40 mg. Compared with placebo, endoscopically assessed mucosal injury was significantly reduced with omeprazole at doses of 20 mg and 40 mg daily (P<.001), with the 20-mg dose associated with the greatest reduction of injury (~80%). (*From* Cryer B, Lapuerta P, Jernamo, et al. Omeprazole can prevent the gastroduodenal mucosal injury associated with combined use of clopidogrel and aspirin. Am J Gastroenterol 2008;103(Suppl 1):S49, data presented in reference.)

treatment were similar in the aspirin and placebo groups (19% and 11%, respectively; $P = .25$). However, 30-day mortality was much higher in patients in whom aspirin had been withheld (placebo users) when compared with patients in whom aspirin was restarted (15% vs 2%; $P = .01$), with the majority of the deaths in the placebo group attributable to cardiovascular reasons. This study's results suggest that it may be more dangerous to withhold aspirin for 1 month in patients with cardiovascular disease than to restart it immediately after successful endoscopic treatment of their bleeding ulcers followed by continuous intravenous infusion of PPI.[51]

With regard to management of acute GI bleeding in patients on dual antiplatelet therapy, clinicians need to balance the increased cardiovascular risks that prompted the indication for dual antiplatelet therapy against the risks of recurrent GI bleeding. Recent guidelines recommend that endoscopic therapy may be performed in high-risk cardiovascular patients on dual antiplatelet therapy and that collaboration between the cardiologist and gastroenterologist should balance the risks for bleeding against the risk of cardiovascular thrombosis on an individual basis.[42,52] In patients in whom individualized cardiac and GI risk stratification suggests that antiplatelet therapies could be withheld for control of acute GI bleeding, the optimum period before reintroduction of antiplatelet therapy has not been established in clinical trials.[42,52]

POTENTIAL PROTON PUMP INHIBITOR INTERACTION WITH CLOPIDOGREL

Given the growing evidence that a PPI might decrease risk for GI bleeding in patients taking clopidogrel, this risk reduction strategy is seemingly a reasonable recommendation for high GI risks patients taking clopidogrel either alone or in combination with low-dose aspirin. However, recent evidence suggests that clopidogrel may be less effective when taken with a PPI. Clopidogrel is a prodrug that must be activated by the CYP2C19 enzyme in the liver to its biologically active metabolite that inhibits platelet activity. The prodrug has no intrinsic antiplatelet activity without activation. Confirmation that activation of the CYP2C19 pathway is clinically relevant to clopidogrel's therapeutic effect comes from several lines of evidence. First, patients with genetic polymorphisms of the CYP2C19 enzymes, by virtue of this polymorphism, have less effective hepatic metabolism of clopidogrel and show a marked decrease in their platelet responsiveness to clopidogrel.[53] Furthermore, patients receiving clopidogrel with a history of coronary artery disease without a functioning CYP2C19 gene have higher rates of coronary stent thrombosis and myocardial infarction than those of patients without genetic mutations.[54,55]

Omeprazole is a potent inhibitor of CYP2C19, but all PPIs may inhibit CYP2C19 to some extent.[56] Studies assessing the short-term effects of omeprazole on the intermediate end point of clopidogrel's inhibition of platelet activation in blood samples from patients demonstrate that after 7 days of use, omeprazole decreases clopidogrel's antiplatelet efficacy.[57] Other studies of other PPIs, lansoprazole, pantoprazole and esomeprazole, do not demonstrate this effect on the intermediate end point of platelet responsiveness.[58,59] Consistent with the hypothesis, observational studies indicate a higher cardiovascular event rate in patients taking PPIs along with clopidogrel and aspirin compared with that of patients undergoing dual antiplatelet therapy without PPIs.[60,61] However, in these observational studies, PPIs were used in a greater number of patients with cardiovascular risk factors. Thus, it is not yet clear whether the perceived increased rate of cardiovascular events in those taking PPIs is the result of channeling of higher cardiovascular risk patients to receive PPI treatment. The question of whether PPI treatment diminishes the antiplatelet efficacy of clopidogrel would ideally be best evaluated by a randomized, placebo-controlled trial. Currently, there is no evidence that other acid inhibitory agents such as the H_2RAs or antacids interfere with the antiplatelet activity of clopidogrel. Whether concurrent use of a PPI with clopidogrel represents a safety concern or not is currently being evaluated by the US Food and Drug Administration.[62] Until more specific regulatory guidance is available, current recommendations are that patients taking both PPIs and clopidogrel concurrently should probably continue to do so until more data become available.[63]

REFERENCES

1. Yusuf S, Zhao F, Mehta SR, et al. Effects of clopidogrel in addition to aspirin in patients with acute coronary syndromes without ST-segment elevation. N Engl J Med 2001;345:494–502.
2. Mehta SR, Yusuf S, Peters RJ, et al. Effects of pretreatment with clopidogrel and aspirin followed by long-term therapy in patients undergoing percutaneous coronary intervention: the PCI-CURE study. Lancet 2001;358:527–33.
3. Steinhubl SR, Berger PB, Mann JT III, et al. Clopidogrel for the Reduction of Events During Observation. Early and sustained dual oral antiplatelet therapy following percutaneous coronary intervention: a randomized controlled trial (CREDO). JAMA 2002;288:2411–20.
4. Antman EM, Hand M, Armstrong PW, et al. 2007 focused update of the ACC/AHA 2004 guidelines for the management of patients with ST-elevation myocardial infarction: a report of the American College of Cardiology/American Heart Association Task Force on Practice Guidelines (Writing Group to Review New Evidence and Update the ACC/AHA 2004 Guidelines for the Management of Patients With ST-Elevation Myocardial Infarction). J Am Coll Cardiol 2008;51:210–47.
5. Sacco RL, Adams R, Albers G, et al. Guidelines for prevention of stroke in patients with ischemic stroke or transient ischemic attack: a statement for healthcare professionals from the American Heart Association/American Stroke Association Council on Stroke: co-sponsored by the Council on Cardiovascular Radiology and Intervention: the American Academy of Neurology affirms the value of this guideline. Stroke 2006;37:577–617.
6. Duffy B, Bhatt DL. Antiplatelet agents in patients undergoing percutaneous coronary intervention: how many and how much? Am J Cardiovasc Drugs 2005;5:307–18.
7. Patrono C, Rodriguez LA, Landolfi R, et al. Low-dose aspirin for the prevention of atherothrombosis. N Engl J Med 2005;353:2373–83.
8. Cryer B, Feldman M. Effects of very low doses of daily, long-term aspirin therapy on gastric, duodenal and rectal prostaglandins and on mucosal injury in healthy humans. Gastroenterology 1999;117:17–25.
9. CAPRIE Steering Committee. A randomized, blinded, trial of clopidogrel versus aspirin in patients at risk of ischaemic events (CAPRIE). Lancet 1996;348:1329–39.
10. Fort FT, Lafolie P, Tóth E, et al. Gastroduodenal tolerance of 75 mg clopidogrel versus 325 mg aspirin in healthy volunteers. Scand J Gastroenterol 2000;35:464–9.
11. Ibáñez L, Vidal X, Vendrell L, et al. Spanish-Italian Collaborative Group for the Epidemiology of Gastrointestinal Bleeding. Upper gastrointestinal bleeding associated with antiplatelet drugs. Aliment Pharmacol Ther 2006;23(2):235–42.
12. Wiviott SD, Braunwald E, McCabe CH, et al. Prasugrel versus clopidogrel in patients with acute coronary syndromes. N Engl J Med 2007;357:2001–15.
13. Chan FKL, Ching JYL, Hung LCT, et al. Clopidogrel versus aspirin and esomeprazole for the prevention of recurrent ulcer bleeding. N Engl J Med 2005;352(3):238–44.

14. Cryer B. Reducing the risks of gastrointestinal bleeding with antiplatelet therapies. N Engl J Med 2005;352(3):287–9.
15. Ma L, Elliott SN, Cirino G, et al. Platelets modulate gastric ulcer healing: role of endostatin and vascular endothelial growth factor release. Proc Natl Acad Sci U S A 2001;98(11):6470–5.
16. Kabbinovar F, Hurwitz HI, Fehrenbaacher L, et al. Phase II, randomized trial comparing bevacizumab plus fluorouracil (FU)/leucovorin (LV) with FU/LA alone in patients with metastatic colorectal cancer. J Clin Oncol 2003;21:60–5.
17. Sheikh RA, Romano PS, Prindiville TP, et al. Endoscopic evidence of mucosal injury in patients taking ticlopidine compared with patients taking aspirin/nonsteroidal antiinflammatory drugs and controls. J Clin Gastroenterol 2002; 34:529–32.
18. McQuaid KR, Laine L. Systematic review and meta-analysis of adverse events of low-dose aspirin and clopidogrel in randomized controlled trials. Am J Med 2006; 119:624–38.
19. Derry S, Loke YK. Risk of gastrointestinal haemorrhage with long-term use of aspirin: meta-analysis. BMJ 2000;321:1183–7.
20. Chan FK. Long-term incidence of ulcer bleeding with low-dose aspirin after eradication of H pylori: A 4- year prospective cohort study. Gastroenterology 2005; 128:A133.
21. Kahn R, Robertson RM, Smith R, et al. The impact of prevention on reducing the burden of cardiovascular disease. Circulation 2008;118(5):576–85.
22. Hernandez-Diaz S, Garcia Rodriguez L. Cardioprotective aspirin users and their excess risk of upper gastrointestinal complications. BMC Med 2006;4:22.
23. Grines CL, Bonow RO, Casey DE Jr, et al. Prevention of premature discontinuation of dual antiplatelet therapy in patients with coronary artery stents: a science advisory from the American Heart Association, American College of Cardiology, Society for Cardiovascular Angiography and Interventions, American College of Surgeons, and American Dental Association, with representation from the American College of Physicians. Circulation 2007;115:813–8.
24. Diener HC, Bogousslavsky J, Brass LM, et al. Aspirin and clopidogrel compared with clopidogrel alone after recent ischaemic stroke or transient ischaemic attack in high-risk patients (MATCH): randomised, double-blind, placebo controlled trial. Lancet 2004;364:331–7.
25. Bhatt DL, Fox KA, HackeW, et al. Clopidogrel and aspirin versus aspirin alone for the prevention of atherothrombotic events. N Engl J Med 2006;354:1706–17.
26. Hallas J, Dall M, Andries A, et al. Use of single and combined antithrombotic therapy and risk of serious upper gastrointestinal bleeding: population based case-control study. BMJ 2006;333:726–8.
27. Lanas A, Scheiman J. Low-dose aspirin and upper gastrointestinal damage: epidemiology, prevention and treatment. Curr Med Res Opin 2007;23:163–73.
28. Lai KC, Lam SK, Chu KM, et al. Lansoprazole for the prevention of recurrences of ulcer complications from long-term low-dose aspirin use. N Engl J Med 2002;346: 2033–8.
29. Yeomans N, Lanas A, Labenz J, et al. Efficacy of esomeprazole (20 mg once daily) for reducing the risk of gastroduodenal ulcers associated with continuous use of low-dose aspirin. Am J Gastroenterol 2008;103(10):2465–73.
30. Lanas A, Yeomans N, Junghard O. Svedberg on behalf of the ASTERIX Investigators. Risk factors for gastroduodenal ulcer during treatment with acetylsalicylic acid for cardiovascular risk management. *European Heart Journal* 2008;29 (suppl 1):402.

31. Lanas A, Fuentes J, Benito R, et al. *Helicobacter pylori* increases the risk of upper gastrointestinal bleeding in patients taking low-dose aspirin. Aliment Pharmacol Ther 2002;16:779–86.

32. Chan FK, Chung SC, Suen BY, et al. Preventing recurrent upper gastrointestinal bleeding in patients with Helicobacter pylori infection who are taking low-dose aspirin or naproxen. N Engl J Med 2001;344:967–73.

33. de Abajo FJ, Garcia Rodriguez LA. Risk of upper gastrointestinal bleeding and perforation associated with low-dose aspirin as plain and enteric-coated formulations. BMC Clin Pharmacol 2001;1:1.

34. Kelly JP, Kaufman DW, Jurgelon JM, et al. Risk of aspirin associated major upper-gastrointestinal bleeding with enteric-coated or buffered product. Lancet 1996; 348:1413–6.

35. Sørensen HT, Mellemkjaer L, Blot WJ, et al. Risk of upper gastrointestinal bleeding associated with use of low-dose aspirin. Am J Gastroenterol 2000 Sep;95(9):2218–24.

36. Lanas A, Garcia-Rodriguez LA, Arroyo MT, et al. Risk of upper gastrointestinal ulcer bleeding associated with selective cyclo-oxygenase-2 inhibitors, traditional non-aspirin non-steroidal anti-inflammatory drugs, aspirin and combinations. Gut 2006;55:1731–8.

37. Collins R, MacMahon S, Flather M, et al. Clinical effects of anticoagulant therapy in suspected acute myocardial infarction: systematic overview of randomised trials. BMJ 1996;313:652–9.

38. Andreotti F, Testa L, Biondi-Zoccai GG, et al. Aspirin plus warfarin compared to aspirin alone after acute coronary syndromes: an updated and comprehensive meta-analysis of 25,307 patients. Eur Heart J 2006;27:519–26.

39. Ng FH, Wong SY, Chang CM, et al. High incidence of clopidogrel-associated gastrointestinal bleeding in patients with previous peptic ulcer disease. Aliment Pharmacol Ther 2003;18:443–9.

40. Lai KC, Chu KM, Hui WM, et al. Esomeprazole with aspirin versus clopidogrel for prevention of recurrent gastrointestinal ulcer complications. Clin Gastroenterol Hepatol 2006;4:860–5.

41. Khurram Z, Chou E, Minutello R, et al. Combination therapy with aspirin, clopidogrel and warfarin following coronary stenting is associated with a significant risk of bleeding. J Invasive Cardiol 2006;18:162–4.

42. Bhatt DL, Scheiman J, Abraham NS, et al. American College of Cardiology Foundation Task Force on Clinical Expert Consensus Documents. ACCF/ACG/AHA 2008 expert consensus document on reducing the gastrointestinal risks of antiplatelet therapy and NSAID use: a report of the American College of Cardiology Foundation Task Force on Clinical Expert Consensus Documents. J Am Coll Cardiol 2008;52(18):1502–17.

43. Chey WD, Wong BC. American College of Gastroenterology guideline on the management of Helicobacter pylori infection. Am J Gastroenterol 2007;102:1808–25.

44. Donnelly MT, Goddard AF, Filipowicz B, et al. Low-dose misoprostol for the prevention of low-dose aspirin induced gastroduodenal injury. Aliment Pharmacol Ther 2000;14:529–34.

45. Watanabe T, Sugimori S, Kameda N, et al. Small bowel injury by low-dose enteric-coated aspirin and treatment with misoprostol: a pilot study. Clin Gastroenterol Hepatol 2008;6(11):1279–82.

46. Goldstein JL, Huang B, Amer F, et al. Ulcer recurrence in high-risk patients receiving nonsteroidal anti-inflammatory drugs plus low-dose aspirin: results of a post HOC subanalysis. Clin Ther 2004;26:1637–43.

47. Fiorucci S, Santucci L, Gresele P, et al. Gastrointestinal safety of NO-aspirin (NCX-4016) in healthy human volunteers: a proof of concept endoscopic study. Gastroenterology 2003;124:600–7.
48. Lanas A, Bajador E, Serrano P, et al. Nitrovasodilators, low-dose aspirin, nonsteroidal anti-inflammatory drugs, and the risk of upper gastrointestinal bleeding. N Engl J Med 2000;343:834–9.
49. Lanas A, García-Rodríguez LA, Arroyo MT, et al. Effect of antisecretory drugs and nitrates on the risk of ulcer bleeding associated with nonsteroidal anti-inflammatory drugs, antiplatelet agents, and anticoagulants. Am J Gastroenterol 2007;102:507–15.
50. Cryer B, Lapuerta P, Jernamo, et al. Omeprazole can prevent the gastroduodenal mucosal injury associated with combined use of clopidogrel and aspirin. Am J Gastroenterol 2008;103(Suppl 1):S49.
51. Sung J, Lau J, Ching J, et al. Can aspirin be reintroduced with PPI inhibitor INFUSION after endoscopic hemostasis: a double-blinded randomized controlled trial. Gastroenterology 2008;130:A44.
52. Eisen GM, Baron TH, Dominitz JA, et al. Guidelines on the management of anticoagulation and anti-platelet therapy for endoscopic procedures. Gastrointest Endosc 2002;55:775–9.
53. Hulot JS, Bura A, Villard E, et al. Cytochrome P450 2C19 loss-of-function polymorphism is a major determinant of clopidogrel responsiveness in healthy subjects. Blood 2006;108:2244–7.
54. Collet JP, Hulot JS, Pena A, et al. Cytochrome P450 2C19 polymorphism in young patients treated with clopidogrel after myocardial infarction: a cohort study. Lancet 2008;10.1016/S0140-6736(08)61845-0.
55. Simon T, Verstuyft C, Mary-Krause M, et al. Genetic determinants of response to clopidogrel and cardiovascular events. N Engl J Med 2009;360:363–75.
56. Li XQ, Andersson TB, Ahlstrom M, et al. Comparison of inhibitory effects of the proton pump-inhibiting drugs omeprazole, esomeprazole, lansoprazole, pantoprazole, and rabeprazole on human cytochrome P450 activities. Drug Metab Dispos 2004;32:821–7.
57. Gilard M, Arnaud B, Cornily JC, et al. Influence of omeprazole on the antiplatelet action of clopidogrel associated with aspirin: the randomized, double-blind OCLA (Omeprazole CLopidogrel Aspirin) study. J Am Coll Cardiol 2008;51:256–60.
58. Small DS, Farid NA, Payne CD, et al. Effects of the proton pump inhibitor lansoprazole on the pharmacokinetics and pharmacodynamics of prasugrel and clopidogrel. J Clin Pharmacol 2008;48:475–84.
59. Siller-Matula JM, Spiel AO, Lang IM, et al. Effects of pantoprazole and esomeprazole on platelet inhibition by clopidogrel. Am Heart J 2009;157:148 e1–5.
60. Pezalla E, Day D, Pulliadath A. Initial assessment of clinical impact of a drug interaction between clopidogrel and proton pump inhibitors. J Am Coll Cardiol 2008; 52(12):1038–9.
61. Aubert RE, Epstein RS, Teagarden JR, et al. Understanding variability in antiplatelet drug effects in acute coronary syndromes. Abstract 3998: proton pump inhibitors effect on clopidogrel effectiveness: the clopidogrel medco outcomes study. Circulation 2008;118:S815.
62. Early Communication about an Ongoing Safety Review of clopidogrel bisulfate (marketed as Plavix). Available at: http://www.fda.gov/cder/drug/early_comm/clopidogrel_bisulfate.htm. Accessed January 20, 2009.
63. PPI interactions with clopidogrel. The Medical Letter Inc 2009;51(1303):1–3.

Balancing Risks and Benefits of Cyclooxygenase-2 Selective Nonsteroidal Anti-Inflammatory Drugs

James M. Scheiman, MD

KEYWORDS

- Peptic ulcer disease • Gastrointestinal bleeding
- Anti-inflammatory therapy • Thrombosis
- Myocardial infarction • Aspirin

"The whole imposing edifice of modern medicine is like the celebrated tower of Pisa - slightly off balance."

—Charles, Prince of Wales

The recognition that users of nonsteroidal anti-inflammatory drugs (NSAIDs) experience an increased likelihood of cardiovascular (CV) adverse events has led patients and clinicians to steer clear from their use.[1] This astonishing recognition of an unexpected side effect, from such a commonly used medication class, may never have been discovered had novel compounds not been developed to reduce their well-documented gastrointestinal (GI) complications. NSAIDs provide important benefits by controlling pain and inflammation for many patients. The alternatives, undertreatment of pain or use of narcotic analgesics, have their own significant adverse consequences. As weighing risks and benefits of any medical intervention is an essential component of clinical decision making, it has become increasingly complex to decide in whom the use of any NSAID—with/without a gastroprotective agent or with/without concomitant aspirin—is appropriate. Given the multiplicity, and in many cases rarity, of adverse events, it is unlikely that a single "megatrial" will adequately address the numerous safety and effectiveness issues. In the meantime, careful synthesis of the literature—not complete reliance on individual studies that address one outcome—is required to inform medication selection. This step-wise approach is crucial, since appropriate NSAID choice should

Division of Gastroenterology, Department of Internal Medicine, University of Michigan School of Medicine, 3912 Taubman Center SPC 5362, University of Michigan Medical Center, Ann Arbor, MI 48109, USA
E-mail address: jscheima@umich.edu

Gastroenterol Clin N Am 38 (2009) 305–314
doi:10.1016/j.gtc.2009.03.006
0889-8553/09/$ – see front matter © 2009 Elsevier Inc. All rights reserved.

gastro.theclinics.com

be driven by an individual patient's CV and/or GI risk assessment rather than a medication's reported adverse event rate in a study of a heterogeneous population.[2]

Clinicians are faced with a real challenge, as they must estimate each patient's baseline risk for both GI and CV adverse events independent of drug therapy and then multiply the impact of various risk modifiers (individual drugs and doses) to estimate the overall patient risk. For example, reducing an otherwise healthy 25-year-old patient's risk of a GI bleed on anti-inflammatory therapy by 50% by selecting a safer drug translates to absolute risk change of less than 1/1000. Compare this to the impact in a 70-year-old with a history of peptic ulcer, in whom the risk of recurrent bleeding at 1 year on an NSAID is at least 10%—two orders of magnitude greater. The same concepts apply to the confirmed but less well-understood increased risk of adverse CV events. This review provides clinicians a framework to implement a rational approach to these competing risks by providing prescribers a simplified method of individualized medication selection.

WHAT ARE THE CARDIOVASCULAR RISKS OF NONSTEROIDAL ANTI-INFLAMMATORY DRUGS?

Both nonselective and cyclooxygenase (COX)-2–selective NSAIDs have been associated with an increased incidence of hospitalization for congestive heart failure and elevated blood pressure.[3,4] Their specific effect on other serious CV events, including myocardial infarction (MI) and death, has been more controversial. Although there are theoretical reasons why COX-2 selective agents may be prothrombotic, such as decreased production of the vasodilator prostacyclin (which also inhibits platelet activation) with concomitant unimpeded COX-1–mediated production of platelet thromboxane A2, the mechanistic relationship to CV events remains incompletely understood.[5]

The CV risk of certain NSAIDs may be aggravated due to a clinically important interaction with low-dose aspirin that has been identified for some, but not all, drugs. Catella-Lawson and colleagues[6] investigated the potential interactions between aspirin and several different NSAIDs and found that ibuprofen could mitigate the cardioprotective effects of aspirin by interfering with aspirin's platelet inhibition. This interaction, thought to be due to ibuprofen blocking aspirin's access to the COX-1 enzyme, was not seen with COX-2 selective inhibitors as well as diclofenac. Platelet aggregation studies support preserved antiplatelet activity in patients taking naproxen, which may override any competition the drug may have at the platelet-binding site.[7,8]

The Vioxx GI Outcomes Research Study (VIGOR) trial studied rheumatoid arthritis patients (who are at increased CV risk due to their chronic inflammatory disease) and showed a higher rate of adverse CV events (nonfatal MI, nonfatal stroke, and death) on 50 mg rofecoxib every day compared with 500 mg naproxen twice daily (0.8% vs 0.4%, $P<.05$).[9] These results were largely due to differences in MI (0.4% vs 0.1%; $P<.01$). No low-dose aspirin was allowed in this study. Although debate centered on whether these findings were due to a cardioprotective effect of naproxen or a deleterious effect of rofecoxib, the adenomatous Polyp Prevention on Vioxx (APPROVe) trial, a randomized, placebo-controlled study that enrolled 2600 patients with a history of colorectal adenomas, confirmed an increased incidence of MI or stroke for those taking 25 mg rofecoxib daily (3.5% vs 1.9%; $P<.001$). The manufacturer subsequently withdrew rofecoxib from the market.[10]

Valdecoxib was withdrawn on request of the Food and Drug and Administration in April 2005. Two trials in patients undergoing coronary artery bypass grafting showed that there was an increase in CV and thromboembolic events.[11] A systematic review and meta-analysis of CV risk with etoricoxib therapy have also been undertaken, and, although the data are limited, there is evidence of an increased CV risk (odds ratio [OR], 1.49) as well.[12]

Celecoxib is the only COX-2 selective inhibitor remaining on the US market. The Adenoma Prevention with Celecoxib trial included 2026 patients who were assigned to one of three groups: placebo, celecoxib 200 mg twice daily, or celecoxib 400 mg twice daily. Like APPROVe, it was designed to assess the impact of celecoxib in preventing the recurrence of polyps. The study was stopped early by the National Cancer Institute after a mean follow-up of 33 months due to a significantly higher number of celecoxib-treated patients experiencing a MI, stroke, or CV death compared with those receiving placebo (OR, 2.5 for celecoxib 400 mg daily; 95% confidence interval [CI], 1.0–7.0; P = .06, and OR, 3.4 for celecoxib 800 mg daily 95% CI, 1.4–9.3; P = .009).[13] In the Prevention of Spontaneous Adenomatous Polyps (PreSAP) trial, no increase in CV events was found for those patients assigned 400 mg celecoxib daily compared with placebo.[14] Although there are no data to implicate celecoxib 200 mg daily with adverse CV outcomes, we must await a large CV outcome trial in progress.[15] A patient-level pooled analysis of adjudicated data from 7950 patients in 6 placebo-controlled trials comparing celecoxib with placebo for conditions other than arthritis was recently published. With 16,070 patient years of follow-up, the hazard ratio overall was 1.6 (95% CI, 1.1–2.3). The risk, increased with dose, was lowest for the 400 mg every day dose (hazard ratio, 1.1; 95% CI, 0.6–2.0), intermediate for the 200 mg twice a day dose (hazard ratio, 1.8; 5% CI, 1.1–3.1), and highest for the 400 mg twice a day dose (hazard ratio, 3.1; 95% CI, 1.5–6.1). Celecoxib was associated with increased risk regardless of baseline aspirin use—suggesting that the mechanism of CV toxicity is more complex than unopposed COX-2 inhibition.[16] Patients at highest baseline risk demonstrated disproportionately greater risk of celecoxib-related adverse events, strongly emphasizing the issue of appropriate patient selection. This has been emphasized by a recent observational study of Medicare beneficiaries as well.[17] The patient characteristics that were found to increase the risk of cardiovascular disease (CVD) events in that study included age greater than 80 years, hypertension, prior MI, prior CVD, rheumatoid arthritis, chronic renal disease, and chronic obstructive pulmonary disease.

WHAT ARE THE CARDIOVASCULAR RISKS OF NONSELECTIVE NONSTEROIDAL ANTI-INFLAMMATORY DRUGS?

In a widely quoted meta-analysis of randomized, controlled trials, performed by the antiplatelet trialist collaboration, the authors concluded that COX-2 NSAIDs *as a class* were associated with a two-fold greater risk of MI, a 1.5-fold greater risk of vascular death, and no increased risk of stroke.[18] However, compared with placebo, nonselective NSAIDs other than naproxen were also associated with an increased risk and may be associated with a higher risk of stroke than COX-2 NSAIDs. For patients at higher risk for CV events, switching from a COX-2 NSAID to a nonselective NSAID may not decrease treatment-related CV risk, but it is likely to increase GI risk. This meta-analysis suggests, however, that for patients with higher CV risks, naproxen may be the safest NSAID. A large systematic review of observational studies confirmed these results as well.[19] Among nonselective drugs, diclofenac had the highest risk with a summary relative risk (RR) of 1.40 (95% CI, 1.16–1.70). The other drugs had summary RRs close to one: naproxen, 0.97 (95% CI, 0.87–1.07); piroxicam, 1.06 (95% CI, 0.70–1.59); and ibuprofen, 1.07 (95% CI, 0.97–1.18).

Although a small, single study, the Alzheimer Disease Anti-inflammatory Prevention Trial[20] reported an excess number of unadjudicated CV events among those assigned naproxen (at over-the-counter low doses) compared with those in the placebo group.

Methodological limitations limit this trial from reversing the evidence provided by meta-analysis.[19]

The overall conclusion is that an increase in overall CV risk is not confined to COX-2 NSAIDs and may be shared by a number of nonselective NSAIDs. It is likely that dose and duration of COX-2 inhibition are important, which may explain why celecoxib at twice-daily dosing has been associated with adverse CV events but every day dosing has not. A further mechanism that may underlie differences between medications is their variable effect on endothelial function, supported by recent data, demonstrating marked intra- and inter-individual responses to COX-2 NSAIDs.[21]

GASTROINTESTINAL ADVERSE EVENTS ASSOCIATED WITH NONSTEROIDAL ANTI-INFLAMMATORY DRUG THERAPY

The pathophysiological basis for NSAID-induced GI injury is that a relative deficiency of gastroduodenal mucosal prostaglandin initiates ulceration. This promotes disruption of the protective mucus layer, inhibition of protective bicarbonate secretion, vasoconstriction (causing local tissue hypoxia), and a topical effect, in which the NSAIDs are "trapped" within cell membranes, leading to superficial epithelial necrosis. Most of the mucosal prostaglandins are derived from COX-1 in the upper GI tract.[22] The "COX-2 hypothesis," that sparing COX-1 can eliminate ulcer risk, was challenged by animal studies that indicated that both COX-1 and COX-2 must be inhibited for gastric ulceration to occur. Thus, the explanation for the reduced GI toxicity of COX-2–specific inhibitors appears to be their lack of dual COX inhibition, rather than COX-1 sparing effects.[23] This explains why in patients taking both cardioprotective aspirin (primarily a COX-1 inhibitor) and a COX-2 inhibitor, the ulcer risk of a dual COX inhibitor would be predicted. The large outcome studies support these predictions.[24,25]

The serious complications of NSAIDs include symptomatic gastric and duodenal ulcers and their complications—perforation and hemorrhage—which may occur during acute or chronic therapy. Ulcer bleeding is a composite of both medication-related injury and drug-induced increased propensity for bleeding. Thus, drugs with more prolonged and complete COX-1 inhibition will not only produce more ulcers but, due to their antiplatelet action, also promote bleeding. This is particularly magnified by the use of aspirin in addition to any chronic NSAID treatment regimen.

Although NSAID use may be accompanied by dyspeptic symptoms, many patients have no antecedent symptoms, particularly the elderly, whose first presentation of NSAID damage may be GI hemorrhage or perforation. Endoscopic surveys indicate that up to 20% to 30% of regular NSAID users develop ulcers, most never becoming clinically apparent, although symptoms—dyspepsia and heartburn—may occur in up to 60% of patients taking NSAIDs. The annual incidence of NSAID-related clinical upper GI events (complicated and symptomatic ulcers) lies between 2.5% and 4.5%, and the annual incidence of serious NSAID complications (perforation, hemorrhage, and obstruction) amounts to 1% to 1.5%.[26]

The risk of developing complications of NSAID therapy is related to a number of factors, which include the type and dose of NSAID used, whether or not aspirin is coprescribed, the use of multiple NSAIDs, the duration of NSAID use, and concomitant drug prescription, such as antiplatelet, anticoagulant, or selective serotonin reuptake inhibitor therapy. Nondrug risk factors include the patient's age, whether there is a history of peptic ulcer, uncomplicated or complicated, or of dyspepsia, particularly if it persists on antisecretory therapy, Helicobacter pylori infection status, and the presence of concurrent diseases. For example, the RR of developing clinically significant adverse events rises to 4.4 with concomitant use of corticosteroids at doses above 10 mg/d and to 12.7 with concomitant anticoagulant prescription. There are similar substantial increases in the RR of ulcer complications for patients aged over 75 years (RR, 10.6) and those with a history of complicated peptic ulceration (RR, 12.5–15.4).[27]

GASTROPROTECTION STRATEGIES

NSAID therapy leads to a prostaglandin-depleted mucosa vulnerable to continuous exposure to acid with impaired response to injury. Strategies for gastroprotection therefore include supplementation with a synthetic prostaglandin analog, gastric acid suppression, or the selective use of those NSAIDs least likely to inhibit gastric prostaglandins. When balancing the CV risks and GI benefits of COX-2 inhibitors, an understanding of the value of alternative GI risk-reducing strategies is essential.

CYCLOOXYGENASE-2 NONSTEROIDAL ANTI-INFLAMMATORY DRUGS VERSUS CONVENTIONAL NONSTEROIDAL ANTI-INFLAMMATORY DRUGS

A Cochrane systematic review (search date, May 2002) with ulcer complications and symptomatic ulcers as primary endpoints identified 17 trials comparing COX-2–specific NSAIDs with nonselective NSAIDs.[28] There was a significant reduction in risk of symptomatic ulcers with COX-2–specific NSAIDs (RR, 0.49; 95% CI, 0.4–0.6). There was also an apparent benefit for serious GI complications (RR, 0.55; 95% CI, 0.4–0.8). One trial published after this review compared lumiracoxib 400 mg daily with ibuprofen 800 mg thrice daily or naproxen 500 mg twice daily in patients with osteoarthritis older than 50 years, with upper GI complications as the end point, and found a significant advantage for lumiracoxib HR 0.34 (95% CI, 0.22–0.53).[24] Although lumiracoxib is not currently available due to serious hepatotoxicity, subanalyses suggested that the benefit of the drug was markedly reduced for patients concurrently taking aspirin (as was seen in a celecoxib trial as well[25]). In summary, COX-2 NSAIDs carry less risk of symptomatic peptic ulcers than conventional NSAIDs and probably less risk of serious GI complications. This benefit is lost when patients are concurrently taking aspirin.

PROTON PUMP INHIBITORS

Proton pump inhibitors (PPIs) are widely used to reduce the ulcer risk of NSAID therapy. One Cochrane review (search date August 2004) identified five studies (1216 patients) on the prevention of NSAID ulcers at 3 to 12 months. All used endoscopic ulceration as the primary outcome. Four of these studies also used a composite symptom end point. PPIs reduced the risk of endoscopic duodenal ulcer (RR, 0.19, 95% CI, 0.09–0.37) and gastric ulcer (RR, 0.40; 95% CI, 0.32–0.51). Dyspeptic symptoms were significantly reduced by PPI in all four trials that used this as an end point. An earlier systematic review (search date May 2002), using Cochrane methodology with serious ulcer complications and symptomatic ulcers as primary endpoints, identified two additional trials. It concluded that it was not possible to draw conclusions on the effect on these outcomes but that endoscopic ulcers seemed to be reduced in patients taking PPI.[28]

Comparative studies were few, but the limited evidence from these is that misoprostol and PPIs are superior to ranitidine and that, in two trials for secondary prophylaxis, PPIs are superior to misoprostol for prevention of duodenal ulcer (RR, 0.29; 95% CI, 0.15–0.56) but not gastric ulcer. One study, in patients with previously documented gastric ulcer, compared lansoprazole 15 mg and 30 mg daily and found both doses equally effective in preventing ulcer recurrence.[29] Recent studies with esomeprazole 20 and 40 mg have confirmed success in treatment of NSAID-induced dyspepsia as well as prevention of ulcer development among *H pylori* negative patients at increased risk of developing ulcers (age >60 years or recent gastric ulcer or duodenal ulcer).[30]

In summary, PPIs are effective in reducing endoscopic ulceration and dyspepsia symptoms. There is evidence that they are more effective than standard doses of H2RAs, and they are as effective as, but better tolerated than, misoprostol in preventing ulcers. There is limited randomized, controlled evidence that long-term PPIs reduce the risk of symptomatic and complicated ulcers.

CYCLOOXYGENASE-2 NONSTEROIDAL ANTI-INFLAMMATORY DRUGS VERSUS CONVENTIONAL NONSTEROIDAL ANTI-INFLAMMATORY DRUGS PLUS PROTON PUMP INHIBITORS

Two trials asked this question directly. In the first, of 287 *H pylori* negative patients whose bleeding peptic ulcers had recently healed, recurrent bleeding occurred in 4.9% (95% CI, 3.1–6.7) of those randomized to celecoxib 200 mg twice a day plus placebo, and in 6.4% (95% CI, 4.3–8.4) of those given diclofenac 75 mg daily plus omeprazole 20 mg daily, during 6 months.[31] The second, in a comparable population over the same period, found that recurrent ulcer complications occurred in 3.7% (95% CI, 0.0–7.3) of those given celecoxib 200 mg daily compared with 6.3% (95% CI, 1.6–11.1) of those given naproxen 750 mg daily plus lansoprazole 30 mg daily; celecoxib was statistically noninferior to lansoprazole cotherapy.[32]

Observational trials have provided support for the value of PPI gastroprotection as an alternative approach to the use of a COX-2–specific inhibitor. In a multicenter study of hospitalized patients in Spain, PPI cotherapy was associated with a marked and consistent relative RR (RR, 0.33; 95% CI, 0.27–0.39) in ulcer bleeding.[33] In a large Tennessee Medicaid database, investigators found similar results. Concurrent users of NSAIDs and PPIs had a 54% (27%–72%) risk reduction, very similar to the 50% (27%–66%) reduction for concurrent users of PPIs and coxibs.[34]

Coxibs alone may not provide sufficient ulcer risk reduction for very high-risk patients. This was recently established by Chan and colleagues, who studied individuals at highest risk of a GI complication: those with previous GI bleeding. They report that the twice-daily addition of a PPI to twice-daily celecoxib lowered the 13-month recurrence of ulcer bleeding to 0% in the combined treatment group compared with 8·9% with celecoxib alone (95% CI for the difference, 4.1–13.7).[35] In summary, in high-risk patients, the risks of further ulcer complications with conventional NSAIDs plus PPI cotherapy and COX-2 NSAIDs are comparable. The combination of COX-2 NSAID and PPI cotherapy can further reduce this risk.

BALANCING THE RISKS AND BENEFITS IN CLINICAL PRACTICE

For individuals with documented CV risks, the selection of an NSAID is not straightforward. Recent position statements, guidelines, and an international working party report,[36,37] supported by collective but not conclusive data, suggest that naproxen is differentiated from other NSAIDs that may increase CV risk. For those with competing CV and GI risks, the trade-offs between reducing GI adverse events (COX-2 instead of a nonselective NSAID) must be explicitly weighed against concerns regarding CV side effects (naproxen instead of other agents).[2] For example, when modeling the impact of GI versus CV risk benefits among users of COX-2 inhibitors in the General Practice Database in the UK, there appeared to be net harm, emphasizing the importance of targeted therapy.[38]

In addition to individual patient characteristics, drug dose, administration, and duration of NSAID use should also be considered. On examination of the existing data, NSAID adverse effects should not be attributed simply by drug classification (ie, COX-2 selective inhibitor or nonselective inhibitors) but instead by the dose and duration of COX-2 inhibition. Although the ongoing CV outcome trial, in which naproxen, ibuprofen, and celecoxib are being compared, will be informative, the lack of a placebo control arm and the years of data collection necessary require timely decisions to be made with available data. Finally, a comment regarding economic considerations is warranted, since it may not be feasible to recommend the "safest" regimen in every circumstance. It has been well documented that cost effectiveness of risk-reducing therapies is intimately related to the patients' underlying risk.[39]

To synthesize current treatment approaches, we have developed a 2x2 table to guide appropriate selection of an NSAID driven by assessment of an individual's CV and GI risk (**Table 1**).[2] The following illustrates how this can guide NSAID selection based on GI and CV risk factors, together with assessments for efficacy and/or drug intolerance. Inherent to the table is the appropriate use of aspirin—clearly of benefit for secondary prevention of CV events. For primary prevention, we advocate the use of Framingham risk calculation and restriction of aspirin to those who meet 10-year risk high enough to justify therapy, 6% to 10% based on US national guidelines.[40]

Patients with no cardiovascular risk (not receiving aspirin) and low gastrointestinal risk. A reasonable option for initial therapy would be a nonselective NSAID. The use of the more expensive but GI safer COX-2 inhibitor is not advocated due to the issue of increased cost.

Patients with no cardiovascular risk (not receiving aspirin), with moderate to high gastrointestinal risk. For patients with moderate GI risk, therapy might begin with a COX-2 selective NSAID, where the evidence for its benefit is strongest. The combination of a nonselective NSAID with a PPI appears to provide similar GI benefits. For patients with a history of GI bleeding, the addition of a PPI is an evidence-based recommendation.

Table 1
Clinicians' guide to anti-inflammatory therapy in 2007

	No or Low-NSAID Gastrointestinal Risk	NSAID Gastrointestinal Risk
No CV risk (without aspirin)	Nonselective NSAID (cost consideration)	COX-2 selective inhibitor or nonselective NSAID + PPI COX-2 selective inhibitor + PPI for those with prior GI bleeding
CV risk (with aspirin)	Naproxen[a] Addition of PPI if gastrointestinal risk of aspirin/NSAID combination warrants gastroprotection	PPI irrespective of NSAID Naproxen if CV risk outweighs GI risk; COX-2 selective inhibitor + PPI for those with previous GI bleeding

Misoprostol at full dose (200 μg 4 times a day) may be substituted for PPI.
Abbreviations: COX, cyclooxygenase; GI, gastrointestinal; PPI, proton pump inhibitor.
[a] Nonselective or selective (low-dose) inhibitor without established aspirin interaction if naproxen is ineffective.
Data from Sukel MP, van der Linden MW, Chen C, et al. Large-scale stopping and switching treatment with COX-2 inhibitors after the rofecoxib withdrawal. Pharmacoepidemiol Drug Saf 2008; 17:9–19.

Patients with no gastrointestinal risk and cardiovascular risks (receiving aspirin). For patients with CV risk but low GI risk, naproxen may offer advantages not present in other NSAIDs. If the patient is intolerant or finds naproxen ineffective, selection of an NSAID that does not interact with aspirin is essential. Thus, ibuprofen is contraindicated. Choices include low-dose celecoxib, which has not been implicated as carrying the CV concerns of higher or multiple daily doses. Diclofenac may be considered as well. Concomitant treatment with a PPI as appropriate should be strongly considered in patients taking any NSAID and aspirin, since the risk of ulcer bleeding in patients taking multiple agents is increased.

The patient with both increased GI and CV risks (on aspirin). Low-dose celecoxib together with a PPI should be used for patients who have both GI and CV risks but in whom the GI risk, such as a recent ulcer bleed, is of greater relevance. If the CV risk is of greater concern, naproxen + PPI is favored.

SUMMARY

Choosing NSAID therapy remains confusing and controversial—the challenge for the clinician is to sum all the risks as well as analgesic and anti-inflammatory efficacy. COX-2 inhibitors are an important scientific advance in pain therapy, and using them in a safe and cost-effective manner is possible when all the competing risks are carefully weighed.

REFERENCES

1. Sukel MP, van der Linden MW, Chen C, et al. Large-scale stopping and switching treatment with COX-2 inhibitors after the rofecoxib withdrawal. Pharmacoepidemiol Drug Saf 2008;17:9–19.
2. Scheiman JM, Fendrick AMF. Summing the risks of NSAID therapy. Lancet 2007; 369:1580–1.
3. McGettigan P, Han P, Jones L, et al. Selective COX-2 inhibitors, NSAIDs and congestive heart failure: differences between new and recurrent cases. Br J Clin Pharmacol 2008;65:927–34.
4. Johnson AG, Nguyen TV, Day RO. Do nonsteroidal anti-inflammatory drugs affect blood pressure: a meta-analysis. Ann Intern Med 1994;121:289–300.
5. Warner TD, Mitchell JA. COX-2 selectivity alone does not define the cardiovascular risks associated with non-steroidal anti-inflammatory drugs. Lancet 2008; 371:270–3.
6. Catella-Lawson F, Reilly MP, Kapoor SC, et al. Cyclooxygenase inhibitors and the antiplatelet effects of aspirin. N Engl J Med 2001;345:1809–17.
7. Brune K, Hochberg M, Schiff M, et al. The platelet inhibitory effects of the combination of naproxen sodium or acetaminophen with low-dose aspirin [abstract]. Arthritis Rheum 2007;56(Suppl):S359.
8. Gladding P, Webster M, Farrell H, et al. The antiplatelet effect of six non-steroidal anti-inflammatory drugs and their pharmacodynamic interaction with aspirin in healthy volunteers. Am J Cardiol 2008;101:1060–3.
9. Bombardier C, Laine L, Reicin A, et al. Comparison of upper gastrointestinal toxicity of rofecoxib and naproxen in patients with rheumatoid arthritis. VIGOR Study Group. N Engl J Med 2000;343:1520–8.
10. Bresalier RS, Sandler RS, Quan H, et al. Cardiovascular events associated with rofecoxib in a colorectal adenoma chemoprevention trial. N Engl J Med 2005; 352(11):1092–102.

11. Aldington S, Shirtcliffe P, Weatherall M, et al. Increased risk of cardiovascular events with parecoxib/valdecoxib: a systematic review and meta-analysis. N Z Med J 2005;18:U1755.
12. Aldington S, Shirtcliffe P, Weatherall M, et al. Systematic review and meta-analysis of the risk of major cardiovascular events with etoricoxib therapy. N Z Med J 2005;118:U1684.
13. Solomon SD, McMurray JJ, Pfeffer MA, et al. Cardiovascular risk associated with celecoxib in a clinical trial for colorectal adenoma prevention. N Engl J Med 2005; 352(11):1071–80.
14. Arber N, Eagle CJ, Spicak J, et al. PreSAP Trial Investigators. Celecoxib for the prevention of colorectal adenomatous polyps. N Engl J Med 2006;355(9): 885–95.
15. PRECISION: Prospective Randomized Evaluation of Celecoxib Integrated Safety vs Ibuprofen Or Naproxen. ClinicalTrials.gov Identifier: NCT00346216.
16. Solomon S, Wittes J, Finn P, et al. Cardiovascular risk of celecoxib in 6 Randomized Placebo-Controlled Trials. The cross trial safety analysis. Circulation 2008; 117:2104–13.
17. Solomon D, Glynn R, Rothman K, et al. Subgroup analyses to determine cardiovascular risk associated with non-steroidal anti-inflammatory drugs and coxibs in specific patient groups. Arthritis Rheum 2008;59:1097–104.
18. McGettigan P, Henry D. Cardiovascular risk and inhibition of cyclooxygenase: a systematic review of the observational studies of selective and nonselective inhibitors of cyclooxygenase. JAMA 2006;296:1633–44.
19. Kearney PM, Baigent C, Godwin J, et al. Do selective cyclo-oxygenase-2 inhibitors and traditional non-steroidal antiinflammatory drugs increase the risk of atherothrombosis? Meta-analysis of randomised trials. BMJ 2006;332: 1302–8.
20. ADAPT Research Group. Cardiovascular and cerebrovascular events in the randomized, controlled Alzheimer's Disease Anti-inflammatory Prevention Trial (ADAPT). PLoS Clin Trials 2006;1:e33. Available at: http://dx.doi.org/10.1371/journal.pctr.0010033.
21. Fries S, Grosser T, Price TS, et al. Marked interindividual variability in the response to selective inhibitors of cyclooxygenase-2. Gastroenterology 2006; 130:55–64.
22. Scheiman JM. NSAIDs, cytoprotection, and gastrointestinal injury. Gastroenterol Clin North Am 1996;25:279–98.
23. Wallace JL, McKnight W, Reuter BK, et al. NSAIDs-induced gastric damage in rats: requirement for inhibition of both cyclooxygenase 1 and 2. Gastroenterology 2000;119:706–14.
24. Silverstein FE, Faich G, Goldstein JL, et al. Gastrointestinal toxicity with celecoxib vs nonsteroidal anti-inflammatory drugs for osteoarthritis and rheumatoid arthritis: the CLASS study: a randomized controlled trial. Celecoxib Long-term Arthritis Safety Study. JAMA 2000;284:1247–55.
25. Schnitzer TJ, Burmester GR, Mysler E, et al. Comparison of lumiracoxib with naproxen and ibuprofen in the Therapeutic Arthritis Research and Gastrointestinal Event Trial (TARGET), reduction in ulcer complications: randomised controlled trial. Lancet 2004;364:665–74.
26. Jones R, Rubin G, Berenbaum F, et al. Gastrointestinal and cardiovascular risks of nonsteroidal anti-inflammatory drugs. Am J Med 2008;121:464–74.
27. Rostom A, Dube C, Wells G, et al. Prevention of NSAID-induced gastroduodenal ulcers. Cochrane Database Syst Rev 2002;(4):CD002296.

28. Hooper L, Brown TJ, Elliott R, et al. The effectiveness of five strategies for the prevention of gastrointestinal toxicity induced by nonsteroidal anti-inflammatory drugs: a systematic review. BMJ 2004;329:948.

29. Graham DY, Agrawal NM, Campbell DR, et al. Ulcer prevention in long term users of non-steroidal anti-inflammatory drugs: results of a double-blind randomized, multicenter, active and placebo-controlled study of misoprostol versus lansoprazole. Arch Intern Med 2002;162:169–75.

30. Scheiman JM, Yeomans ND, Talley NJ, et al. Prevention of ulcers by esomeprazole in at-risk patients using non-selective NSAIDs and COX 2 inhibitors. Am J Gastroenterol 2006;101:701–10.

31. Chan FK, Hung LC, Suen BY, et al. Celecoxib versus diclofenac and omeprazole in reducing the risk of recurrent ulcer bleeding in patients with arthritis. N Engl J Med 2002;347:2104–10.

32. Lai KC, Chu KM, Hui WM, et al. Celecoxib compared to lansoprazole and naproxen to prevent gastrointestinal ulcer complications. Am J Med 2005;118:1271–8.

33. Lanas A, García-Rodríguez LA, Arroyo MT, et al. Effect of antisecretory drugs and nitrates on the risk of ulcer bleeding associated with nonsteroidal anti-inflammatory drugs, antiplatelet agents, and anticoagulants. Am J Gastroenterol 2007;102: 507–15.

34. Ray WA, Chung CP, Stein CM, et al. Risk of peptic ulcer hospitalizations in users of NSAIDS within gastroprotective cotherapy versus coxibs. Gastroenterology 2007;133:790–8.

35. Chan FKL, Wong VWS, Suen BY, et al. Combination of a cyclooxygenase-2 inhibitor and a proton pump inhibitor for the prevention of recurrent ulcer bleeding in patients with very high gastrointestinal risk: a double-blind, randomized trial. Lancet 2007;369:1621–6.

36. Zhang W, Moskowitz RW, Nuki G, et al. OARSI recommendations for the management of hip and knee osteoarthritis, part II: OARSI Evidence-based, Expert Consensus Guidelines. Osteoarthritis Cartilage 2008;16:137–62.

37. Chan FKL, Abraham N, Scheiman JM, et al. Management of patients on nonsteroidal anti-inflammatory drugs: a clinical practice recommendation from the First International Working Party on Gastrointestinal and Cardiovascular Effects of Nonsteroidal Anti-Inflammatory Drugs and Anti-Platelet Agents. Am J Gastroenterol 2008;103:2908–18.

38. van Staa TP, Smeeth L, Persson I, et al. What is the harm-benefit ratio of Cox-2 inhibitors? Int J Epidemiol 2008;37:405–13.

39. Fendrick AM, Bandekar RR, Chernew ME, et al. Role of initial NSAID choice and patient risk factors in the prevention of NSAID gastropathy: a decision analysis. Arthritis Rheum 2002;47:36–43.

40. Bhatt D, Scheiman JM, Abraham N, et al. ACCF/ACG/AHA clinical expert consensus document on reducing the gastrointestinal risks of antiplatelet therapy and NSAID use. Circulation 2008;118:1894–909.

Prevention of Nonsteroidal Anti-Inflammatory Drug-Induced Ulcer: Looking to the Future

Stefano Fiorucci, MD

KEYWORDS

- Aspirin • CINOD • Cyclooxygenase • COX-2 inhibitors
- Hydrogen sulfide • Naproxen • Nitric oxide

Nonsteroidal anti-inflammatory drugs (NSAIDs) are among the most widely used medications in the world because of their demonstrated efficacy in reducing pain and inflammation.[1] Musculoskeletal pain affects millions of people of all ages around the world, and it is estimated that each year health care providers write approximately 60 million prescriptions for various forms of NSAIDs in North America, many of which are for the treatment of osteoarthritis in the elderly.[1] Acute or chronic pain limit physical and mental activity, have a major impact on quality of life, and may increase the risk of diseases different from those that cause pain. Treatment of pain is essential to medical clinical practice and should be considered a human right.

Although ancillary mechanisms have been demonstrated, the basic mode of action of aspirin and nonaspirin NSAIDs lies in the inhibition of COX, an enzyme involved in prostaglandin generation.[2,3] Prostaglandins are produced by the gastric mucosa, exert a "cytoprotective function," and mediate key mechanisms of what has been termed the "gastric mucosal barrier."[4] This includes the maintenance of gastric blood flow during exposure to a noxious substance, secretion of bicarbonate and mucus by the surface epithelial cells, and the rapid repair of superficial injury through the process of epithelial restitution.

The COX exists at least in two isoforms, COX-1 and COX-2, with prostaglandins mediating inflammation at the site of the injury generated by COX-2, whereas the prostaglandins involved in protecting the GI tract derive from COX-1.[2,3] Traditional NSAIDs

Conflict of interest: Stefano Fiorucci, is a share holder of a company, ANTIBE THERAPEUTICS SA, that holds patents for H₂S-releasing NSAIDs.
Dipartimento di Medicina Clinica e Sperimentale, Università di Perugia, Via E. dal Pozzo, 06122 Perugia, Italy
E-mail address: fiorucci@unipg.it

Gastroenterol Clin N Am 38 (2009) 315–332
doi:10.1016/j.gtc.2009.03.001
0889-8553/09/$ – see front matter © 2009 Elsevier Inc. All rights reserved.

(tNSAIDs) nonspecifically inhibit both COX-1 and COX-2, and their adverse events in the GI tract are attributed to the inhibition of COX-1-derived prostaglandins.

Indeed, although effective at relieving pain and inflammation, nonselective NSAIDs (ns-NSAIDs) are associated with a significant risk of serious GI adverse events.[1] Long-term NSAID therapy generates adverse GI complications ranging from stomach erosions and submucosal hemorrhages to life-threatening complications, such as bleeding and perforation.[5] The average relative risk (RR) of developing a serious GI complication in patients exposed to NSAIDs, as a group, is five- to six-fold that of those not taking NSAIDs. NSAIDs are the leading cause of bleeding peptic ulcers; when sensitive biochemical assays are used, NSAIDs, including low-dose aspirin, may have been used in more than 90% of patients with bleeding ulcers. It is estimated that peptic ulcer bleeding and perforation occur with a frequency of 1% to 3% per 100-year patient treatment, with a mortality of 6% to 10%.[5,6] Deaths related to NSAID-induced GI complications have been estimated to be as high as 16,500 per year in the United States. Recent observational data from the Spanish National Health System indicate a much lower frequency of 15.3 deaths per 100,000 NSAID users.[1,5,6]

The growing public awareness of GI complications associated with the use of NSAIDs and aspirin has prompted a search for safer alternatives (**Table 1**). These include adoption of cotherapies with the prostaglandin analog misoprostol[7,8] or a proton pump inhibitor (PPI)[9,10] and development of new NSAIDs that carry on a reduced risk of GI damage.

In the last decade, several strategies have emerged as state-of-the-art approaches to improve the NSAID safety profile. These are (a) the development of selective inhibitors of the COX-2, the coxibs;[2,3] (b) the development of new chemical agents obtained by the combination of NO-releasing moieties coupled with aspirins[11,12] and ns-NSAIDs,[11,13,14] the so-called NO-NSAIDs or CINOD;[11] and (c) new formulations of tNSAIDs. The latter approach combines in a single pill a fixed dose of a tNSAID, mostly naproxen, with a fixed dose of a PPI (lansoprazole, omeprazole, and, more recently, esomeprazole).

In addition, we and other researchers have reported in 2007 on the generation of another class of NSAID derivatives, the hydrogen sulfide (H_2S)-releasing NSAIDs,[14–16] which exploits the protective effect of H_2S in the gastric mucosa.[17]

Additional approaches have also been described over the years and are listed in **Table 1**.[18]

THE PRESENT AND THE FUTURE OF COXIBS

The development of coxibs was grounded on the hypothesis that COX-2 was the source of prostaglandins E_2 and I_2, which mediate inflammation, and that COX-1

Table 1
COX inhibitors that have demonstrated increased gastrointestinal safety

Drug	Manufacturer	Stage
Coxibs	Various	On the market
Naproxcinod and CINOD	Nicox SA	Phase III
Dual COX-LOX inhibitors	Merckle	Phase III[a]
H_2S-releasing NSAIDs	Antibe Therapeutics, CTG	Preclinical
Lipid-conjugated NSAIDs		Preclinical
Coformulation of naproxen with PPI	Astra-Zeneca	Phase III

Abbreviation: LOX, lipooxygenase.
[a] Program on shadow because of failure in efficacy.

was the source of the same prostaglandins in gastric epithelium, where they afford cytoprotection.[2,3] Three coxibs—celecoxib, rofecoxib, and valdecoxib—have been approved for use by the Food and Drug Administration (FDA); a fourth, etoricoxib, has been approved by the European regulatory authority, and a fifth, lumiracoxib, has been withdrawn from the market on August 11, 2007, by Australia's Therapeutic Goods Administration (TGA, the Australian equivalent of the FDA and the European Medicines Agency) due to concerns that it may cause liver failure. According to the TGA, the agency had received eight reports of serious adverse liver reactions to the drug, including two deaths and two liver transplants (see on http://www.tga.gov.au/media/2007/070811-lumiracoxib.htm). Coxibs are significantly better tolerated than NSAIDs in the GI tract. However, although coxibs produce severe GI complications less frequently than ns-NSAIDs, GI bleeding still develops in approximately 1% patient years.[3] This "residual" damage may be a consequence of the fact that COX-2 is rapidly expressed in response to GI injury and contributes significantly to mucosal defense and repair by generating lipoxins, a lipid mediator involved in gastric adaptation.[19]

Shortly after their introduction into the market, it was clear that coxibs might cause adverse effects in the renal and cardiovascular systems. Rofecoxib and celecoxib suppress the formation of prostacyclin (PGI_2) in healthy volunteers (see[2] for a review). Prostaglandin I_2 had previously been shown to be the predominant COX product in endothelium, inhibiting platelet aggregation, causing vasodilatation, and preventing the proliferation of vascular smooth-muscle cells in vitro. Studies in mice and humans have shown that COX-2 is the dominant source of PGI_2. The individual cardiovascular effects of PGI_2 in vitro contrast with those of thromboxane $(TX)A_2$, the major COX-1 product of platelets, which causes platelet aggregation, vasoconstriction, and vascular proliferation. Whereas aspirin and tNSAIDs inhibit both TXA_2 and PGI_2, the coxibs leave TXA_2 generation unaffected, reflecting the absence of COX-2 in platelets. Thus, a unique mechanism, that is, depression of PGI_2 formation, might predispose patients receiving coxibs to an exaggerated thrombotic response perhaps through the rupture of an atherosclerotic plaque.

Rofecoxib was then withdrawn from the market by Merck, following the premature cessation of the Adenomatous Polyp Prevention on Vioxx study,[20] which was designed to determine the drug's effect on benign sporadic colonic adenomas. This study demonstrated a significant increase by a factor of 3.9 in the incidence of serious thromboembolic adverse events in the group receiving 25 mg of rofecoxib per day compared with the placebo group.[20] Blood pressure was elevated in patients in the rofecoxib group early in the course of the study, but the incidence of myocardial infarction and thrombotic stroke in the two groups began to diverge progressively after a year or more of treatment.

Celecoxib, rofecoxib, and valdecoxib were approved by the FDA on the basis of trials that typically lasted 3 to 6 months and in which the end point was a clinical surrogate—endoscopically visualized gastric ulceration. After the drugs were approved, the results of two studies of GI outcomes were reported: the Vioxx Gastrointestinal Outcomes Research (VIGOR)[21] trial and the Celecoxib Long-Term Arthritis Safety Study (CLASS) trial.[22] In the VIGOR trial,[20] the rate of serious GI events among those receiving rofecoxib was half that among those receiving a tNSAID, naproxen—2% compared with 4%. However, a significant increase by a factor of 5 in the incidence of myocardial infarction was observed. Although this increase was a source of concern, it was argued that the small number of events reflected the play of chance or that naproxen was actually cardioprotective. However, epidemiologic studies of the possible cardioprotection afforded by naproxen have proved inconclusive.

In the CLASS trial,[22] celecoxib was compared with ibuprofen or diclofenac. In the original report, celecoxib appeared to have a more favorable GI -side-effect profile, and no increase in cardiovascular risk was revealed. However, this report contained only half the data (from only 6 months of a 1-year study): when the full data set became available, it was clear that celecoxib did not differ from the tNSAIDs in its effect on the predefined GI end points. Indeed, the most powerful evidence supporting claims of celecoxib's superiority over tNSAIDs in terms of GI effects rests on a post hoc analysis of the CLASS data for patients who did not use aspirin. However, a similar retrospective approach to the data also reveals signs of increased cardiovascular risk. The Therapeutic Arthritis Research and Gastrointestinal Event Trial is a large GI -outcome study that compared lumiracoxib with naproxen or ibuprofen.[23] The primary end point was the incidence of serious GI events, which was reduced significantly among patients receiving lumiracoxib. This difference was observed only in patients who were not taking aspirin. Although the trial, much like the CLASS trial,[22] was not powered to detect a difference in the rates of cardiovascular events in nonaspirin users, more such events occurred in the lumiracoxib group than those in the other group (0.26 vs. 0.18 per 100 patient years; hazard ratio, 1.47), although the difference was not significant. Further, in a study of patients undergoing coronary-artery bypass grafting, treatment with parecoxib, a valdecoxib prodrug, was associated with a cluster of cardiovascular events, and the drug was rejected by the FDA.[23–25] Finally, a series of epidemiologic analyses have also raised questions about the cardiovascular safety of the coxibs.[26,27] Although the epidemiologic approach has commonly relied on databases of prescriptions and is particularly subject to bias due to the over-the-counter consumption of NSAIDs and aspirin, these studies broadened the context of the available evidence by relating risk to the dose of rofecoxib used.

LOWER GASTROINTESTINAL SAFETY OF COXIBS

Increased mucosal permeability and mucosal inflammation are often silent but occur with most tNSAIDs.[28] Anemia, occult blood loss, GI bleeding and perforation, diverticulitis and strictures due to fibrous diaphragms may also occur,[25] although the frequency of these events has not been well studied. Indirect data from outcome trials estimate that serious GI events from the lower GI tract may represent 25% to 50% of all GI complications associated with NSAIDs.[28] Coxibs have a better safety profile in the lower GI tract when compared with that of tNSAIDs, although the data are still scarce. Compared with classic NSAIDs, coxibs do not increase mucosal permeability and inflammation or are linked to occult bleeding. Studies with video capsule endoscopy in healthy volunteers have shown that the incidence of small-bowel lesions with naproxen plus omeprazole is higher than that observed with either celecoxib[29] alone. Data obtained from different studies have shown that celecoxib is associated with risk reduction and a lower proportion of anemia than tNSAIDs. A post hoc analysis of the VIGOR trial revealed a lower incidence of serious lower GI events with rofecoxib when compared with that with naproxen. Consistent results were reported from a meta-analysis of lower GI events favoring rofecoxib/etoricoxib over ns-NSAIDs (RR, 0.55; 95% CI, 0.36–0.84).[28] No clinical trial has specifically evaluated the lower GI tract adverse effects with NSAIDs or coxibs.

ASPIRIN COMEDICATION

Both the CLASS and TARGET[21,22] studies have demonstrated that coxibs lose their protective effects on the GI tract when administered to patients taking aspirin. We have shown that the cause of this detrimental interaction might be the suppression of the generation of a class of lipid mediators produced by the interaction of aspirin with the COX-2 isoenzyme[30] and named the aspirin-triggered lipoxin (ATL). ATLs are generated in the gastric mucosa in response to aspirin and appear to be involved in gastric adaptation to aspirin.[31,32] Inhibition of COX-2 activity by ns-NSAIDs and cox-ibs interferes with the adaptation of the gastric mucosa to aspirin[32] and exacerbates the mucosal injury. A similar mechanism has been demonstrated to take part in the human stomach.[32]

NITRIC OXIDE, HYDROGEN SULFIDE AND NONSTEROIDAL ANTI-INFLAMMATORY DRUGS

NO is now recognized as one of the most important of such mediators in the human body,[12] mediating blood flow, neurotransmission, immune reactions, and muscle contraction (**Table 2**). The importance of NO in this regard was recognized by the award of a Nobel Prize to Furchgott, Murad and Ignarro in 1998.[33] H_2S is the latest gas to be recognized as an important endogenous mediator.[17] In the context of the digestive system, roles for H_2S in the maintenance of mucosal integrity, regulation of blood flow, and modulation of inflammatory reactions are rapidly emerging. Since the early 1990s, a body of evidence supports the notion that acute gastric injury in animal models of NSAID gastropathy is a neutrophil-dependent process.[34] Rats that had been immunodepleted of their circulating neutrophils develop very little gastric damage when given NSAIDs at doses that, in normal rats, caused widespread hemorrhagic lesions.[34] Moreover, interfering with the adherence of neutrophils to the vascular endothelium, through the administration of monoclonal antibodies directed against leukocyte or endothelial adhesion molecules, also greatly reduced the severity of NSAID-induced gastric damage. We were the first in the middle of the 1990s to demonstrate that NSAIDs trigger leukocyte adherence to the vascular endothelium though a mechanism that requires the release of tumor necrosis factor alpha (TNF-α), and administration of TNF-α antagonists or inhibitors protects against the gastric toxicity induced by ns-NSAIDs.[35] In the same period of time, NO was demonstrated to be an important modulator of adhesive interactions between leukocytes and the vascular endothelium (reviewed in[12]). This raised the possibility that the protective

Table 2
Mucosal protective effects of gastric prostaglandin E_2 and gaseous mediators—Nitric oxide and Hydrogen sulfide

	Prostaglandin E_2	Nitric Oxide (NO)	Hydrogen Sulfide (H_2S)
Expression of key enzymes in the stomach	COX-1 and COX-2[a]	eNOS and iNOS[b]	CSE and CBS[c]
Mucosal blood flow	Increased	Increased	Increased
Bicarbonate production	Increased	Increased	Unknown
Mucus secretion	Increased	Increased	Unknown
Cytoprotection	Yes	Yes	Yes
Regulation of mucosal barrier integrity	Yes	Unknown	Unknown
Epithelial cell proliferation	Yes	No	Yes

[a] Cyclooxygenase 1 and 2.
[b] Endothelial NO synthase (eNOS) and inducible NO synthase (iNOS).
[c] Cystathionine-γ-lyase (CSE) and cystathionine-β-synthase (CBS).

effects of NO that had been observed in experimental models of gastric damage might be in part due to its ability to inhibit leukocyte-endothelial adhesion. This lead to the generation by Del Soldato[11] of a new class of anti-inflammatory drugs, the CINOD, that exploit the functional role of NO in gastric protection.

COX-INHIBITING NO-DONATING DRUG

Cox-inhibiting no-donating drugs (CINODs) (**Fig. 1** and **Table 3**) were developed exploiting the concept that NO and/or NO-derived compounds endorsed by NO biological activity, released in the body circulation and gastric mucosa, would enhance the mucosal blood flow and reduce leukocyte-endothelial cell adherence into the gastric microcirculation.[11–14] Aspirin and several ns-NSAIDs, including naproxen, diclofenac, and flurbiprofen (see **Table 3**), have since then been coupled to a nitroxybutyl or a nitrosothiol moiety to generate new chemical entities that, while maintaining the COX-inhibiting activity of parental NSAID, release a discrete amount of NO. On the other hand, CINODs show a substantially different pharmacokinetic in comparison with parent NSAIDs, including a delayed peak of plasma concentration, which could be explained by lower permeability of biological barriers to these agents and/or slower dissolution of the CINOD formulation.[14] The full pharmacokinetic of CINODs is not completely understood yet. It is still unclear whether CINODs are absorbed intact or are metabolized by GI fluids, the GI wall, or during their first pass through the liver. The site of NO formation is also only partially known. This is an important issue, since the exact amount and the site where NO is released are of relevance for the biological effects. Although, it is unlikely that the different kinetic explains the reduced GI toxicity of CINODs, it may account for the absent hypotensive effect of these compounds with respect to an equimolecular dose of NO donors.[14,36–38]

PRECLINICAL PHARMACOLOGY

So far, only the NO-releasing derivative of naproxen has been investigated in clinical trials. This compound originally named HCT-3012 was then christened AZ3582 and, more recently, naproxcinod (see **Fig. 1**). Naproxcinod, like naproxen, inhibits both

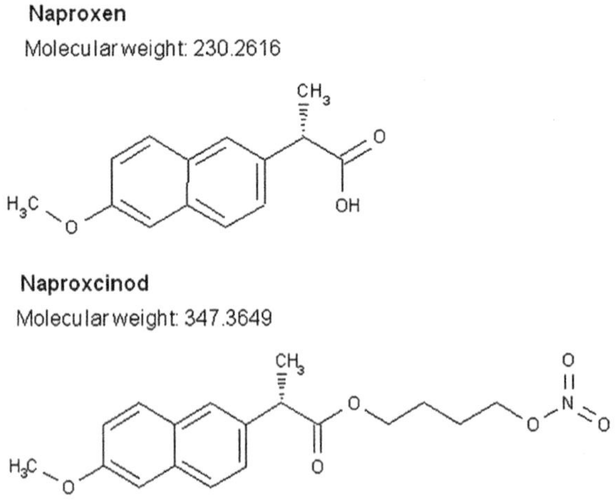

Naproxen
Molecular weight: 230.2616

Naproxcinod
Molecular weight: 347.3649

Fig. 1. Chemical structure of naproxcinod.

Table 3
List of available CINODs and companies involved in their development

Drug	Company	Status
NO-aspirin (NCX-4016)	NicOx[a]	Program abandoned
NO-diclofenac	NicOx	Preclinical
NO-naproxen"NaproCINOD"	NicOx	Two phase III trials ongoing[b]
NO-ketoprofen	NicOx	Preclinical
NO-ibuprofen	NicOx	Preclinical
S-NO-diclofenac	Nitromed	Pre-clinical
Selective COX-2 inhibitors: NO-rofecoxib	Nitromed/Merck Sharp and Dohme	Phase II[c]

[a] One of the metabolites was found to be mutagenic (www.Nicox.com).
[b] Results expected in the third to fourth quarter 2008.
[c] Trials stopped because rofecoxib was withdrawn from the market.

COX-1 and COX-2, thereby suppressing the synthesis of proinflammatory prostanoids.[39,40] CINODs inhibit prostaglandin E2 (PGE_2) generation from human monocytes/macrophages both in resting cells (COX-1-dependent activity) or after endotoxin challenge (COX-2-dependent activity).[36,37,39] CINODs also inhibit PGE_2 production in relevant models of inflammation, such as the adjuvant-induced arthritis in rats.[33] In the case of aspirin, its NO-releasing derivative (NCX-4016, see **Table 1**) inhibits platelet aggregation and thromboxane B2 generation in animals and in human studies.[41] There is a wealth of evidence that CINODs release NO when added to biological fluids (blood, liver homogenates, and others), whereas they are stable in an inert medium. This has raised the concept that CINODs release NO through the effect of a class of, as yet not well-defined, "esterases." In addition, NCX-4016 and possibly other CINODs, requiring the intervention of cellular esterases, release NO with a different kinetic with respect to conventional NO donors, such as sodium nitroprusside or S-nitroso-N-acetylpenicillamine.[42] Available data demonstrate that NO-releasing CINODs cause less GI injury than the parent compound, at least in rodents. Animal data demonstrate that at any different dosage NO-diclofenac, naproxcinod, NO-flubiprofen, NO-ketoprofen or NO-aspirin cause significantly less gastric mucosal injury than parent NSAIDs.[14,41,43] A similar reduction of GI toxicity is observed if the compounds are administered systemically rather than orally, suggesting that the reduced injury is not simply due to reduced topical irritant properties. Animal studies have also demonstrated that CINODs spare the stomach but inhibit gastric mucosal COX activity. Despite CINODs' effect on gastric microcirculation, it is noteworthy that, in experimental animals, they do not alter systemic arterial blood pressure even when administered intravenously, in large doses, or when administered during an experimental model of endotoxic shock.

The enthusiastic findings emerging from animal data were partially confirmed by human studies.[43] Two phase 1 trials have investigated the GI safety profile of naproxcinod and NCX-4016. In one of these studies, twice-daily administration of 800 mg NCX-4016, an NO-releasing derivative of aspirin, for 1 week did not produce gastric injury (ie, the endoscopic scores were not different from those of the placebo-treated group), whereas an equimolar dose of aspirin produced extensive gastric injury.[41] This degree of gastric safety was observed despite the fact that NCX-4016 suppressed whole-blood TXA_2 synthesis as effectively as did aspirin. Although NCX4016 was certainly better tolerated than aspirin in the GI tract, its development was stopped in 2007, because one of the main metabolites (NCX4015) was found to be mutagenic in vitro.

In the case of naproxcinod, one study has tested the gastric safety of this compound in a randomized, double-blind, three-crossover, proof-of-concept study carried out in 31 healthy volunteers.[43] The rate of GI events following oral administration of naproxcinod was compared to naproxen and placebo (naproxen 500 mg twice daily and naproxcinod 750 mg twice daily). The mean total number of gastroduodenal erosions over the 12-day study period was 11.5 for naproxen compared with 4.1 for naproxcinod (differences were seen for both the stomach and duodenum), and more than half of the latter group did not display any erosions. Studies on intestinal permeability indicated that there were no changes during placebo or naproxcinod treatment. In contrast, naproxen caused a significant rise in small intestinal permeability. A 95% bioconversion of naproxcinod to naproxen was noted.[43] Confirming these findings, another study conducted in healthy volunteers demonstrated that Naproxcinod causes significantly less gastroduodenal lesions than does plain naproxen.[44]

The results of a phase II trial, named STAR, are also available.[45] This study was designed to evaluate the GI safety and efficacy of the COX-inhibiting NO donor naproxcinod in patients with hip or knee osteoarthritis. About 970 patients were randomized (7:7:2) to naproxcinod 750 mg twice daily, naproxen 500 mg twice daily, or placebo twice daily in a double-blind study. The primary end point was the 6-week incidence of endoscopic gastroduodenal ulcers (diameter > or = 3 mm). The overall damage measured on the Lanza scale was a secondary end point. The incidence of gastric and duodenal ulcers was reduced by 40% with naproxcinod in comparison with naproxen (9.7% vs 13.7%; $P = .07$) versus 0% on placebo. The incidence of Lanza scores greater than 2 was higher with naproxen (43.7%) than that with naproxcinod (32.2%) ($P<.001$). Compared with baseline, significantly fewer ulcers and erosions developed in stomach and stomach/duodenum combined and fewer erosions developed in stomach, duodenum, and both combined on naproxcinod than on naproxen. The pain killer activity of naproxcinod was also evaluated in this study.[45] Naproxcinod (375 mg twice a day and 750 mg twice a day) is superior to placebo and as effective as rofecoxib 25 mg/d in treating the signs and symptoms of osteoarthritis of the knee.

The conclusions of this study indicate that at doses with similar efficacy in relieving osteoarthritis symptoms, the primary end point of 6-week endoscopic gastroduodenal ulcer incidence was not significantly different between naproxcinod and naproxen, although most secondary endoscopic GI end points favored naproxcinod.[45]

The interpretation of the results of this study has raised a number of controversies, but despite positive results on a number of secondary endpoints, the company that was running the project (Astra Zeneca) reached the conclusion that naproxcinod would not match the GI safety of a coxib and dropped the project in 2003.

The GI safety of another CINOD, NO-flurbiprofen, HCT-1026, has also been evaluated in a double-blind, placebo-controlled, endoscopic study. The study was conducted in 32 healthy subjects, randomly allocated to receive 7 days' treatment with HCT-1026 (100 and 150 mg twice a day), flurbiprofen (100 mg twice a day), or placebo. In this study, administration of HCT-1026 resulted in a significant attenuation of GI damage with respect to flurbiprofen (Fiorucci S., unpublished data, 2003), although a significant gastric injury was detected (Fiorucci S., unpublished data, 2003).

COX-INHIBITING NO-DONATING DRUGS AND THE CARDIOVASCULAR SYSTEM

Since 2003, naproxcinod has been developed directly by Nicox SA, the company that owned the original patent, along with a number of NO-releasing derivatives of NSAIDs.

At the time when the program was abandoned by Astra Zeneca, approximately 3000 patients were administered naproxcinod at various dosages in several proof-of-concept studies designed to investigate effects of this compound on cardiac and renal safety as well as efficacy in various settings of pain and on blood pressure. The results of these studies demonstrate that in contrast to naproxen, naproxcinod does not increase systemic blood pressure. This generated that idea that naproxcinod, despite inhibiting COXs, will release NO in the systemic circulation, preventing one of the most common side effects of NSAIDs, that is, worsening of hypertension. It is well recognized that long-term use of NSAIDs might cause renal injury and reduction of renal perfusion in patients in whom there is a greater dependency on local vasodilator prostaglandin synthesis for maintenance of renal blood flow.[46,47] In a parallel, randomized, double-blind study, a total of 60 healthy subjects (age range, 20–44 years) received two single doses of 750 mg naproxen, 1500 mg naproxcinod (AZD3582), 50 mg rofecoxib, 500 mg naproxen, or placebo. The first dose was given under a normal-sodium diet, and the second dose was given under a low-sodium diet. In this study, the effects of naproxcinod on renal function in terms of reduction in sodium excretion and glomerular filtration rates seem to be qualitatively similar to those of NSAIDs, under normal sodium intake and sodium depletion. It can be speculated that in humans the NO derived from naproxcinod does not reach relevant levels in the kidney to obtain a pharmacologic effect in terms of renal vasodilation.[39] Moreover, it is well known that NSAIDs can exacerbate hypertension and interfere with the antihypertensive effects of some agents.[46]

CINODs can be clearly distinguished from conventional and COX-2 selective NSAIDs in terms of cardiovascular toxicity. In contrast to COX-2 inhibitors, in healthy subjects naproxcinod (AZD3582) causes a transient decrease in systolic blood pressure (SBP), with peak effects approximately 2 hours after dosing. The same hypotensive effect was observed in osteoarthritic patients treated with naproxcinod (AZD3582) after repeated administration of the compound.[47] This cardiovascular safety of NO-NSAIDs is now seen as particularly attractive with respect to their prospects of gaining regulatory approval for the treatment of arthritis. Phase III clinical trials of "naproxcinod" (see **Table 3**) are currently underway and aimed particularly at further demonstrating a safer cardiovascular profile of this drug compared with older NSAIDs and selective COX-2 inhibitors (**Table 4**). Thus, naproxcinod seems to have a rather unique pharmacological profile, in that it inhibits COX but has an intrinsic cardiovascular safety in comparison with tNSAIDs. The effect of naproxcinod on blood pressure has been reported in a study where 118 patients were randomized on a 1:1 basis to receive naproxcinod or naproxen, with escalating doses every 3 weeks. The trial included three doses of naproxcinod (375 mg twice a day, 750 mg twice a day, and a supratherapeutic dose of 1125 mg twice a day), which were compared to naproxen (250, 500, and 750 mg twice a day). Twenty-four–hour blood pressure monitoring was conducted at baseline and at the end of each 3-week dose escalation (ie, at the end of week 3, 6, and 9), using an ambulatory blood pressure monitoring (ABPM) device. The primary objective of the study was to characterize the 24-hour arterial blood pressure profile of the three doses of naproxcinod, as measured by ABPM after each dose, compared to naproxen. At all time points, naproxcinod showed a decrease in the mean 24-hour SBP and diastolic blood pressure (DBP) from baseline in contrast to naproxen. In terms of the overall treatment effect, as an average over week 3, 6, and 9, naproxen raised systemic blood pressure by 1.5 mm Hg from baseline, whereas naproxcinod lowered it by 2.3 mm Hg, resulting in a difference between the two treatments of 3.8 mm Hg ($P = .011$) in favor of naproxcinod. The results of this study were released on November 4, 2008. Furthermore, in contrast to naproxen, naproxcinod

Table 4
Naproxcinodand osteoarthritis

Title	ClinicalTrials. Gov. Identifier	Study Phase	Status	Detailed Description
Efficacy and Safety Study of Naproxcinod in Subjects with Osteoarthritis of the Knee	NCT00504127	III	Active, not recruiting	This is a 53-wk study consisting of a 26-wk, randomized, double-blind, parallel-group, multicenter study comparing the efficacy and safety of naproxcinod, naproxen (375 mg bid and 750 mg bid), and placebo. The first 26 wk will be followed by a naproxen-controlled treatment period up to 52 wk and a 1-wk posttreatment safety follow-up.
Efficacy and Safety Study of Naproxcinod in Subjects with Osteoarthritis of the Hip	NCT00541489	III	Active, not recruiting	This is a 13-wk randomized, double-blind, parallel-group, multicenter study comparing the efficacy and safety of naproxcinod (750 mg, bid), placebo, and naproxen (500 mg, bid).
Analgesic Efficacy and Safety Study of Naproxcinod in Subjects with Osteoarthritis of the Knee.	NCT00542555	III	Completed	This is a 13-wk, double-blind study followed by a 52-wk, open-label, treatment study. These are randomized, parallel group, multicenter studies comparing efficacy and safety of naproxcinod, placebo, and naproxen.

Reference: http://clinicaltrials.gov.

reduced the mean 24-hour SBP and DBP from baseline at every dose comparison. Three large studies are currently ongoing to evaluate the efficacy of naproxcinod in comparison with plain naproxen in osteoarthritic patients. These studies are summarized in (**Table 5**) studies 301, 302, and 303 have been designed to investigate the efficacy of naproxcinod in patients with osteoarthritis of the knee (study 303) and the hip (study 301 and 302). Overall, the results of the 302 studies support naproxcinod's non-detrimental effect on blood pressure and are consistent with those observed in the 301 study, with naproxcinod 750 mg twice a day showing a numerical reduction in SBP and DBP at weeks 13 and 26, compared with baseline and naproxen 500 mg twice a day. In addition, a post hoc pooled analysis of the blood pressure data from studies 301 and 302 showed a statistically significant reduction for naproxcinod 750 mg twice a day, compared with naproxen 500 mg twice a day, in terms of the mean change from baseline at week 13, of 2.3 mm Hg ($P = .004$) for SBP and 1.1 mm Hg ($P = .034$) for DBP. In the planning of the phase III program, NicOx had foreseen the pooling of office blood pressure measurements from more than one study to obtain the necessary statistical power to correctly assess the effects of naproxcinod on blood pressure compared with those of naproxen.

THE CLINICAL POSITIONING OF NAPROXCINOD

The combination of slightly enhanced GI safety (a reduced risk of formation of GI ulcers was detected in the STAR study[45]) and enhanced cardiovascular safety makes naproxcinod an effective alternative to ns-NSAIDs and coxibs in a subset of patients that require NSAIDs although carrying an enhanced risk for cardiovascular events. CINODs are likely to be the first-choice therapy for those patients. However, since CINODs still causes GI injury at a rate that is superior to coxib and in theory will cause the same damage of tNSAIDs to the lower GI tract, it is predicted that a comedication therapy with a PPI will be required. In addition, it is likely that naproxcinod will be an interesting alternative to coxibs in patients who also take low doses of aspirin. However, because the risk for GI bleeding in the two treatments is cumulative, a comedication with a PPI will also be required.

HYDROGEN SULFATE-RELEASING NONSTEROIDAL ANTI-INFLAMMATORY DRUGS

H_2S has until recently been better known as an industrial pollutant than as an endogenous mediator of numerous physiological processes.[17] H_2S is produced through a number of pathways, the most common being related to the metabolism of L-cysteine, cystine, and homocysteine by a group of widely expressed enzymes, the cystathionine-β synthase and the cystathionine-γ lyase.[17,48,49] Endogenous levels of H_2S have been reported to be as high as 160 μM in the brain, with serum levels of 30 to 100 μM.[50] Even after administration of H_2S donors in doses that produce pharmacological effects, the concentration of H_2S in plasma seldom exceeded the normal range or did so for a very brief period of time[50] because of the highly efficient systems for metabolizing, scavenging, and sequestering H_2S.[17,50] Toxic effects of H_2S are observed in the lung with concentrations in excess of 250 μM, and coma and death can occur with concentrations above 1000 μM.[49] As is the case with NO, physiological concentrations of H_2S are likely to be beneficial, whereas concentrations many times greater than the physiological range would tend to be detrimental. Recent studies suggest that H_2S is an inorganic substrate for mammalian mitochondria, and the mitochondria of colonic epithelial cells may be particularly well adapted for the use of the substrate.[44]

Table 5
PN400 phase III trials

Title	Study Phase	Status	Detailed Description
A 12-Month, Phase III, Open-Label, Multi-Center Study to Evaluate the Long-Term Safety of PN400	III	Active, not recruiting	To evaluate the long-term safety of PN400 in subjects at risk for developing NSAID-associated upper GI ulcers. Subjects are instructed to take 2 tablets a day, one in the morning and one in the afternoon/evening. The morning tablet should be taken with water, on an empty stomach 30 to 60 min before breakfast or the first meal. The afternoon/evening tablet should be taken with water, on an empty stomach 30 to 60 min before dinner. Tablets should be swallowed whole and not broken, crushed, or chewed.
A 6-Month, Phase III, Randomized, Double-Blind, Parallel-Group, Controlled, Multi-Center Study to Evaluate the Incidence of Gastric Ulcers (PN400 301-302).	III	Completed	Primary: To demonstrate that PN400 is effective in reducing the risk of gastric ulcers in subjects at risk for developing NSAID-associated gastric ulcers Secondary: To determine if PN400 is effective in reducing the risk of duodenal ulcers in subjects at risk for developing NSAID-associated ulcers To compare upper GI symptoms in subjects treated with PN400 vs naproxen as measured by scores on the Severity of Dyspepsia Assessment instrument and the Overall Treatment Evaluation - Dyspepsia To compare heartburn symptoms in subjects treated with PN400 vs naproxen To evaluate the safety and tolerability of PN400 and naproxen
Study Evaluating the Efficacy of PN400 bid and Celecoxib qd in Patients with Osteoarthritis of the Knee	III	Active, not recruiting	Randomized, double-blind, parallel group, placebo-controlled, multi-center study evaluating the efficacy of PN400 bid and Celecoxib qd in patients with osteoarthritis of the knee

| Study to Evaluate the Incidence of Gastric Ulcers with **PN400** (Esomeprazole/Naproxen) Versus Diclofenac/Misoprostol in Subjects Who Are at High Risk for Developing NSAID-Associated Ulcers | III | Terminated | Primary:
 To determine the incidence of gastric ulcers following administration of **PN400** in a high-risk population over 6 mo Diclofenac/misoprostol used as a positive control

 Secondary:
 To determine the incidence of duodenal ulcers during treatment with **PN400** and diclofenac/misoprostol in a high-risk population
 To evaluate the degree of upper GI injury as measured by Lanza scores (1991) during treatment with **PN400** and diclofenac/misoprostol in a high-risk population
 To compare GI symptoms in subjects treated with **PN400** vs diclofenac/misoprostol as measured by scores on the Gastrointestinal Symptoms Rating Scale instrument
 To evaluate the safety and tolerability of **PN400** and diclofenac/misoprostol in a high-risk population |
| Study Evaluating the Efficacy of **PN400** bid and Celebrex qd in Patients with Osteoarthritis of the Knee | III | Active, not recruiting | Randomized, double-blind, parallel-group, placebo-controlled, multi-center study evaluating the efficacy of **PN400** bid and Celecoxib qd in patients with osteoarthritis of the knee. Inclusion criteria: male or nonpregnant female subjects ≥ 50 y of age with history of OA of the knee as well as other standard inclusion criteria for a study of this nature |

http://clinicaltrials.gov.

H_2S acts at least in part by activation of ATP-sensitive K+ channels (K+ATP).[17,48–51] Recently, potent anti-inflammatory effects of H_2S were demonstrated. For example, H_2S donors suppressed leukocyte adherence to the vascular endothelium and reduced leukocyte extravasation and edema formation.[52] Inhibition of endogenous H_2S synthesis, on the other hand, triggered leukocyte adherence to the vascular endothelium and enhanced edema formation.[46] These actions of H_2S also appeared to be mediated via activation of K+ATP channels.[52] H_2S has also been shown to reduce visceral pain perception, which may also be mediated via activation of K+ATP channels.[50] This might have relevance in the field of NSAID-induced analgesia, since analgesic effects of NSAIDs have been suggested to be mediated, at least in part, via K+ATP channels.[50]

H_2S is also produced by the gastric mucosa (see **Table 2**), and, like NO, contributes to the ability of this tissue to resist the damage induced by luminal substances.[15] Notably, we have shown that H_2S synthesis was found to be significantly reduced following administration of NSAIDs, apparently through suppression of the expression of cystathionine-μ-lyase, one of the key enzymes for conversion of L-cysteine into H_2S.[17] Thus, suppression of mucosal H_2S synthesis may represent another mechanism, aside from suppression of COX activity, through which NSAIDs produce GI damage. Administration of H_2S donors could prevent the decrease in gastric blood flow induced by NSAIDs as well as diminish NSAID-induced leukocyte adherence. It also decreased the NSAID-induced accumulation of leukocytes in the gastric mucosa as well as expression of endothelial and leukocyte adhesion molecules.[53] Several of these H_2S-induced effects were produced via activation of K+ATP channels.

The synthesis of H_2S-releasing derivatives of NSAIDs has been reported recently.[17] As was the case with CINODs, an H_2S-releasing derivative of diclofenac was substantially better tolerated, in terms of gastric damage than the parent drugs.[17] With administration of this same dose of the compound three times during 24 hours, very low levels of intestinal damage were also observed, at least 90% less than that observed in rats administered diclofenac at an equimolar dose.[12] Moreover, there was no change in hematocrit in the rats treated with the H_2S-releasing derivative, whereas diclofenac administration resulted in a decrease in hematocrit of 50%, consistent with the widespread bleeding that was evident in the GI tract.[17] The anti-inflammatory action of H_2S has been exploited recently in the design of novel derivatives of mesalamine for the treatment of inflammatory bowel disease. A mesalamine derivative that includes an H_2S-releasing moiety (ATB-429) was recently shown to exhibit markedly enhanced anti-inflammatory actions in experimental colitis.[51]

NEW FORMULATIONS OF NAPROXEN

Results from several clinical trials have shown that comedication with PPI significantly reduced the severity of GI damage associated with the use of tNSAIDs. The benefit of this cotherapy in patients with risk factors for GI bleeding is similar to that of shifting from an NSAID to a coxib. Recently, these results have been exploited with the generation of a single pill containing a fixed combination of PPI with naproxen. These tablets are designed to provide a release of the PPI component in the stomach while the NSAID component contained in a pH-sensitive layer is released in an environment with decreased presence of acid. Several formulation-development and clinical studies have been carried out to support two combinations designated as PN100 (lansoprazole/naproxen) and PN200 (omeprazole/naproxen). In two, 14-day, proof-of-concept studies in human volunteers, both PN100 and PN200 were shown to be effective in preventing gastric mucosal injury when compared with enteric-coated naproxen alone. The phase III trials of a fixed dose combination of esomeprazole with naproxen (PN400) were targeted to be completed by the end of 2008. In addition, a combination of aspirin with a PPI for cardiovascular protection, along with the potential reduction in the risk of colorectal cancer and adenomas, is also under evaluation.

SUMMARY

The great challenge for those attempting to develop safer NSAIDs is shifting from a focus on GI toxicity to the increasingly more appreciated cardiovascular toxicity.

At present, coxib shows an unmatched GI safety and appears to be a rational choice for patients at a low cardiovascular risk who have had serious GI events. In these patients, however, a cost-effective alternative is the use of tNSAIDs associated with comedication with a low-cost PPI or PN400.

Because it seems prudent to avoid coxibs in patients who have cardiovascular disease or who are at risk for it, naproxcinod will be an appealing alternative to coxibs and tNSAIDs. However, because naproxcinod carries a significant risk of GI bleeding, a comedication therapy with a PPI inhibitor will be required if these patients also present risk factors for GI events.

Although the development of H_2S-releasing anti-inflammatory drugs is in its infancy, the preclinical data available thus far provide cause for optimism. The quest for the development of NSAIDs devoid of cardiovascular toxicity and that spare the gastric mucosa to the same extent as that of a coxib, however, is still open.

REFERENCES

1. Wolfe MM, Lichtenstein DR, Singh G. Gastrointestinal toxicity of nonsteroidal anti-inflammatory drugs. N Engl J Med 1999;340:1888–99.
2. FitzGerald GA. COX-2 and beyond: approaches to prostaglandin inhibition in human disease. Nat Rev Drug Discov 2003;2:879–90.
3. FitzGerald GA, Patrono C. The coxibs, selective inhibitors of cyclooxygenase-2. N Engl J Med 2001;345:433–42.
4. Wallace JL, Granger DN. The cellular and molecular basis of gastric mucosal defense. FASEB J 1996;10:731–40.
5. Lanas A, Perez-Aisa MA, Feu F, et al. A nationwide study of mortality associated with hospital admission due to severe gastrointestinal events and those associated with nonsteroidal anti-inflammatory drug use. Am J Gastroenterol 2005; 100:1685–93.
6. Lanas A, García Rodríguez LA, Arroyo MT, et al. Risk of upper gastrointestinal ulcer bleeding associated with selective COX-2 inhibitors, traditional non-aspirin NSAIDs, aspirin, and combinations. [May 10, 2006, E-pub ahead of print]. Gut 2006;55:1731–8.
7. Lazzaroni M, Battocchia A, Bianchi Porro G. Coxibs and non-selective NSAIDs in the gastrointestinal setting: what should patients and physicians do. Dig Liver Dis 2007;39:589–96.
8. Silverstein FE, Graham DY, Senior JR, et al. Misoprostol reduces serious gastrointestinal complications in patients with rheumatoid arthritis receiving nonsteroidal anti-inflammatory drugs. A randomized, double-blind, placebo-controlled trial. Ann Intern Med 1995;123:241–9.
9. Hawkey CJ, Karrasch JA, Szczepanski L, et al. Omeprazole compared with misoprostol for ulcers associated with nonsteroidal antiinflammatory drugs. Omeprazole versus Misoprostol for NSAID-induced Ulcer Management (OMNIUM) Study Group. N Engl J Med 1998;338:727–34.

10. Yeomans ND, Tulassay Z, Juhasz L, et al. A comparison of omeprazole with ranitidine for ulcers associated with nonsteroidal antiinflammatory drugs. Acid Suppression Trial: Ranitidine versus Omeprazole for NSAID-associated Ulcer Treatment (ASTRONAUT) Study Group. N Engl J Med 1998;338:719–26.

11. Fiorucci S, Del Soldato P. NO-aspirin: mechanism of action and gastrointestinal safety. Dig Liver Dis 2003;35(Suppl 2): S9–19.

12. Wallace JL, Ignarro LJ, Fiorucci S. Potential cardioprotective actions of nitric oxide-releasing aspirin. Nat Rev Drug Discov 2002;1:375–82.

13. Fiorucci S, Antonelli E. NO-NSAIDs: from inflammatory mediators to clinical readouts. Inflamm Allergy Drug Targets 2006;5:121–31.

14. Fiorucci S, Distrutti E, Santucci L. NSAIDs, Coxibs CINOD and H_2S -releasing NSAIDs, what lies beyond the horizon? Dig liver Dis 2007;39:1043–51.

15. Wallace JL, Caliendo G, Santagada V, et al. Gastrointestinal safety and anti-inflammatory effects of a hydrogen sulphide-releasing diclofenac derivative in the rat. Gastroenterology 2007;132:261–71.

16. Li L, Rossoni G, Sparatore A, et al. Anti-inflammatory and gastrointestinal effects of a novel diclofenac derivative. Free Radic Biol Med 2007;42:706–19.

17. Fiorucci S, Distrutti E, Cirino G, et al. The emerging roles of hydrogen sulphide in the gastrointestinal tract and liver. Gastroenterology 2006;131:259–71.

18. Bias P, Buchner A, Klesser B, et al. The gastrointestinal tolerability of the LOX/COX inhibitor, licofelone, is similar to placebo and superior to naproxen therapy in healthy volunteers: results from a randomized, controlled trial. Am J Gastroenterol 2004 Apr;99(4):611–8.

19. Fiorucci S, de Lima OM Jr, Mencarelli A, et al. Cyclooxygenase-2-derived lipoxin A4 increases gastric resistance to aspirin-induced damage. Gastroenterology 2002;123:1598–606.

20. Bresalier RS, Sandler RS, Quan H, et al. Adenomatous Polyp Prevention on Vioxx (APPROVe) Trial Investigators. Cardiovascular events associated with rofecoxib in a colorectal adenoma chemoprevention trial. N Engl J Med 2005;352: 1092–102.

21. Bombardier C, Laine L, Reicin A, et al. VIGOR Study Group. Comparison of upper gastrointestinal toxicity of rofecoxib and naproxen in patients with rheumatoid arthritis. VIGOR Study Group. N Engl J Med 2000;343:1520–8.

22. Silverstein FE, Faich G, Goldstein JL, et al. Gastrointestinal toxicity with celecoxib vs nonsteroidal anti-inflammatory drugs for osteoarthritis and rheumatoid arthritis: the CLASS study: a randomized controlled trial. Celecoxib Long-term Arthritis Safety Study. JAMA 2000;284:1247–55.

23. Schnitzer TJ, Burmester GR, Mysler E, et al. Comparison of lumiracoxib with naproxen and ibuprofen in the Therapeutic Arthritis Research and Gastrointestinal Event Trial (TARGET), reduction in ulcer complications: randomised controlled trial. Lancet 2004;364:665–74.

24. Farkouh ME, Kirshner H, Harrington RA, et al. Comparison of lumiracoxib with naproxen and ibuprofen in the Therapeutic Arthritis Research and Gastrointestinal Event Trial (TARGET), cardiovascular outcomes: randomised controlled trial. Lancet 2004;364:675–84.

25. Nussmeier NA, Whelton AA, Brown MT, et al. Complications of the COX-2 inhibitors parecoxib and valdecoxib after cardiac surgery. N Engl J Med 2005;352: 1081–91.

26. Johnsen SP, Larsson H, Tarone RE, et al. Risk of hospitalization for myocardial infarction among users of rofecoxib, celecoxib, and other NSAIDs: a population-based case-control study. Arch Intern Med 2005;165:978–84.

27. Juni P, Nartey L, Reichenbach S, et al. Risk of cardiovascular events and rofecoxib: cumulative meta-analysis. Lancet 2004;364:2021–9.
28. Laine L, Connors LG, Reicin A, et al. Serious lower gastrointestinal clinical events with nonselective NSAID or coxib use. Gastroenterology 2003;124(2):288–92.
29. Goldstein JL, Eisen GM, Lewis B, et al. Video capsule endoscopy to prospectively assess small bowel injury with celecoxib, naproxen plus omeprazole, and placebo. Clin Gastroenterol Hepatol 2005;3:133–41. 10.1016/S1542-3565(04)00619-6.
30. Wallace JL, Fiorucci S. A magic bullet for mucosal protection and aspirin is the trigger!. Trends Pharmacol Sci 2003;24(7):323–6.
31. Fiorucci S, Distrutti E, de Lima OM, et al. Relative contribution of acetylated cyclo-oxygenase (COX)-2 and 5-lipooxygenase (LOX) in regulating gastric mucosal integrity and adaptation to aspirin. FASEB J 2003;17:1171–3.
32. Fiorucci S, Santucci L, Wallace JL, et al. Interaction of a selective cyclooxyge-nase-2 inhibitor with aspirin and NO-releasing aspirin in the human gastric mucosa. Proc Natl Acad Sci U S A 2003;100:10937–41.
33. Murad F. Shattuck lecture. Nitric oxide and cyclic GMP in cell signaling and drug development. N Engl J Med 2006;355(19):2003–11.
34. Wallace JL, Keenan CM, Granger DN. Gastric ulceration induced by nonsteroidal anti-inflammatory drugs is a neutrophil-dependent process. Am J Phys 1990;259:G462–7.
35. Santucci L, Fiorucci S, Di Matteo FM, et al. Role of tumor necrosis factor alpha release and leukocyte margination in indomethacin-induced gastric injury in rats. Gastroenterology 1995;108(2):393–401.
36. Wallace JL, Reuter B, Cicala C, et al. A diclofenac derivative without ulcerogenic properties. Eur J Pharmacol 1994;257:249–55.
37. Wallace JL, Reuter B, Cicala C, et al. Novel nonsteroidal anti-inflammatory drug derivatives with markedly reduced ulcerogenic properties in the rat. Gastroenter-ology 1994;107:173–9.
38. Stefano F, Distrutti E. Cyclo-oxygenase (COX) inhibiting nitric oxide donating (CI-NODs) drugs: a review of their current status. Curr Top Med Chem 2007;7(3):277–82.
39. Fiorucci S, Di Lorenzo A, Renga B, et al. Nitric oxide (NO)-releasing naproxen (HCT-3012[(S)-6-methoxy-alpha-methyl-2-naphthaleneacetic Acid 4-(nitrooxy)-butyl ester]) interactions with aspirin in gastric mucosa of arthritic rats reveal a role for aspirin-triggered lipoxin, prostaglandins, and NO in gastric protection. J Pharmacol Exp Ther 2004;311(3):1264–71.
40. Fiorucci S, Antonelli E, Santucci L, et al. Gastrointestinal safety of nitric oxide-derived aspirin is related to inhibition of ICE-like cysteine proteases in rats. Gastroenterology 1999;116:1089–106.
41. Fiorucci S, Santucci L, Gresele P, et al. Gastrointestinal safety of NO-aspirin (NCX-4016) in healthy human volunteers: a proof of concept endoscopic study. Gastroenterology 2003;124:600.
42. Fiorucci S, Mencarelli A, Distrutti E, et al. Nitric oxide regulates immune cell bioenergetic: a mechanism to understand immunomodulatory functions of nitric oxide-releasing anti-inflammatory drugs. J Immunol 2004;173:874–82.
43. Hawkey C, Jones JI, Atherton CT, et al. Gastrointestinal safety of AZD3582, a cy-clooxygenase inhibiting nitric oxide donator: proof of concept study in humans. Gut 2003;52:1537–42.
44. Nitronaproxen: AZD 3582, HCT 3012, Naproxen Nitroxybutylester, NO-Naproxen. Drugs R D 2006;7(4):262–6.
45. Lohmander LS, McKeith D, Svensson O, et al. STAR Multinational Study Group. Ann Rheum Dis 2005;64:449–56.

46. Huledal G, Jonzon B, Malmenas M, et al. Renal effects of the cyclooxygenase-inhibiting nitric oxide donator AZD3582 compared with rofecoxib and naproxen during normal and low sodium intake. Clin Pharmacol Ther 2005;77:437–50.

47. Schnitzer TJ, Kivitz AJ, Lipetz RS, et al. Comparison of the COX-inhibiting nitric oxide donator AZD3582 and rofecoxib in treating the signs and symptoms of Osteoarthritis of the knee. Arthritis Rheum 2005;53:827–37.

48. Wang R. Two's company, three's a crowd: can H_2S be the third endogenous gaseous transmitter? FASEB J 2002;16:1792-8.

49. Goubern M, Andriamihaja M, Nubel T, et al. Sulfide, the first inorganic substrate for human cells. FASEB J 2007;21:1699–706.

50. Distrutti E, Sediari L, Mencarelli A, et al. Evidence that hydrogen sulphide exerts antinociceptive effects in the gastrointestinal tract by activating KATP channels. J Pharmacol Exp Ther 2006;316:325–35.

51. Distrutti E, Sediari L, Mencarelli A, et al. 5-Amino-2-hydroxybenzoic acid 4-(5-thioxo-5H-[1, 2]dithiol-3yl)-phenyl ester (ATB-429), a hydrogen sulphide-releasing derivative of mesalamine, exerts antinociceptive effects in a model of postinflammatory hypersensitivity. J Pharmacol Exp Ther 2006;319:447–58.

52. Zanardo RC, Brancaleone V, Distrutti E, et al. Hydrogen sulphide is an endogenous modulator of leukocyte-mediated inflammation. FASEB J 2006;20:2118–20.

53. Fiorucci S, Orlandi S, Mencarelli A, et al. Enhanced activity of a hydrogen sulphide-releasing derivative of mesalamine (ATB-429) in a mouse model of colitis. Br J Pharmacol 2007;150:996–1002.

Nonsteroidal Anti-Inflammatory Drugs and Lower Gastrointestinal Complications

Angel Lanas, MD, DSc*, Federico Sopeña, MD, DSc

KEYWORDS

- Nonsteroidal anti-inflammatory drugs
- Gastrointestinal bleeding • Gastrointestinal ulcers
- Lower gastrointestinal tract • Bacteria • Gut inflammation

Upper gastrointestinal (GI) side effects are the most common adverse events of nonsteroidal anti-inflammatory drugs (NSAIDs). However, other GI side effects are increasingly being recognized in clinical practice. In the last few years, it is becoming clear that NSAIDs can damage the small bowel and the colon and that the magnitude of the damage may be greater than that of NSAID-associated gastropathy.[1–3] In spite of this, awareness of NSAID-induced enteropathy is low in clinical practice. There are several reasons for the low appreciation of NSAID enteropathy. The condition is usually asymptomatic and diagnosis has, until recently, been possible only with the use of tests that are not available in clinical practice. Although case reports, epidemiologic studies, and pathologic series are available for more than 20 years, the current increasing interest in this field may be due to a growing investment on research from pharmaceutical companies with interest in NSAID gastropathy. Now that the safety concern for cardiovascular events seems to settle and this concern is almost similar for traditional NSAIDS (tNSAIDs) and coxibs, the interest is coming back to the GI tract, and the new territory to explore is the lower GI tract.[4,5]

MECHANISMS OF INTESTINAL DAMAGE BY NONSTEROIDAL ANTI-INFLAMMATORY DRUGS

It is not completely clear how NSAIDs initiate damage in the lower GI tract. The widespread view is that upper GI toxicity by NSAIDs is mediated by both a

Funding Support: This manuscript has been supported by funds from the Government of Aragón (B01) and grant from Fondo de Investigaciones Sanitarias (FIS 05/2445).
Service of Digestive Diseases, University Hospital, University of Zaragoza, Instituto Aragonés de Ciencias de la Salud, CIBERehd, C/San Juan Bosco 15, 50009 Zaragoza, Spain
* Corresponding author.
E-mail address: alanas@unizar.es (A. Lanas).

non–prostaglandin-dependent local injury and, overall, by the systemic inhibition of the cyclooxygenase (COX) -1 enzyme.[4,6] This leads to a subsequent reduction in cytoprotective prostaglandins required for an effective mucosal defense.[6] The pathogenic mechanism leading to inflammatory changes in the distal GI tract is less well known at this time. Although mucosal prostaglandin inhibition after NSAID use is present in all parts of the digestive tract, there are significant differences between the distal and the proximal GI tract in the concurrence of other pathogenic factors that may increase the damage.[7] One proposed mode of action is that drug induces changes in local eicosanoid metabolism coupled with a topical toxic effect of the drug, increased by the enterohepatic circulation of the drug.[6–8] These effects compromise the mucosal cell integrity, which translates to increased epithelial permeability. Increased intestinal permeability permits mucosal exposure to toxins and luminal aggressors such as bacteria and their degradation products, bile acids, and pancreatic secretion with a predictable inflammatory reaction.[9] This inflammation varies in intensity from mild to severe, producing erosions and ulcers.[2]

The importance of neutrophils in this process has been emphasized by the finding that NSAID-intestinal damage is almost completely abolished or markedly attenuated in neutropenic rats.[10] As in other body tissues, the neutrophil recruitment in the intestine is a process mainly mediated by β2 integrins CD11/CD18 on stimulation of several cytokines. Tumor necrosis factor-alpha (TNF-α) acts as a relevant cytokine promoting NSAID-induced neutrophil recruitment in the mucosa.[11] Intestinal bacteria appear to be the main neutrophil chemoattractant. In this connection, a recent study found an unbalanced growth of gram-negative bacteria in the ileum of NSAID-treated animals and showed that heat-killed *Escherichia coli* cells, and their purified lipopolysaccharide caused deterioration of NSAID-induced ulcers. Indeed, lipopolysaccharide, a major cell wall component of gram-negative enterobacteria, was found capable of aggravating NSAID-induced intestinal injury.[12]

Antimicrobials, such as tetracycline, kanamycin, metronidazole, or neomycin plus bacitracin, attenuate NSAID enteropathy, thus giving further support to the pathogenic role of enteric bacteria. An additional, although indirect, proof of the role exerted by gut bacteria in the pathogenesis of NSAID enteropathy is represented by the similarities between indomethacin-induced intestinal damage and Crohn's disease. Not only are these lesions anatomically (both macro- and microscopically) similar but they are also sensitive to the same drugs, for example, sulfasalazine, steroids, immunosuppressive compounds, and antibiotics.[13,14]

A recent study by Watanabe and colleagues[15] extended these findings by adding another important piece to the puzzle. In particular, they showed experimentally that only a decrease in gram-negative but not gram-positive organisms lessens indomethacin-induced intestinal damage. These data have suggested a pathogenic mechanism of NSAID-induced enteropathy. Once the mucosal barrier has been disrupted by NSAIDs, luminal gram-negative bacteria enter the cell and are then recognized by the transmembrane toll-like receptor (TLR4) thanks to their lipopolysaccharides component. Activation of TLR4 induces cytokine mucosal expression, which triggers neutrophil recruitment with subsequent release of proteases and reactive oxygen species, leading ultimately to mucosal injury. The bacteria-induced inflammatory cascade could, therefore, be blunted either via manipulation of microbial ecology or through blockade of TLR4.[13]

Enterohepatic recirculation of NSAIDs may be an important factor.[16] NSAID-induced damage to the intestinal epithelium is therefore derived from a direct or local effect after oral administration, a recurrent local effect due to the enterohepatic recirculation of the drug, and the systemic effects after absorption. Supportive of this hypothesis is the fact that ligation of the bile duct prevents/reduces small intestinal damage by NSAIDs.[17]

The degree of increase in permeability is related to the potency of inhibition of COX activity and is diminished by the administration of prostaglandins COX-2 selective inhibitors.[18] There also are data suggesting that inhibition of both COX-1 and COX-2 is required as well as possible interference with mitochondrial energy metabolism of intestinal cells.[19] Taken together, these data are consistent with the notion that the effect of intestinal permeability is primarily a local intestinal event and that COX-1 and/or dual COX-1 and COX-2 inhibition plays a role in this initial event. Once intestinal permeability is increased, a cascade of events, driven by toxin and bacteria, induce inflammation and mucosal ulceration, which could eventually progress to bleeding, perforation, or gut stricture due to fibrosis involved in the healing repair process.[1,4,6] Why some lesions in some patients progress to more severe side effects and some others do not is not known. Recent studies have started to unravel risk factors that may help the clinician in the proper management of patients who need NSAID under this perspective.[20]

LESIONS INDUCED BY NONSTEROIDAL ANTI-INFLAMMATORY DRUGS IN THE DISTAL GASTROINTESTINAL TRACT

The prevalence of NSAID-associated lower GI side effects, including both clinical and subclinical side effects, may exceed those detected in the upper GI tract and include a wide spectrum of lesions (**Table 1**).[1,4]

Increased Permeability and Inflammation

Subclinical mucosal damage is very frequent in the distal GI tract since at least 60% to 70% of patients taking NSAIDs develop enteropathy.[1,4] The two most frequent abnormalities are the presence of increased gut permeability and mucosal inflammation. Increased gut permeability can be seen as soon as 12 hours after the ingestion of single doses of most tNSAIDs.[21] The process is rapidly reverted in 12 hours, but it takes longer with continued NSAID use. The administration of prostaglandins reduces or eliminates the damage initially, but this effect is rapidly overcome by the enterohepatic circulation of the NSAIDs.[21]

The increase in gut permeability is not observed with all NSAIDs, because those that do not undergo enterohepatic recirculation may not have this effect. It is now clear that long-term ingestion of most conventional NSAIDs (indomethacin, piroxicam, naproxen, ibuprofen, sulindac), except nabumetone and probably aspirin, increase intestinal

Table 1
Occurrence of main adverse effects of NSAIDs in the lower GI tract with NSAID use

Adverse Effect	Frequency (%)	References
Increased gut permeability	44–70	6,8,22,23,44
Gut inflammation	60–70	24,25
Blood loss and anemia	30	25,26,28,29
Malabsorption	40–70	18,25,30
Protein loss	10	25
Mucosal ulceration	30–40	34,35,40
Complications requiring hospitalizations	0.3–0.9	20,50,52,57
Diaphragms of the small bowel	<1	47

permeability.[4,16,21,22] The possible reasons for the lack of small intestinal inflammation associated with nabumetone and aspirin may relate to their site of absorption and lack of excretion in bile. Aspirin, an acidic NSAID, is mostly absorbed through the gastroduodenal mucosa, whereas nabumetone is nonacidic and therefore not trapped within enterocytes during drug absorption. Short-term studies with COX-2 selective inhibitors have shown that these agents do not increase intestinal permeability,[8,23] suggesting that either dual COX or COX-1 inhibition is a requisite to induce damage to the small bowel.

Animal data have shown an increase in intestinal TNF-α production soon after NSAID administration, which suggests that the presence of intestinal inflammation is rapid following increased gut permeability. Different studies have shown that NSAIDs increase fecal calprotectin (a nondegraded neutrophil cytosolic protein) in patients with rheumatoid arthritis or osteoarthritis taking NSAIDs.[24] These tests have shown that intestinal inflammation is present in 60% to 70% of patients taking NSAIDs and that, once established, it may be detected up to 1 to 3 years after the NSAID has been stopped. An initial increase in small intestine permeability is a prerequisite of the subsequent development of small intestine inflammation, which is associated with blood and protein loss, but it is often silent.[25]

Blood Loss and Anemia

NSAID enteropathy is associated with continuous and mild bleeding. In the longer term, this may result in iron deficiency and anemia. Although anemia is frequent in patients taking NSAIDs, no studies have been performed to determine the exact burden and clinical impact of this problem in patients taking NSAIDs or aspirin. Furthermore, in many instances, there is no close relationship between demonstrable lesions on the upper GI tract and GI blood loss.[26]

In other situations, patients taking NSAIDs or aspirin may develop anemia, with or without positive fecal occult blood test, but the usual upper or lower GI endoscopic procedures do not show mucosal lesions, suggesting that the small bowel could be the cause of the blood loss. The significance of the presence of isolated mucosal lesions in the small bowel and anemia has not, however, been properly defined. Using enteroscopy, Morris and colleagues[27] investigated the site of blood loss in patients on NSAIDs for rheumatoid arthritis with chronic iron deficiency anemia who had negative gastroscopy and colonoscopy findings. They showed that 47% of these patients had small bowel ulcerations and concluded that this contributed to their anemia. The amount of blood loss from the small intestine is in most cases modest, between 2 and 10 mL/d. The study of subclinical blood loss has methodological problems (long transit times, collection of stool samples, methods for measuring radioactivity in blood and stool, etc) that have not yet been solved.[8]

In a systematic review including 1162 individuals in 47 trials conducted over 5 decades, Moore and colleagues[28] found that most NSAIDs and low-dose (325 mg) aspirin resulted in a small average increase in fecal blood loss of 1 to 2 mL/d from about 0.5 mL/d at baseline (**Fig. 1**). Some individuals lost much more blood than average, at least for some of the time, with 5% of those taking NSAIDs having a daily blood loss of 5 mL or more and 1% having a daily blood loss of 10 mL or more; rates of daily blood loss of 5 mL/d or 10 mL/d were 31% and 10%, respectively, for aspirin at daily doses of 1800 mg or greater. A small comparative study of misoprostol and no treatment in 21 patients with small bowel enteropathy and iron deficiency anemia showed a rise of 15 g/L in hemoglobin with misoprostol compared with no change without treatment.[29]

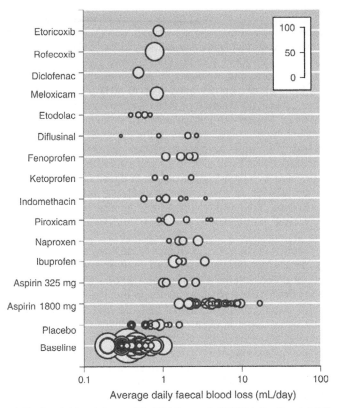

Fig. 1. Mean daily fecal blood loss with NSAIDs and COX-2–selective inhibitors in individual treatment arms. Daily fecal blood loss is shown on a logarithmic scale for aspirin, cyclo-oxygenase-2 selective inhibitors (coxibs), and NSAIDs with more than 20 participants. The size of the symbol is proportional to the number of individuals (inset scale). (*From* Moore RA, Derry S, Henry J, et al. Faecal blood loss with aspirin, nonsteroidal anti-inflammatory drugs and cyclo-oxygenase-2 selective inhibitors: systematic review of randomized trials using autologous chromium-labelled erythrocytes. Arthritis Res Ther 2008;10:R7.)

Malabsorption, Protein Loss, and Ileal Dysfunction

Patients with NSAID enteropathy may have a protein-losing enteropathy, which can lead to hypoalbuminemia. Some studies have shown a loss of proteins labeled with [51]chromium in patients on long-term NSAID therapy at the ileum level, demonstrating the presence of a protein-losing enteropathy. Low serum albumin is found in about 10% of hospitalized patients with rheumatoid arthritis.[30]

NSAIDs do not cause malabsorption when given short term, but malabsorption of D-xylose has been documented in patients on long-term NSAID treatment. Some studies suggest that up to 40% to 70% of patients using NSAIDs may have some degree of intestinal malabsorption.[18,25] The use of sulindac and fenamates has been associated with severe malabsorption and atrophic mucosa similar to that seen in celiac sprue.[31] NSAID use increases the risk of acute diarrhea, which can be the factor responsible for many episodes seen in general practice.[32]

Mucosal Ulceration

Capsule endoscopy studies have now shown that NSAIDs induce intestinal ulceration in the small bowel, confirming previous autopsy data.[33] Enteroscopic detection of NSAID damage is very frequent and includes edema, erythema, villous denudation, mucosal hemorrhage, erosions, or ulcers.[34] Some reports suggest that this type of lesions are very frequent and can be seen in up to 40% of rheumatic patients taking NSAIDs.[34,35] The clinical significance of these findings are not yet clear, since most endoscopic mucosal lesions are just petechia or erosions. It is very possible that the clinical considerations usually referred to the upper GI tract, where erosions and acute mucosal lesions are often seen in patients taking NSAIDs but have very little clinical consequences, can also be applied to lesions seen in the small bowel. In any case, it may well be possible that ulcers and erosions of the small bowel could explain why some patients on NSAIDs or low-dose acetylsalicylic acid (ASA) (asprin) develop bleeding of "unknown" source, iron deficiency anemia, hypoalbuminemia, or even abdominal symptoms, particularly if the upper and lower endoscopy studies are normal.[2,4]

Colonoscopy studies have also shown that NSAID use is associated with isolated colonic ulcers, diffuse colonic ulceration that may or may not be associated with occult bleeding, or complications such as major GI bleeding and or perforation.[36–38] Diffuse colitis has been observed after the use of mefenamic acid, ibuprofen, piroxicam, naproxen, or aspirin.[39] Up to 30% of patients who receive NSAID therapy via the rectum may show some kind of discomfort. More rarely, proctitis, ulceration, bleeding, or rectal stricture have also been described.[40]

NSAIDs may exacerbate pre-existing lesions, including diverticulitis, reactivation of inflammatory bowel diseases (IBDs), and intestinal bleeding from angiodysplastic lesions.[4,40–42] Patients with IBD frequently have extraintestinal manifestations, including colitis-associated arthritis, sacroileitis, and ankylosing spondylitis The treatment of these rheumatologic conditions with nonselective NSAIDs has been reported to lead to frequent disease exacerbation.[4,42] It should be acknowledged that these data are of poor quality and therefore the exact effect of tNSAIDs in the exacerbation of IBD is unclear based on the available evidence. Whether the selective COX-2 inhibitors can be used safely in the setting of IBDs is controversial. A 2006 study has shown that therapy with celecoxib for up to 14 days did not have a greater relapse rate than placebo in patients with ulcerative colitis in remission.[43]

To spare gastroduodenal damage, some NSAIDs have been formulated as enteric-coated compounds and are released in the small bowel. Endoscopic studies have shown that these compounds are associated either with reduced or no damage to the gastroduodenal mucosa but can increase the exposure and toxicity of the active drug to the distal intestine.[44–46]

Diaphragms

Another rare and unique complication of NSAID use is the development of multiple, concentric, luminal protrusions of fibrotic mucosa and submucosa, nearly occluding the lumen. The term "diaphragm disease" was coined by Lang and colleagues,[47] who were the first to describe the entity, and is considered by many to be pathognomonic for NSAID-related injury, although a case report not finding a relationship with NSAID use has been published.[48] The strictures are diaphragm-like rings of scar tissue and are a distinguishable pathologic entity, which may have a silent clinical evolution or more often induce obstruction, anemia, and/or diarrhea and require surgery for treatment and/or diagnosis. Due to the potential existence of several concomitant rings in other parts of the intestine, it is important to perform a full examination of the small and large intestine, including an intraoperative enteroscopy.

The diaphragms are about 2- to 4-mm thick and can significantly reduce the small bowel lumen diameter, resulting in different degrees of bowel obstruction. Kessler and colleagues[49] reported that 17% of patients with NSAID-induced small bowel ulceration developed intestinal obstruction. There are also numerous case reports of NSAID-induced small bowel and colonic strictures.[4] With the capsule enteroscopy technique, new cases are being discovered, and today, this complication may well overcome other GI complications related to NSAID use (eg, gastric outlet obstruction).

LIFE-THREATENING COMPLICATIONS FROM THE LOWER GASTROINTESTINAL TRACT

Although increased permeability, inflammation, or even GI ulceration is the most common manifestation of NSAID toxicity, GI bleeding and perforation are the most clinically relevant side effects, since they contribute significantly to the increased risk of morbidity and mortality associated with these drugs. There is evidence that NSAIDs and/or aspirin are associated with complications from the lower GI tract since the early 1990s.[37,50,51] Current evidence suggests that NSAIDs increase the risk of lower GI bleeding and perforation to a similar extent to that seen in the upper GI tract. One study evaluated both nonaspirin NSAIDs and aspirin use in all consecutive patients admitted to hospital because of GI bleeding and in addition to clinical history; aspirin use was assayed by estimating platelet COX activity and aspirin plasma levels.[37] The study found that 86% of patients with lower GI bleeding had evidence of recent aspirin or NSAID use. Other studies[38,51] confirmed later that the risk of developing a lower GI bleeding event is increased with NSAID use. Using a similar methodology to that mentioned here,[37] a similar picture was found later for intestinal perforations.[38] The proportion of perforations resulting in death is high (around 30%) when compared with other NSAID-associated side effects.[37,38,52] A formulation that released indomethacin in the small bowel was associated with intestinal perforation and withdrawn from the market.[53] Epidemiologic studies have shown that the risk of major upper GI bleeding is not reduced with enteric-coated NSAID compounds, which suggests that they do not solve the problem of NSAID-induced GI damage.[54]

Apart from observational studies, post hoc analysis of randomized, controlled trials designed to evaluate the incidence of upper GI complications with NSAIDs have confirmed that these compounds are also associated with severe lower GI clinical events. The Vioxx Gastrointestinal Outcomes Research (VIGOR) study evaluated 8076 rheumatoid patients who were randomized to receive either naproxen or rofecoxib. The results showed that in the naproxen group, the rate of serious events beyond the duodenum was 0.89/100 patient years, which accounted for 39.4% of all serious GI events.[55] In a smaller trial designed to evaluate the incidence of recurrent upper GI bleeding in high-risk patients who had developed a recent ulcer bleeding episode required NSAID treatment, celecoxib was as effective as diclofenac plus omeprazole, with respect to the prevention of recurrent bleeding.[56] A post hoc analysis of the data showed that lower GI events, including a fatal small bowel perforation, anemia, colitis, and bleeding due to angiodysplasia, accounted for one-third of all GI clinically relevant bleeding events.

A report in 2008,[20] which summarized the results of the Multinational Etoricoxib and Diclofenac Arthritis Long-term (MEDAL) program, a trial designed to evaluate the incidence of CV events in patients taking either diclofenac or etoricoxib, evaluated the occurrence of upper and lower GI severe events in 34,701 osteoarthritis or rheumatoid arthritis patients older than 50 years of age with a mean duration of therapy of 18 months. GI clinical events were confirmed by a blinded adjudication committee. Lower GI complications rates, which included perforation or obstruction requiring hospitalization or bleeding, were 0.32 and 0.38 per 100 patient years for etoricoxib and diclofenac, respectively. Bleeding was the most common event (rates of 0.19 and 0.23 per 100 patient years, respectively).[49] It was of interest to note that the incidence of lower GI complications was similar to that observed in the upper GI tract (**Fig. 2**).[20,57]

The burden of lower GI complications associated with NSAID use has to be defined. In a nationwide study on the mortality associated with NSAID use in 2001 in Spain, it was shown that the frequency of life-threatening complications due to the lower GI tract represented no less than a third of all GI complications due to NSAIDs with similar complication rates.[53] In this study, the case fatality rate was almost identical for both upper and lower GI complications (**Fig. 3**). A new study of this group has shown that the time trends of hospitalization due to GI complications is decreasing for upper GI complications and increasing for lower GI complications. In fact, the ratio of upper/lower was 4.1 in 1996 and only 1.4 in 2005. Extensive validation of cases also showed that hospitalizations due to lower GI events were associated with increased mortality and consumed more resources than those for upper GI complications.[58]

One study from Canada[59] in 2008 has reported lower figures for GI events in the distal tract than those in the upper tract. They conducted a population-based, retrospective cohort study, which included 644,183 elderly patients who received 1,778,541 prescriptions for NSAIDs (315,222; 17.7% with a proton pump initiator [PPI]). Among users of tNSAIDs without PPIs, the crude rates of hospitalization were 0.7 cases/1000 patient years for complications in the lower GI tract compared with 4.4/1000 patient years for complications in the upper GI tract. Among users of NSAIDs and PPIs, the rates were of 1.4/1000 patient years for the lower GI tract compared with

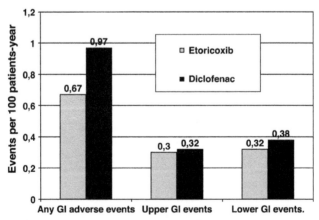

Fig. 2. Upper and lower GI complications rates in the MEDAL program, which included bleeding, perforation, or obstruction requiring hospitalization. It was interesting to note that the incidence of lower GI complications was similar to those observed in the upper GI tract and that there were no differences between diclofenac and etoricoxib. (*Data from* Laine L, Curtis SP, Langman M, et al. Lower gastrointestinal events in a double-blind trial of the cyclo-oxigenase–2 selective inhibitor etoricoxib and the traditional nonsteroidal anti-inflammatory drug diclofenac. Gastroenterology 2008;135:1517–25 and Laine L, Curtis SP, Cryer B, et al. MEDAL Steering Committee. Assessment of upper gastrointestinal safety of etoricoxib and diclofenac in patients with osteoarthritis and rheumatoid arthritis in the Multinational Etoricoxib and Diclofenac Arthritis Long-term (MEDAL) programme: a randomised comparison. Lancet 2007;369(9560):465–73.)

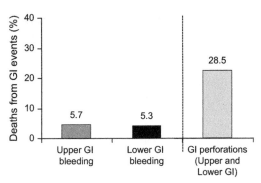

Fig. 3. In a nationwide study on the mortality associated with NSAID use, it was shown that the frequency of life-threatening complications due to the lower GI tract represented no less than a third of all GI complications due to NSAIDs. In this study, the case fatality rate was almost identical for both upper and lower GI complications and was much higher in GI perforation than in GI bleeding events. (*From* Lanas A, Perez-Aisa MA, Feu F, et al. A nationwide study of mortality associated with hospital admission due to severe gastrointestinal events and those associated with nonsteroidal antiinflammatory drug use. Am J Gastroenterol 2005;100:1685–93.)

2.0/1000 patient years for the upper GI tract, suggesting that PPIs reduced hospitalizations for upper but not lower GI complications associated with NSAIDs. Interestingly, they confirmed that NSAIDs increased the risk of hospitalization from lesions of either the upper or the lower GI tract when compared with acetaminophen at less than 3 g/d.

Another clinical manifestation of side effects associated with NSAID use in the lower GI tract is complicated diverticular disease. Apart from isolated case reports, a systematic review of the literature[5] in 2006 identified seven studies that have examined this association. According to this review, four case-control studies found increased risk of complicated diverticular disease with tNSAID use when compared with controls with no disease, with odds ratios (ORs) ranging from 1.8 to 11.2; another one had a strong trend toward an association (adjusted OR, 1.8; 95% confidence interval [CI], 0.96–3.4). A prospective cohort study found that tNSAID users were significantly more likely than nonusers to develop symptomatic diverticular disease (relative risk, 1.5; 95% CI, 1.1–2.1), and finally, a randomized, controlled, 10-day trial reported acute diverticulitis in 1 subject taking ibuprofen versus none in the placebo group. Use of ASA and NSAIDs may increase the risk of bleeding through previous lower GI condition, in particular, diverticular disease of the colon.[40]

Foutch reported on 13 patients with diverticular bleeding and found that three of four with more severe bleeding had been taking a combination of ASA and NSAIDs, whereas zero of nine patients with less severe bleeding had taken this combination.[60] Wilcox and colleagues reported on 105 patients with lower GI bleeding and 1895 non-bleeding controls and found that, after adjusting for age, race, and gender, the risk for lower GI bleeding among those taking NSAIDs was 2.6 times of those not taking them (95% CI, 1.7–3.9). Specifically, the reported risk of diverticular bleeding was increased by 3.4 (95% CI, 1.9–6.2) if taking NSAIDS.[51]

It has been suggested[61] that the use of NSAIDs and other drugs such as opioids and corticosteroids increases the risk of colonic diverticular perforation. However, low-dose ASA did not seem to affect the risk of diverticular perforation, whereas calcium channel blockers were associated with a reduced risk of perforation.

LOWER GASTROINTESTINAL DAMAGE WITH COX-2 SELECTIVE INHIBITORS

COX-2 selective NSAIDs could be safer than tNSAIDS for the lower GI tract. The lack of intestinal damage with this type of agents in some animal experiments[62] has been confirmed in preclinical study and, in 2000 and 2001, in clinical studies in humans.[8,63] In the short term, these agents do not increase mucosal permeability and have displayed a 50% reduction of serious lower GI side effects compared with tNSAIDS in some but not all post hoc analysis of outcome studies.[20,55]

Smecuol and colleagues,[8] demonstrated that gastric permeability was significantly affected by naproxen but not by slow-releasing indomethacin, meloxicam, or celecoxib. Intestinal permeability was significantly increased by the first three NSAIDs but not by celecoxib. Colonic permeability was not significantly increased by any of the four drugs. Similar results have been obtained with etoricoxib in one study considering fecal occult blood.[64] Daily fecal red blood cell loss was measured in 62 subjects receiving etoricoxib (120 mg once daily), ibuprofen (800 mg thrice daily), or placebo for 28 days. The between-treatment ratio of fecal blood loss for etoricoxib versus placebo (1.06) was not significantly different from unity; however, the ratios for ibuprofen versus placebo (3.26) and etoricoxib (3.08) were significantly greater than unity ($P<.001$).

Capsule endoscopy studies have shown that COX-2 selective inhibitor agents perform better than tNSAIDs and PPIs in the small bowel in healthy volunteers. There are several studies with similar methodological design that have shown that short-term celecoxib treatment in healthy volunteers is associated with less damage to the small bowel than that with naproxen or ibuprofen plus a PPI.[65,66] Similar results have recently confirmed that lumiracoxib 100 mg once daily induces less damage to the small bowel than naproxen 500 mg twice daily and omeprazole 20 mg once daily.[67] It is unclear whether these results with short-term treatment obtained in healthy volunteers will be reproduced in patients suffering from different rheumatic conditions in long-term treatments. A capsule enteroscopy study performed in 140 patients on long-term NSAIDs and COX-2 selective agents in 60 healthy volunteers has shown that 62% of patients on conventional NSAIDs had abnormal studies (reddened folds, 13%; denuded areas, -39%; and mucosal breaks, 29%), which differed significantly ($P<.001$) from controls. The main pathology was related to 2% of patients with diaphragm-like strictures and 3% who had bleeding without an identifiable lesion. Similar damage was also seen in 50% of patients on selective COX-2 inhibitors (reddened folds, 8%; denuded areas, 18%; and mucosal breaks, 22%), which did not differ significantly ($P>.5$) from that seen with NSAIDs. Since this study was not a randomized, controlled trial and it is unclear whether patients on COX-2 inhibitors had previously used NSAID, these data must be taken with care, but more data need to be collected before we claim that coxibs are safer to the GI tract than tNSAIDs.[68]

When looking at mores serious GI events, some case reports have communicated acute colitis or lower intestinal complication associated with COX-2 inhibitor use.[69] Post hoc analyses of the VIGOR and MEDAL trials have come out with different results. In VIGOR, lower GI events were as frequent as upper GI events, and the benefits of rofecoxib 50 mg/d over naproxen (500 mg twice a day) were present in both the upper and the lower GI tract, with a similar risk reduction of 50% and 60%, respectively (**Fig. 4**).[55] However, in MEDAL although the incidence of lower GI events barely exceeded that seen in the upper GI tract (patients were advised to take PPI if they had risk factors), there were no benefits of etoricoxib over diclofenac when looking at the incidence of lower GI complications (see **Fig. 3**).[20]

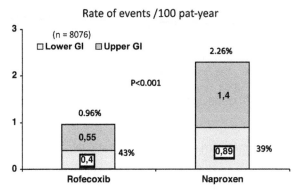

Fig. 4. Post hoc analyses of the VIGOR trial. Serious GI lower events were as frequent as upper GI events, and the benefits of rofecoxib (50 mg/d) over naproxen (500 mg bid) were present in both the upper and the lower GI tract, with a similar risk reduction of 50% and 60%, respectively. (*Data from* Langman MJ, Morgan L, Worrall A. Use of anti-inflammatory drugs by patients admitted with small or large bowel perforations and haemorrhage. Br Med J (Clin Res Ed) 1985;290(6465):347–49.)

Based on current data, one cannot conclude that the available COX-2 selective inhibitors show a demonstrated safer profile in clinically relevant endpoints in the lower GI tract when compared with tNSAIDS. It is possible that differences may depend on the dose used and the type of tNSAID used as a comparator, since these agents may carry different intrinsic toxicity to the lower GI tract, for example, naproxen may be more toxic than diclofenac, as shown in different epidemiologic studies in the upper GI tract.[70] One important piece of information may be available this year on completion of the CONDOR trial (the celecoxib versus. Omeprazole and Diclofenac for at-risk Osteoarthritis and Rheumatoid arthritis patients). This ongoing trial is testing the hypothesis that celecoxib is safer for the entire GI tract when compared with diclofenac associated to omeprazole. To do this, the study is assessing all potential serious GI events occurring either in the upper or the lower GI tract, including acute bleeding, perforation, obstruction, or hemoglobin decreased greater than or equal to 2 gm/dL from baseline, in a new composite endpoint called "clinically significant upper and lower GI events."[71]

LOWER GASTROINTESTINAL DAMAGE BY LOW-DOSE ASPIRIN

It is generally believed that low-dose ASA does not cause any small bowel damage, since the drug is largely absorbed before reaching the intestine, and this would limit the topical action on the intestinal mucosa. GI injury by ASA therapy is the result of both local topical effects and a decrease in mucosal COX-1–derived prostaglandins, which could be a systemic effect. Very little clinical information is available so far. A recent study has evaluated the effect of low-dose enteric-coated aspirin on the small bowel. Twenty healthy volunteers underwent videocapsule endoscopy (VCE), fecal calprotectin, and permeability tests (sucrose and lactulose/mannitol [lac/man] ratio) before and after ingestion of 100 mg of enteric-coated ASA daily for 14 days. Half of the healthy volunteers showed some degree of mucosal damage in the VCE studies, including erosions and two ulcers in one patient.[72] The median baseline lac/man ratio increased after ASA use and the post-ASA lac/man ratio was above the upper end of normal in 10 out of 20 volunteers. The median baseline fecal calprotectin concentration also increased significantly after ASA use, although only three patients had values above the cutoff (>50 μg/g).[72] These data should be taken with care since the clinical significance of this is unclear. It must be remembered that low-dose aspirin is associated with acute gastric damage, but very few patients develop serious adverse events. However, the data show that low-dose enteric-coated aspirin may induce damage to the small bowel and could be the responsible agent in some patients with anemia or GI bleeding taking this drug, although they had no clear gastric or colonic cause.

DIAGNOSIS OF NONSTEROIDAL ANTI-INFLAMMATORY DRUG ENTEROPATHY

Probably the single most important reason for underestimating the clinical importance of NSAID enteropathy is the difficulty in making a diagnosis. Barium radiologic examination of the small-bowel mucosa is very deficient in detecting flat lesions. A number of noninvasive tests have been developed to evaluate indirect parameters of mucosal damage. Inflammatory markers (fecal calprotectin excretion) and permeability tests (urinary recovery of orally administered probes) assess the functional integrity of the intestinal epithelium. The presence of abnormal intestinal permeability is considered an important marker of NSAID enteropathy. More recently, VCE has allowed the assessment of the macroscopic morphology in the entire small bowel.[35,65–68]

Small Bowel Permeability and Inflammation Assessment

The rationale for using permeability tests in the diagnosis of NSAID enteropathy is based on the knowledge that NSAIDs disrupt the intercellular integrity of intestinal epithelial cells. Different probes have been used.[73,74] The reported prevalence of permeability changes in patients on NSAID treatment is wide, which may be explained by differences in the sensitivity of test procedures and other aspects including dose and osmolarity of the probe.[73–75] Administration of site-specific permeability probes detecting defects at different levels of the GI tract may allow, in a single screening test, the assessment of the functional integrity of the GI mucosa.[8,72] Thus, simultaneous use of sucrose, lactulose/mannitol, and sucralose probes allows noninvasive detection of gastric, enteric, or colonic damage, respectively. The choice of intestinal permeability tests for clinical testing is wide, but their availability in hospitals and clinical biochemical laboratories is limited. The disadvantage of using intestinal permeability tests for the diagnosis of NSAID enteropathy is that they are nonspecific and may be abnormal in a variety of other conditions.[8,25,67,68]

Intestinal inflammation is the defining feature of NSAID enteropathy. NSAID enteropathy was initially shown in humans by [111]indium-labeled leukocyte technique, which involves abdominal scintigraphy as well as a 4-day fecal collection. This technique detects inflammation in 50% to 70% of patients taking long-term NSAIDs with all conventional NSAIDs except with aspirin and nabumetone. The method is expensive, and the need for radioactive probes will make its use in clinical practice difficult.[44] Calprotectin is a protein of the cytosol of neutrophils, monocytes, and macrophages. The amount in feces, determined by ELISA, reflects the traffic of these cells into the intestine. Single stool fecal concentrations of calprotectin correlate with the 4-day fecal excretion of [111]indium-labeled leucocytes and histopathological parameters of inflammation in IBD. Enteropathy is evident within 7 days of NSAID ingestion in volunteers. The prevalence of NSAID enteropathy in long-term users, using this method, is variously reported as 44% to 70%.[1,8] However, as with the intestinal permeability tests, this method is not disease specific (it is specific for inflammation), and raised levels of fecal calprotectin are consistently evident in IBD and colorectal cancer.

Nevertheless, it may have a role as the first line of noninvasive investigation before other more invasive tests are ordered.

Role of Endoscopy in the Detection of Nonsteroidal Anti-inflammatory Drug-Induced Enteropathy or Major Gastrointestinal Complications

The wireless capsule endoscopy technology has improved the visualization of the small bowel, and the burden of NSAID-induced damage at this level is being better defined, including the detection of mucosal breaks, erosions, and ulcers. Capsule endoscopy has been shown to provide painless and superior visualization of the small intestine compared with enteroscopy.[76] Double- or single-balloon enteroscopy should only be used if endoscopy treatment is expected to be necessary during the procedure. Capsule endoscopy studies that have also used fecal calprotectin tests have not found significant correlation between the two tests.[62,67] This may well prove that inflammation is not always associated with mucosal breaks, and the opposite, that isolated mucosal breaks may not be associated with diffuse inflammation. Capsule endoscopy technique is expensive and time consuming, but it is now progressively available to clinicians and becoming the test of choice to diagnose NSAID enteropathy. However, there are reports suggesting the existence of a high number of false positives[77] and significant lesions missed.[78]

In case of major GI bleeding events, the initial choice should be standard upper GI and lower GI endoscopy, if the first was negative. Capsule endoscopy may be necessary for diagnosis purposes, when the other procedures have been negative or the small bowel is the first area of interest.[79] Capsule endoscopy may also be the technique of choice in patients who develop anemia when taking NSAIDs, and other causes have been ruled out with hemodilution, anemia of chronic diseases, lesions in the gastroduodenal or colonic mucosa, or when lesions found in the stomach or the colon are not considered relevant to induce anemia. Finally, it must be pointed out that angiography is another well-defined technique that can be used for both diagnosis and therapy in cases of NSAID-induced major GI bleeding.[80]

PREVENTION AND TREATMENT
Misoprostol, COX-2 Selective Inhibitors, and NO-Donating Agents

At present, effective means to prevent NSAID-associated intestinal lesions in patients are not available. The efforts to generate safer NSAIDs, including ASA, have followed different routes such as the development of enteric-coated or slow-release formulations. As commented here, these formulations could shift the problem to a more distal site within the digestive tract. Since all conventional NSAIDs appear to cause NSAID enteropathy, there is little sense to switch from one to another. The only exception could be the switch to a COX-2 selective agent, since these drugs have been found in some studies to be safer to the lower GI tract compared with tNSAIDs.[55,64–68] However, their long-term safety requires appropriate studies.

So far, two main strategies have been developed to minimize the GI effects of NSAIDs in the upper GI tract. PPI inhibit gastric acid secretion and reduce NSAID-associated dyspepsia and gastric injury, but they do not protect the small intestine. In contrast, selective (COX)-2 inhibitors spare COX-1–dependent prostaglandin synthesis throughout the GI tract and should lack the harmful effects of NSAIDs on the GI tract, including the small bowel and the colon.

VCE investigations have shown that the combination of a PPI with a tNSAID is not capable of preventing the intestinal damage associated with short-term administration of naproxen or ibuprofen.[64–68] If NSAID enteropathy is to be prevented, it is reasonable to coadminister misoprostol with the NSAID, as this reduces the permeability changes caused by NSAIDs. Misoprostol may also be effective in established cases of NSAID enteropathy. However, although misoprostol improves anemia in patients with proven NSAID enteropathy,[29] its ability to reverse intestinal permeability changes induced by indomethacin or naproxen is controversial.[4] Davies and colleagues[30] performed a double-blind, placebo-controlled, randomized study that showed that there was no reduction in intestinal permeability of ^{51}Cr-EDTA after treatment with indomethacin and misoprostol, but they used comparatively low doses of misoprostol. A recent uncontrolled report from Watanabe and colleagues[81] in 11 patients who had developed gastric ulcers when taking low-dose aspirin showed that misoprostol but not PPI therapy improved the mucosal lesions found in the small bowel by capsule. In any case, specifically designed clinical trials to evaluate this indication are lacking.

COX-2 selective inhibitors may be one alternative to tNSAIDs to prevent GI damage in the lower GI tract. In this report, we have previously summarized available data that indicate that these agents induce less damage to the small bowel in healthy volunteers and are associated with less severe side effects in the lower GI tract than tNSAIDs in some reports. While we wait for new data in the ongoing outcome trial (CONDOR) that will evaluate outcomes for the entire GI tract and compare celecoxib with diclofenac plus omeprazole,[71] some attention is being focused on nitric oxide (NO) donating NSAIDs. Preclinical studies with these compounds have demonstrated reduced intestinal adverse effects (ie, ulceration and bleeding) compared with those of parent compounds.[82] Although NO-naproxen failed to increase intestinal permeability in healthy volunteers,[83] no clinical data regarding the lower GI tract are available in patients. A good number of other potential approaches are being tested, but they are still in preclinical development.[84,85]

Sulphasalazine

Pathologic similarities between NSAID enteropathy and IBD led to the suggestion that *sulphasalazine* may be a possible therapeutic option in NSAID enteropathy. Hayllar and colleagues[86] assessed the use of disease-modifying, antirheumatic drugs including sulphasalazine in patients taking NSAIDs. Sulphasalazine significantly reduced intestinal inflammation and blood loss, whereas other second-line antirheumatic drugs did not.

Antibiotics

Several studies have suggested that intraluminal bacteria play a significant role in the pathogenesis of small bowel damage induced by NSAIDs and that enterobacterial translocation into the mucosa represents the first step that sets in motion a series of events leading to gross lesion formation.[4,12–17,87,88] Experimental and clinical investigations indicate that in the short term, antibacterial agents either reduce or abolish NSAID enteropathy.[13,14] The evidence from animal experiments has been confirmed in human studies, showing that metronidazole, an antimicrobial mainly targeted against anaerobic organisms, significantly prevented indomethacin-induced increase in intestinal permeability in healthy volunteers and reduced inflammation and blood loss in rheumatic patients taking NSAIDs.[89] However, potential adverse effects of systemic antimicrobials and the occurrence of drug resistance have so far precluded this approach. Antibiotics may also be used cyclically to eliminate certain enteric bacterial populations, followed by exogenous probiotics or prebiotics to fill the open ecologic niche, thereby improving the balance of enteric microbiota for long-term efficacy. The availability to modulate the innate immune system may break the link between anti-inflammatory activity and intestinal toxicity of NSAIDs.[13] The availability of poorly absorbed and effective antibiotics (eg, rifaximin) should open new thera-peutic options to limit the extent of intestinal damage in some patients.[13,14] Despite all the above evidence, no clinical trials have been formally performed in humans to evaluate the effect of antibiotics in the prevention of intestinal damage induced by NSAIDs.

Finally, other treatments may be required for some of the complications of NSAID enteropathy, including endoscopy or surgical therapy in case of open bleeding lesions, surgical or endoscopic balloon dilatation for accessible strictures, surgery and or antibiotics for diverticulitis, and surgical intervention for most, if not all, cases of obstruction or perforation.

SUMMARY

In addition to the upper GI tract, NSAIDs can damage the small bowel and the colon. NSAID enteropathy is frequent and may be present in more than 60% of patients taking these drugs long term. In most cases, damage is subclinical, including increased mucosal permeability, inflammation, erosions, ulceration, but other more serious clinical outcomes such as anemia, and overall bleeding, perforation, obstruc-tion, diverticulitis and deaths have also been described. The magnitude of these serious outcomes from the lower GI tract is not well defined, but recent data suggest that they may be as frequent and severe as upper GI complications. Contrary to what happens in the upper GI tract, treatment and prevention of NSAID enteropathy is diffi-cult, since the pathogenic mechanisms are different and not well understood. Among other options, misoprostol, antibiotics, and sulphasalazine have been proved to be effective in animal models, but they have not been properly tested in humans. Selec-tive COX-2 inhibition is emerging as a potential alternative to tNSAIDs in the prevention of damage in the lower GI tract in rheumatologic patients. Preliminary studies in healthy volunteers have shown that these drugs are associated with no or less small bowel damage than tNSAIDs plus PPI, although their long-term effects in patients need to be properly tested. Post hoc analysis of previous outcome studies focused on complications of upper GI tract or cardiovascular events have shown contradictory results. Data from one ongoing trial comparing celecoxib versus diclofenac plus PPI and examining serious outcomes from the whole GI tract will probably provide new insights in this area.

REFERENCES

1. Adebayo D, Bjarnason I. Is non–steroidal anti-inflammatory drug (NSAID) enter-opathy clinically more important than NSAID gastropathy? Postgrad Med J 2006;82:186–91.
2. Bjarnason I, Hayllar J, Macpherson AJ, et al. Side effects of nonsteroidal anti-inflammatory drugs on the small and large intestine in humans. Gastroenterology 1993;104:1832–47.
3. Tibble JA, Sigthorsson G, Foster R, et al. High prevalence of NSAID enteropathy as shown by a simple faecal test. Gut 1999;45:362–6.
4. Lanas A, Panés J, Piqué JM. Clinical implications of COX-1 and/or COX-2 inhibi-tion for the distal gastrointestinal tract. Curr Pharm Des 2003;9(27):2253–66.
5. Laine L, Smith R, Min K, et al. Systematic review: the lower gastrointestinal adverse effects of non–steroidal anti-inflammatory drugs. Aliment Pharmacol Ther 2006;24:751–67.

6. Bjarnason I, Fehilly B, Smethurst P, et al. Importance of local versus systemic effects of non–steroidal anti-inflammatory drugs in increasing small intestinal permeability in man. Gut 1991;32:275–7.

7. Whittle BJR. Mechanisms underlying intestinal injury induced by anti-inflammatory COX inhibitors. Eur J Pharmacol 2004;500:427–39.

8. Smecuol E, Bai JC, Sugai E, et al. Acute gastrointestinal permeability responses to different non–steroidal anti-inflammatory drugs. Gut 2001;49:650–5.

9. Sigthorsson G, Simpson RJ, Walley M, et al. COX–1 and 2, intestinal integrity and pathogenesis of NSAID-enteropathy in mice. Gastroenterology 2002;122: 1913–23.

10. Chmaisse HM, Antoon JS, Kvietys PR, et al. Role of leukocytes in indomethacin-induced small bowel injury in the rat. Am J Phys 1994;266:G239–46.

11. Stadnyk AW, Dollard C, Issekutz TB, et al. Neutrophil migration into indomethacin induced rat small intestinal injury is CD11a/CD18 and CD11b/CD18 codependent. Gut 2002;50:629–35.

12. Hagiwara M, Kataoka K, Arimochi H, et al. Role of unbalanced growth of gram-negative bacteria in ileal ulcer formation in rats treated with a nonsteroidal anti-inflammatory drug. J Med Invest 2004;51:43–51.

13. Scarpignato C. NSAID-induced intestinal damage: are luminal bacteria the therapeutic target? Gut 2008;57:145–8.

14. Lanas A, Scarpignato C. Microbial flora in NSAID induced intestinal damage: a role for antibiotics? Digestion 2006;73(Suppl 1):36–50.

15. Watanabe T, Higuchi K, Kobata A, et al. Nonsteroidal anti-inflammatory drug-induced small intestinal damage is toll-like receptor 4 dependent. Gut 2008;57: 181–7.

16. Fortun PJ, Hawkey CJ. Nonsteroidal anti-inflammatory drugs and the small intestine. Curr Opin Gastroenterol 2005;21:169–75.

17. Reuter BK, Davies NM, Wallace JL. Nonsteroidal anti-inflammatory drug enteropathy in rats: role of permeability, bacteria, and enterohepatic circulation. Gastroenterology 1997;112:109–17.

18. Bjarnason I, Zanelli G, Smith T, et al. The pathogenesis and consequence of non steroidal anti-inflammatory drug induced small intestinal inflammation in man. Scand J Rheumatol Suppl 1987;64:55–62.

19. Somasundaram S, Rafi S, Hayllar J, et al. Mitochondrial damage: a possible mechanism of the "topical" phase of NSAID induced injury to the rat intestine. Gut 1997;41:344–53.

20. Laine L, Curtis SP, Langman M, et al. Lower gastrointestinal events in a double-blind trial of the cyclo-oxigenase-2 selective inhibitor etoricoxib and the traditional nonsteroidal anti-inflammatory drug diclofenac. Gastroenterology 2008;135: 1517–25.

21. Bjarnason I, Williams P, Smethurst P, et al. Effect of non–steroidal anti-inflammatory drugs and prostaglandins on the permeability of the human small intestine. Gut 1986;27:1292–7.

22. Bjarnason I, Smethurst P, Macpherson A, et al. Glucose and citrate reduce the permeability changes caused by indomethacin in humans. Gastroenterology 1992;102:1546–50.

23. Sigthorsson G, Crane R, Simon T, et al. COX-2 inhibition with rofecoxib does not increase intestinal permeability in healthy subjects: a double blind crossover study comparing rofecoxib with placebo and indomethacin. Gut 2000;47:527–32.

24. Bjarnason I, Zanelli G, Smith T, et al. Nonsteroidal anti-inflammatory drug-induced intestinal inflammation in humans. Gastroenterology 1987;93:480–9.

25. Bjarnason I, Zanelli G, Prouse P, et al. Blood and protein loss via small intestinal inflammation induced by nonsteroidal antiinflammatory drugs. Lancet 1987;2: 711–4.
26. Hedenbro JL, Wetterberg P, Vallengren S, et al. Lack of correlation between fecal blood loss and drug-induced gastric mucosal lesions. Gastrointest Endosc 1998; 34:247–51.
27. Morris AJ, Madhok R, Sturrock RD, et al. Enteroscopic diagnosis of small bowel ulceration in patients receiving non–steroidal antiinflammatory drugs. Lancet 1991;337:520.
28. Moore RA, Derry S, Henry J, et al. Faecal blood loss with aspirin, nonsteroidal anti-inflammatory drugs and cyclo-oxygenase-2 selective inhibitors: systematic review of randomized trials using autologous chromium-labelled erythrocytes. Arthritis Res Ther 2008;10:R7.
29. Morris AJ, Murray L, Sturrock RD, et al. Short report: the effect of misoprostol on the anaemia of NSAID enteropathy. Aliment Pharmacol Ther 1994;8:343–6.
30. Davies NM, Saleh JY, Skjodt NM. Detection and prevention of NSAID-induced enteropathy. J Pharm Pharm Sci 2000;3:137–55. (www.ualberta.ca/~csps).
31. Freeman HJ. Sulindac-associated small bowel lesion. J Clin Gastroenterol 1986; 8:569–71.
32. Etienney I, Beaugerie L, Viboud C, et al. Non–steroidal anti-inflammatory drugs as a risk factor for acute diarrhoea: a case cross-over study. Gut 2003;52:260–3.
33. Allison MC, Howatson AG, Torrance CJ, et al. Gastrointestinal damage associated with the use of nonsteroidal antiinflammatory drugs. N Engl J Med 1992;327:749–54.
34. Costamagna G, Shah SK, Riccioni ME, et al. A prospective trial comparing small bowel radiographs and video capsule endoscopy for suspected small bowel disease. Gastroenterology 2002;123:999–1005.
35. Graham DY, Opekun AR, Willingham FF, et al. Visible small-intestinal mucosal injury in chronic NSAID users. Clin Gastroenterol Hepatol 2005;3:55–9.
36. Kurahara K, Matsumoto T, Iida M, et al. Clinical and endoscopic features of nonsteroidal anti-inflammatory drug-induced colonic ulcerations. Am J Gastroenterol 2001;96:473–80.
37. Lanas A, Sekar MC, Hirschowitz BI. Objective evidence of aspirin use in both ulcer and non–ulcer upper and lower gastrointestinal bleeding. Gastroenterology 1992;103:862–9.
38. Lanas A, Serrano P, Bajador E, et al. Evidence of aspirin use in both upper and lower gastrointestinal perforation. Gastroenterology 1997;112:683–9.
39. Hall RI, Petty AH, Cobden Y, et al. Enteritis and colitis associated with mefenamic acid. BMJ 1983;287:1182.
40. Zuccaro G. Epidemiology of lower gastrointestinal bleeding. Best Pract Res Clin Gastroenterol 2008;22:225–32.
41. Felder JB, Korelitz BI, Rajapakse R, et al. Effects of nonsteroidal antiinflammatory drugs on inflammatory bowel disease: a case control study. Am J Gastroenterol 2000;95:1949–54.
42. Forrest K, Symmons D, Foster P. Systematic review: is ingestion of paracetamol or non-steroidal anti-inflammatory drugs associated with exacerbations of inflammatory bowel disease? Aliment Pharmacol Ther 2004;20:1035–43.
43. Sandborn WJ, Stenson WF, Brynskov J, et al. Safety of celecoxib in patients with ulcerative colitis in remission: a randomized, placebo-controlled, pilot study. Clin Gastroenterol Hepatol 2006;4:203–11.
44. Davies NM. Sustained release and enteric coated NSAIDs: are they really GI safe? J Pharm Pharm Sci 1999;2:5–14. (www.ualberta.ca/~csps).

45. Trondstad RI, Aadland E, Holler T, et al. Gastroscopic findings after treatment with enteric-coated and plain naproxen tablets in healthy subjects. Scand J Gastroenterol 1987;20:239–42.

46. Piao ZZ, Lee MK, Lee BJ. Colonic release and reduced intestinal tissue damage of coated tablets containing naproxen inclusion complex. Int J Pharm 2008;350: 205–11.

47. Lang J, Price AB, Levi AJ, et al. Diaphragm disease: pathology of disease of the small intestine induced by non–steroidal anti-inflammatory drugs. J Clin Pathol 1988;41:516–26.

48. Santolaria S, Cabezali R, Ortego J, et al. Diaphragm disease of the small bowel: a case without apparent nonsteroidal anti-inflammatory drug use. J Clin Gastroenterol 2001;32:344–6.

49. Kessler WF, Shires GT, Fahey TJ. Surgical complications of non–steroidal anti-inflammatory drug-induced small bowel ulceration. J Am Coll Surg 1997;185:250–4.

50. Langman MJ, Morgan L, Worrall A. Use of anti-inflammatory drugs by patients admitted with small or large bowel perforations and haemorrhage. Br Med J (Clin Res Ed) 1985;290(6465):347–9.

51. Wilcox CM, Alexander LN, Cotsonis GA, et al. Nonsteroidal antiinflammatory drugs are associated with both upper and lower gastrointestinal bleeding. Dig Dis Sci 1997;42:990–7.

52. Lanas A, Perez-Aisa MA, Feu F, et al. A nationwide study of mortality associated with hospital admission due to severe gastrointestinal events and those associated with nonsteroidal antiinflammatory drug use. Am J Gastroenterol 2005; 100:1685–93.

53. Day TK. Intestinal perforation associated with osmotic slow release indomethacin capsules. Br Med J 1983;287:1671–2.

54. Kelly JP, Kaufman DW, Jurgelon JM, et al. Risk of aspirin-associated major upper-gastrointestinal bleeding with enteric-coated or buffered product. Lancet 1996; 348:1413–6 [see comments].

55. Laine L, Connors LG, Reicin A, et al. Serious lower gastrointestinal clinical events with nonselective NSAID or coxib use. Gastroenterology 2003;124:288–92.

56. Chan FK, Hung LC, Suen BY, et al. Celecoxib versus diclofenac and omeprazole in reducing the risk of recurrent ulcer bleeding in patients with arthritis. N Engl J Med 2002;26:2104–10.

57. Laine L, Curtis SP, Cryer B, et al. MEDAL Steering Committee. Assessment of upper gastrointestinal safety of etoricoxib and diclofenac in patients with osteoarthritis and rheumatoid arthritis in the Multinational Etoricoxib and Diclofenac Arthritis Long-term (MEDAL) programme: a randomised comparison. Lancet 2007;369(9560):465–73.

58. Lanas A, Garcia-Rodriguez LA, Ponce M, et al. Time trends and impact of upper and lower gastrointestinal bleeding and perforation in clinical practice. Am J Gastroenterol, in press.

59. Rahme E, Barkun A, Nedjar H, et al. Hospitalizations for upper and lower GI events associated with traditional NSAIDs and acetaminophen among the elderly in Quebec, Canada. Am J Gastroenterol 2008;103:872–82.

60. Foutch PG. Diverticular bleeding: are nonsteroidal anti-inflammatory drugs risk factors for hemorrhage and can colonoscopy predict outcome for patients? Am J Gastroenterol 1995;90:1779–84.

61. Piekarek P, Israelsson LA. Perforated colonic diverticular disease: the importance of NSAIDs, opioids, corticosteroids, and calcium channel blockers. Int J Colorectal Dis 2008;23:1193–7.

62. Riendeau D, Percival M, Boyce S, et al. Biochemical and pharmacological profile of a tetrasubstituted furanone as a highly selective COX-2 inhibitor. Br J Pharmacol 1997;121:105–17.

63. Hunt RH, Bowen B, Mortensen ER, et al. A randomized trial measuring fecal blood loss after treatment with Rofecoxib, Ibuprofen, or Placebo in healthy subjects. Am J Med 2000;109:201–6.

64. Hunt RH, Harper S, Callegari P, et al. Complementary studies of the gastrointestinal safety of the cyclo-oxygenase-2-selective inhibitor etoricoxib. Aliment Pharmacol Ther 2003;17(2):201–10.

65. Goldstein JL, Eisen GM, Lewis B, et al. Video capsule endoscopy to prospectively assess small bowel injury with celecoxib, naproxen plus omeprazole, and placebo. Clin Gastroenterol Hepatol 2005;3(2):133–41.

66. Goldstein JL, Eise GM, Lewis B, et al. Small bowel mucosal injury is reduced in healthy subjects treated with celecoxib compared with ibuprofen plus omeprazole, as assessed by video capsule endoscopy. Aliment Pharmacol Ther 2007; 25:1211–22.

67. Hawkey CJ, Ell C, Simon B, et al. Less small-bowel injury with lumiracoxib compared with naproxen plus omeprazole. Clin Gastroenterol Hepatol 2008;6: 536–44.

68. Maiden L, Thjodleifsson B, Seigal A, et al. Long-term effects of nonsteroidal anti-inflammatory drugs and cyclooxygenase–2 selective agents on the small bowel: a cross-sectional capsule enteroscopy study. Clin Gastroenterol Hepatol 2007;5: 1040–5.

69. Freitas J, Farricha V, Nascimento I, et al. Rofecoxib: a possible cause of acute colitis. J Clin Gastroenterol 2002;34:451–3.

70. Lanas A, García-Rodríguez LA, Arroyo MT, et al. Risk of upper gastrointestinal ulcer bleeding associated with selective cyclo-oxygenase-2 inhibitors, traditional non-aspirin non–steroidal anti-inflammatory drugs, aspirin and combinations. Gut 2006;55:1731–8.

71. Peura D, Chan FK, Wilcox CM, et al. Response to Ray and colleagues: the called-for large clinical trial is already ongoing. Gastroenterology 2008;134(1): 370–1.

72. Smecuol E, Sanchez P, Ines M, et al. Low dose aspirin affects the small bowel mucosa. Results of a pilot study using a multidimensional assessment. Clin Gastroenterol Hepatol, in press.

73. Bjarnason I, Peters TJ. Intestinal permeability, non–steroidal anti-inflammatory drug enteropathy and inflammatory bowel disease: an overview. Gut 1989;30: 22–8.

74. Davies NM. Non–steroidal anti-inflammatory drug-induced gastrointestinal permeability. Aliment Pharmacol Ther 1998;12:303–20.

75. Bjarnason I, Takeuchi K, Bjarnason A, et al. The G.U.T. of gut. Scand J Gastroenterol 2004;39:807–15.

76. Mylonaki M, Fritscher-Ravens A, Swain P. Wireless capsule endoscopy: a comparison with push enteroscopy in patients with gastroscopy and colonoscopy negative gastrointestinal bleeding. Gut 2003;52:1122–6.

77. Signorelli C, Villa F, Rondonotti E, et al. Sensitivity and specificity of the suspected blood identification system in video capsule enteroscopy. Endoscopy 2005;37: 1170–3.

78. Chong AK, Chin BW, Meredith CG. Clinically significant small-bowel pathology identified by double-balloon enteroscopy but missed by capsule endoscopy. Gastrointest Endosc 2006;64:445–9.

79. Maiden L, Thjodleifsson B, Theodors A, et al. A quantitative analysis of NSAID-induced small bowel pathology by capsule enteroscopy. Gastroenterology 2005;128:1172–8.

80. Barnert J, Messmann H. Management of lower gastrointestinal bleeding. Best Pract Res Clin Gastroenterol 2008;22:295–312.

81. Watanabe T, Sugimori S, Kameda N, et al. Small bowel injury by low-dose enteric-coated aspirin and treatment with misoprostol: a pilot study. Clin Gastroenterol Hepatol 2008;6:1279–82.

82. Lanas A. Role of nitric oxide in the gastrointestinal tract. Arthritis Res Ther 2008; 10(Suppl 2):S4 Epub 2008 Oct 17.

83. Hawkey CJ, Jones JI, Atherton CT, et al. Bjarnason IT Gastrointestinal safety of AZD3582, a cyclooxygenase inhibiting nitric oxide donator: proof of concept study in humans. Gut 2003;52(11):1537–42.

84. Niwa Y, Nakamura M, Ohmiya N, et al. Efficacy of rebamipide for diclofenac-induced small-intestinal mucosal injuries in healthy subjects: a prospective, randomized, double-blinded, placebo-controlled, cross-over study. J Gastroenterol 2008;43(4):270–6.

85. Sivalingam N, Hanumantharaya R, Faith M, et al. Curcumin reduces indomethacin-induced damage in the rat small intestine. J Appl Toxicol 2007;27(6):551–60.

86. Hayllar J, Smith T, Macpherson A, et al. Nonsteroidal antiinflammatory drug-induced small intestinal inflammation and blood loss. Effects of sulfasalazine and other disease-modifying antirheumatic drugs. Arthritis Rheum 1994;37:1146–50.

87. Robert A, Asano T. Resistance of germfree rats to indomethacin-induced intestinal lesions. Prostaglandins 1974;14:333–41.

88. Koga H, Aoyagi K, Matsumoto T, et al. Experimental enteropathy in athymic and euthymic rats: synergistic role of lipopolysaccharide and indomethacin. Am J Phys 1999;273(3 Pt 1):G576–82.

89. Bjarnason I, Hayllar J, Smethurst P, et al. Metronidazole reduces intestinal inflammation and blood loss in non-steroidal anti-inflammatory drug induced enteropathy. Gut 1992;33(9):1204–8.

Helicobacter pylori-Negative Nonsteroidal Anti-Inflammatory Drug-Negative Ulcer

Kenneth E.L. McColl, MD, FMedSci, FRSE

KEYWORDS

- Ulcer • *Heliocobacter pylori*
- Nonsteriodal anti-inflammatory drugs • Negative

The major causes of ulceration of the stomach and duodenum are *Helicobacter pylori* infection and the use of nonsteroidal anti-inflammatory drugs (NSAIDs) or aspirin.[1–5] However, some ulcers are apparently unrelated to those risk factors, and there is considerable variation in the reported proportion of such ulcers. Recent reports from North America suggest that up to 50% of ulcers are *H pylori* negative,[6–8] whereas in other parts of the world, a proportion of *H pylori*-negative ulcers remains much lower at less than 5%.[3,9,10] At least two factors may explain this marked variation in the re-ported proportion of ulcers being unrelated to *H pylori* infection and NSAIDs. The first is the background prevalence of *H pylori* infection in the community being studied, and the second is the robustness of the exclusion of *H pylori* infection and of the use of NSAIDs and aspirin (**Fig. 1**).

The background prevalence of *H pylori* infection varies markedly between different countries, being almost 100% in some regions of the developing world and less than 10% in highly affluent communities. If one assumes that the risk of developing an ulcer in any country is one in four in an *H pylori* infected subject and one in 20 in an unin-fected subject, one can calculate the effect of the background prevalence of the infec-tion on the proportion of ulcers that are *H pylori* negative. This simple mathematical calculation indicates that the proportion of *H pylori*-negative ulcers would be only 5% in a country with a 65% background prevalence of the infection. In contrast, the proportion of *H pylori*-negative ulcers would be 44% in a country with a 20% back-ground prevalence of *H pylori* infection. A relatively small decrease in the prevalence of the infection in the community markedly increases the proportion of *H pylori*-nega-tive to *H pylori*-positive ulcers, as it simultaneously increases the number of *H pylori*-negative ulcers and decreases the number of *H pylori*-positive ulcers. The background

Medical Sciences, Gardiner Institute, Western Infirmary, Glasgow, Scotland, G11 6NT, UK
E-mail address: k.e.l.mccoll@clinmed.gla.ac.uk

Gastroenterol Clin N Am 38 (2009) 353–361
doi:10.1016/j.gtc.2009.03.004
0889-8553/09/$ – see front matter © 2009 Elsevier Inc. All rights reserved.

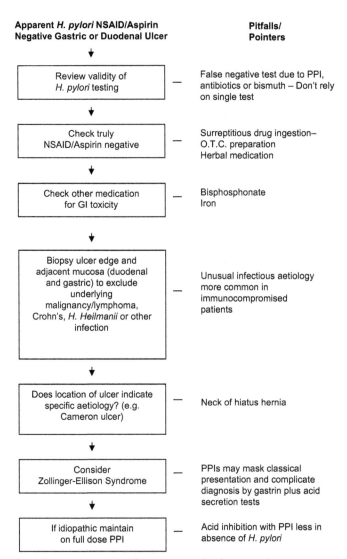

Apparent *H. pylori* NSAID/Aspirin Negative Gastric or Duodenal Ulcer

Pitfalls/ Pointers

Review validity of *H. pylori* testing — False negative test due to PPI, antibiotics or bismuth – Don't rely on single test

Check truly NSAID/Aspirin negative — Surreptitious drug ingestion– O.T.C. preparation Herbal medication

Check other medication for GI toxicity — Bisphosphonate Iron

Biopsy ulcer edge and adjacent mucosa (duodenal and gastric) to exclude underlying malignancy/lymphoma, Crohn's, *H. Heilmanii* or other infection — Unusual infectious aetiology more common in immunocompromised patients

Does location of ulcer indicate specific aetiology? (e.g. Cameron ulcer) — Neck of hiatus hernia

Consider Zollinger-Ellison Syndrome — PPIs may mask classical presentation and complicate diagnosis by gastrin plus acid secretion tests

If idiopathic maintain on full dose PPI — Acid inhibition with PPI less in absence of *H. pylori*

Fig. 1. Flow chart for management of apparent *Helicobacter pylori* NSAID/aspirin negative gastric or duodenal ulcer. (*From* McColl KE. How I manage *H pylori*-negative NSAID/aspirin-negative peptic ulcers. Am J Gastroenterol 2009;104:192; with permission.)

prevalence of *H pylori* infection in Scotland is 65%, which is consistent with 95% of the ulcers occurring in *H pylori*-infected subjects.[11] In the United States, the prevalence of *H pylori* infection is much slower at about 30% in the white population, which is consistent with 20% of the ulcer patients being *H pylori* negative.[12]

If the prevalence of *H pylori* infection falls over the next few decades, so will the prevalence of ulcer disease. However, a proportion of *H pylori*-negative ulcers will progressively increase, and they will become a predominant type of ulcer disease.

The falling prevalence of *H pylori* infection may increase the prevalence of *H pylori*-negative ulcers as well as the proportion of *H pylori*-negative to -positive ulcers. It is quite likely that some patients with *H pylori*-positive ulcers would have developed these ulcers even in the absence of *H pylori* infection, but because of the infection, they are labeled *H pylori*-positive ulcers. Only with the fall in *H pylori* prevalence in the community will these ulcers become apparent as *H pylori*-negative ulcers and thus will increase the number categorized as *H pylori*-negative ulcers.

It is unclear whether ulcers that persist after successful *H pylori* eradication have a similar etiology to ulcers first presenting in the absence of the infection. The proportion of ulcers remaining unhealed following successful eradication of *H pylori* infection is approximately 10%.[13–15] Are these ulcers the same as *H pylori*-negative ulcers with the infection merely having been an innocent bystander due to its high prevalence in the general population? Alternatively, has the infection produced permanent changes to the structure and function of the stomach, which continues to predispose to mucosal ulceration after the organism has been eradicated? The fact that the eradication of *H pylori* infection cures the great majority of patients with even severe ulcer disease, provided they are not NSAID or aspirin related, points against the infection causing a permanent ulcer diathesis. It would therefore seem most likely that ulcers recurring after *H pylori* eradication are equivalent to ulcers in patients without evidence of current or previous *H pylori* infection and should be classified and managed in the same way.

MANAGEMENT OF PATIENTS WITH APPARENT *H PYLORI*-NEGATIVE NONSTREOIDAL ANTI-INFLAMMATORY DRUGS-NEGATIVE ULCERS

If a patient is found to have ulceration of the stomach or duodenum without evidence of *H pylori* infection or a history of NSAID/aspirin ingestion, then it is necessary to undertake further investigations to determine the etiology of the ulcer disease. Such investigations are necessary, because they may reveal causes that lead to the need for specific treatment. Merely treating a patient found to have an *H pylori*-negative NSAID-negative ulcer with acid inhibitory medication is probably inappropriate.

The first consideration in a patient not taking NSAIDs found to have chronic ulceration of the duodenum and stomach and a negative *H pylori* test is that the test result is a false negative. Several medications frequently prescribed for patients with upper gastrointestinal (GI) symptoms or disease result in false-negative *H pylori* tests. The elevation of intragastric pH by proton pump inhibitors or high-dose H_2 antagonists markedly reduces the bacterium's urease activity and may produce false-negative urease tests, including the breath test and the urease strip test.[16–18] Such therapy also reduces the density of colonization in both the gastric antrum and body.[19,20] Though patients are advised to stop such medication 2 to 3 weeks before *H pylori* testing, compliance with this advice is unreliable, particularly in asymptomatic subjects. Many antibiotics, as well as bismuth-containing preparations, will also suppress *H pylori* infection and its urease activity. Even under optimal conditions, most individual *H pylori* tests have a sensitivity less than 95%, which means that 1 in 20 infected subjects may be missed.[21]

One situation where *H pylori* infection is particularly likely to be missed is when a patient presents with acute upper GI bleeding secondary to ulcer disease. The biopsy urease test has a higher false-negative rate in this setting possibly due to the effect of blood in the stomach together with the medications prescribed in the acute clinical situation.[22]

It is extremely important that *H pylori* is not missed in patients with ulcer disease, as this will deny them the chance of long-term cure of the condition by eradicating the infection. It will also leave them at increased risk of developing ulcer complications over subsequent years. To ensure that *H pylori* infection is not missed, it is important to take biopsies from both the antrum and body region of the stomach for both histology and urease tests. In addition, it may also be appropriate to check *H pylori* serology. A recent study has suggested that in some patients with duodenal ulceration, the infection is confined to the duodenal mucosa and eradicating it cures the ulcer disease.[23] Consequently, in patients with duodenal ulceration and no evidence of *H pylori* in the stomach, biopsies should also be taken from the duodenal mucosa for examination for *H pylori* organisms.

In addition to thoroughly excluding *H pylori* infection, it is also important to be certain that the patient is not taking unrecognized NSAIDs or other medication that might be causing the condition. A careful history and examination of recent prescription records are important. Patients should also be carefully questioned about their use of over-the-counter medications including herbal medications, some of which contain salicylates. In some cases, urine and serum analyses to detect surreptitious use of these drugs may be appropriate.[24] Several medications in addition to NSAIDs and aspirin may damage the GI mucosa, including iron, bisphosphonates, and colchicine, and all medicines recently taken by patients should be scrutinized for any potential mucosal-damaging effects. Careful reassessment of the *H pylori* status and NSAID aspirin usage will reduce the number of unexplained ulcers. However, a small proportion of ulcers does occur in the absence of well-established risk factors and may be related to a variety of other conditions. The one condition not to be missed in patients with unexplained gastric or duodenal ulceration is an underlying tumor. Before a routine biopsy is performed on the ulcers of the stomach to exclude cancer, this is not the practice for duodenal ulceration. However, in a patient with *H pylori*-negative NSAID-negative duodenal ulceration, the possibility of underlying carcinoma or lymphoma needs to be considered, and this is one situation where biopsies should also be taken from the duodenal ulcer and surrounding duodenal mucosa.

Another cause of gastric and/or duodenal ulceration in patients without *H pylori* infection and not taking NSAIDs/gastrin is Crohn's disease.[5,25] The pattern of upper GI ulceration associated with Crohn's disease is highly variable. In some patients with Crohn's disease, the disorder may be confined to the stomach and/or duodenum. Consequently, biopsies should be taken from both the duodenum and stomach in patients with unexplained ulcer disease to check for granulomas and other histologic features of Crohn's disease. In certain circumstances, investigations of the more distal GI tract may be indicated.

Patients with ulceration of the upper GI tract have been reported to have infections other than *H pylori*. Goddard and colleagues[26] reported that in duodenal ulceration associated with *Helicobacter Heilmannii* treating the infection with quadruple anti-*H pylori* therapy cured the ulcer disease.[26] There are also a number of case reports of chronic gastric ulcers associated with cytomegalovirus infection in immunocompromised patients.[27,28] The typical inclusion bodies are seen in the gastric biopsies. These ulcers healed following treatment with genciclovir.[27,28] There is also a report of the presence of the herpes simplex virus in *H pylori*-negative ulcers, although the nature of the association is unclear.[29]

Cameron and Higgins[30] reported ulceration of the proximal stomach in patients with hiatus hernia and occurring where the gastric mucosa passes through the diaphragmatic hiatus. These ulcers were associated with iron deficiency anemia, although the nature of the association is unclear. The ulcers may be single or multiple. The authors postulated that these ulcers were related to mucosal trauma or ischemia. These Cameron ulcers were described before *H pylori* infection was recognized, and thus the role of the infection is unclear. However, if ulcers at this site are present in patients with no other explanation or persist after treating *H pylori* infection, they may well be caused by local mucosal trauma or ischemia.

Gastric ulceration has also been reported following high-dose radiotherapy of the upper abdominal region.[31] This is assumed to have been a direct complication of the therapy, although the *H pylori* status of the patients has not been documented.[31] For many years, radiotherapy of the thorax has been used to produce experimental duodenal ulcers in laboratory animals.[32] It is thought to exert its effects by interfering with the protective functions afforded by the vagus nerve.

Ulcers may also occur in patients with severe systemic illness, for example, following extensive burns, and these stress ulcers are likely to be independent of *H pylori* status.[22]

Systemic mastocytosis causes duodenal ulceration due to the histamine stimulating increased acid secretion.[33] Other manifestations of the increased histamine release, including pruritis, flushing, and maculopapular rash, should make one suspect the diagnosis. In addition, a mast cell infiltrate is apparent in gastric and duodenal biopsies. The mechanism of duodenal ulceration in systemic mastocytosis would indicate that it may occur in the absence of *H pylori* infection, although this has not been formally documented.

Most of the causes of *H pylori*-negative NSAIDs/aspirin-negative ulcers can be detected by careful clinical history and upper GI endoscopy, including taking adequate biopsies of the ulcer and surrounding tissue and including both the stomach and the duodenum. If this does not provide a satisfactory explanation for mucosal ulceration, then one has to consider the possibility of Zollinger Ellison syndrome.

The Zollinger Ellison syndrome is due to an underlying gastrin-secreting tumor and effects of the hypergastrinemia on the upper GI tract. The constant high levels of gastric acid secretion stimulated by the persisting hypergastrinaemia usually result in severe and multiple ulcers of the stomach and duodenum, and the ulceration often extends into the more distal duodenum. Ulcer complications, including perforation and bleeding, are common, and reflux esophagitis is also associated with the condition. The syndrome may also cause diarrhea, which is thought to be due to the high levels of acid emptying the duodenum, denaturing the duodenal and pancreatic enzymes necessary for normal and esophageal function. Patients may have a family history of endocrine tumors, as the Zollinger Ellison syndrome is sometimes part of a multiple endocrine neoplasia syndrome. The classical description of the Zollinger Ellison syndrome was made before the age of powerful proton pump inhibitor therapy, which effectively suppresses the acid secretion and thus the severe manifestations of the disease. Patients with upper GI symptoms are usually commenced on acid inhibitory therapy before endoscopic investigation, and this may result in the endoscopic features being similar to patients with more common forms of ulcer disease. Proton pump inhibitor therapy also makes the diagnosis of the Zollinger Ellison syndrome by these additional tests more complicated. Interpretation of pentagastrin-stimulated acid output required discontinuation of proton pump inhibitor therapy, and this may be difficult and probably unwise in patients who may have an underlying gastrinoma. Rebound acid hypersecretion during the first few weeks after discontinuing proton pump inhibitor therapy may further complicate the interpretation of acid secretory tests. Serum gastrin may be difficult to interpret due to its increased concentration as a result of the proton pump inhibitor therapy, which will overlap with values in patients with gastrinoma.[34] The most discriminating test in this situation is probably the secretin test.[35,36] Following intravenous injection of secretin, the serum gastrin increases in patients with gastrinoma but not in control patients. A rise of 120 pg/mL is considered positive.[37] This occurs due to the fact that gastrinomas have secretin receptors.[37] It should, however, be noted that the effects of proton pump inhibitor therapy on the interpretation of the secretin test are not known.

Once all the above investigations have been completed, there remain a very small proportion of patients with apparently idiopathic ulcer disease. Do these patients have a similar unrecognized etiology or are they a heterogeneous group of patients with different unrecognized etiologies? We performed gastric function tests in a small group of subjects with idiopathic gastroduodenal ulceration and observed increased acid output, increased gastrin, and accelerated gastric emptying.[38] Exaggerated gastrin response was also observed by Kamada and colleagues[38] in three of nine idiopathic ulcer patients. These abnormalities resemble those occurring in patients with H pylori infection in whom the exaggerated gastrin caused by the infection leads to increased acid output and thus duodenal ulceration. It was suggested that some unrecognized underlying factor might be reproducing the changes in association with the H pylori infection. However, since then we and others have recognized that discontinuation of proton pump inhibitor therapy can produce the same abnormalities, that is, hypergastrinemia and rebound acid hypersecretion.[39–41] Most of the patients who have been studied with idiopathic ulcer disease have been on powerful acid inhibitory therapy, and it is now unclear whether the abnormalities reported are indeed related to the underlying disease or related to its treatment with powerful acid inhibitory therapy.

The management of patients with idiopathic ulcers is unclear. The published studies of the value of acid inhibitor therapy in healing ulcers have been performed in patients with H pylori-positive ulcers or with NSAID associated ulcers. Proton pump inhibitor therapy has been shown to be more effective at inhibiting acid secretion in H pylori infected versus uninfected subjects.[42,43] This can be explained by the fact that such therapy causes an increase in oxyntic mucosal gastritis, which impairs gastric secretion further and augments the pharmacologic effect of the drug. H pylori-negative ulcers are more difficult to manage and more susceptible to complications than traditional ulcers.[5,22,44] This may be related to their reduced responsiveness to acid inhibitor therapy, and consequently increased doses of proton pump inhibitor therapy may be appropriate. The natural history of idiopathic ulcers is fully documented due to their rarity. In addition, the role of surgery to reduce gastric acid secretion is unclear. However, my personal experience is that these patients can be successfully managed in the long term on adequate proton pump inhibitor therapy.

SUMMARY

The most important clinical point for dyspeptic H pylori-negative NSAID-absent negative ulcers is to adequately ensure that these common risk factors are indeed absent. Once that is done, further investigations to include the rare causes of ulcer disease need to be performed and exclusion of underlying malignancy ensured. The possibility of the Zollinger Ellison syndrome should be considered, remembering that proton pump inhibitor therapy will mitigate its classical, clinical features.

REFERENCES

1. Hyvarinen H, Salmenkyla S, Sipponen P. Helicobacter pylori-negative duodenal and pyloric ulcer: role of NSAIDs. Digestion 1996;57:305–9.
2. Gisbert JP, Blanco M, Mateos JM, et al. H pylori-negative duodenal ulcer prevalence and causes in 774 patients. Dig Dis Sci 1999;44(11):2295–302.
3. Tsuji H, Kohli Y, Fukumitsu S, et al. Helicobacter pylori-negative gastric and duodenal ulcers. J Gastroenterol 1999;34:455–60.
4. Elitsur Y, Lawrence Z. Non-Helicobacter pylori related duodenal ulcer disease in children. Helicobacter 2001;6(3):239–43.

5. McColl KEL, El-Nujumi AM, Chittajallu RS, et al. A study of the pathogenesis of *Helicobacter pylori* negative chronic duodenal ulceration. Gut 1993;34:762–8.
6. Ciociola AA, McSorley DJ, Turner K, et al. *Helicobacter pylori* infection rates in duodenal patients in the United States may be lower than previously estimated. Am J Gastroenterol 1999;94:1834–40.
7. Sprung DJ, Apter M, Allen B, et al. The prevalence of *Helicobacter pylori* in duodenal ulcer disease – a community based study. Am J Gastroenterol 1996; 91:1926.
8. Jyotheeswaran S, Shah AN, Jim HO, et al. Prevalence of *Helicobacter pylori* in peptic ulcer patients in Great Rochester, NY: is empirical triple therapy justified? Am J Gastroenterol 1998;93:574–8.
9. Aoyama N, Shinoda Y, Maisushima Y, et al. *Helicobacter pylori* negative peptic ulcer in Japan: which contributes most to peptic ulcer development, *Helicobacter pylori*, NSAIDs or stress? XII. J Gastroenterol 2000;35:33–7.
10. Arroyo MT, Montse F, deArgila CM, et al. The prevalence of peptic ulcer not related to Helicobacter pylori or non-steroidal anti-inflammatory drugs is negligible in Southern Europe. *Helicobacter* 2004;9:249–54.
11. McDonagh TA, Woodward M, Morrison CE, et al. *Helicobacter pylori* infection and coronary heart disease in the north Glasgow MONICA population. Eur Heart J 1997;18:1257–60.
12. Graham DY, Malaty HM, Evans DG, et al. Epidemiology of *Helicobacter pylori* infection in an asymptomatic population in the United States. Gastroenterology 1991;100:1495–501.
13. Hopkins RJ, Girardi LS, Turney EA. Relationship between *Helicobacter pylori* eradication and reduced duodenal and gastric ulcer recurrence: A review. Gastroenterology 1996;110:1244–52.
14. Penston JG. Review article: Clinical aspects of *Helicobacter pylori* eradication therapy in peptic ulcer disease. Aliment Pharmacol Ther 1996;10:469–86.
15. Laine L, Jopkins RJ, Girardi LS. Has the impact of *Helicobacter pylori* therapy on ulcer recurrence in the United States been overstated? A meta-analysis of rigorously designed trials. Am J Gastroenterol 1998;93(9):1409–15.
16. El-Nujumi A, Hilditch TE, Williams C, et al. Current or recent proton pump inhibitor therapy markedly impairs the accuracy of the [^{14}C] urea breath test. Eur J Gastroenterol Hepatol 1998;10:759–64.
17. Chey WD, Spybrook M, Carpenter S, et al. Prolonged effect of omeprazole on the ^{14}C-urea breath test. Am J Gastroenterol 1996;91:89–92.
18. Chey WD, Woods M, Scheiman JM, et al. Lansoprazole and ranitidine affect the accuracy of the ^{14}C-urea breath test by a pH-dependent mechanism. Am J Gastroenterol 1997;92:446–50.
19. Graham DY, Genta R, Evans D, et al. *Helicobacter pylori* does not migrate from the antrum to the corpus in response to omeprazole. Am J Gastroenterol 1996; 91:2120–4.
20. Dicket W, Kenny BD, McConnell JB. Effect of proton pump inhibitors on the detection of *Helicobacter pylori* in gastric biopsies. Aliment Pharmacol Ther 1996;10:289–93.
21. McNulty C, Teare L, Owen R, et al. Test and treat for dyspepsia – but which test? Urea breath test and stool antigen test are better than serological tests. Br Med J 2005;330(7483):105–6.
22. Chan HL, Wu JC, Chan FK, et al. Is non-*Helicobacter pylori*, non-NSAID peptic ulcer a common cause of upper GI bleeding? A prospective study of 977 patients. Gastrointest Endosc 2001;53:438–42.

23. Pietroiusti A, Forlini A, Magrini A, et al. Isolated *H pylori* duodenal colonization and idiopathic duodenal ulcers. Am J Gastroenterol 2008;103:55–61.
24. Hirschowitz BI. Intractable peptic ulceration due to aspirin abuse in patients who have not had gastric surgery. Gastroenterology 1997;112:A962.
25. Borody T, Byrnes D, George L, et al. How common are duodenal ulcers negative for *Helicobacter pylori*? No. 5. Gastroenterology 1990;98(Pt 2):A23.
26. Goddard AF, Logan RP, Atherton JC, et al. Healing of duodenal ulcer after eradication of *Helicobacter heilmannii*. Lancet 1997;349:1815–6.
27. Fukami T, Akiyama K, Ohbayashi Y, et al. Cytomegalovirus-associated gastric ulcers in immunocompromised patients. Dig Endosc 2001;13:54–60.
28. Orton DI, Orteu CH, Rustin MH. Cytomegalovirus-associated gastric ulcer in an immunosuppressed patient with pemphigus vulgaris. Clin Exp Dermatol 2001; 26(2):170–2.
29. Tsamakidis K, Panotopoulou E, Dimitroulopoulos D, et al. Herpes simplex virus type 1 in peptic ulcer disease: an inverse association with *Helicobacter pylori*. World J Gastroenterol 2005;11(42):6644–9.
30. Cameron AJ, Higgins JA. Linear gastric erosion. Gastroenterology 1986;91:338–42.
31. Streitparth F, Pech M, Bohmig M, et al. *In Vivo* assessment of the gastric mucosal tolerance dose after single fraction, small volume irradiation of liver malignancies by computed tomography-guided, high-dose-rate brachytherapy. Int J Radiat Oncol Boil Phys 2006;65(5):1479–86.
32. Gompertz RH, Michalowski AS, Man WK, et al. Duodenal ulcer – a model of impaired mucosal defence. Gut 1992;33(8):1044–9.
33. Cherner JA, Jensen RT, Dubois A, et al. Gastrointestinal dysfunction in systemic mastocytosis: a prospective study. Gastroenterology 1988;95:657–67.
34. Berna MJ, Hoffman M, Serrano J, et al. Prospective study of fasting serum gastrin in 309 patients from the National Institute of Health and comparison with 2229 cases from the literature. Medicine 2006;85(6):295–330.
35. Metz DC, Buchanan M, Purich E, et al. A randomised controlled crossover study comparing synthetic porcine and human secretins with biologically derived porcine secretin to diagnose Zollinger-Ellison syndrome. Aliment Pharmacol Ther 2001;15:669–76.
36. Berna MJ, Hoffman M, Long SH, et al. Prospective study of gastrin provocative testing in 293 patients from the National Institutes of Health and comparison with 537 cases from the literature. Evaluation of diagnostic criteria, proposal of new criteria, and correlations with clinical and tumoral features. Medicine 2006; 85:331–64.
37. Long SH, Berna MJ, Thil M, et al. Secretin-receptor and secretin-receptor-variant expression in gastrinomas: correlation with clinical and tumoral features and secretin and calcium provocative test results. J Clin Endocrinol Metab 2007; 92(11):4394–402.
38. Kamada T, Haruma K, Kusunoki H, et al. Significance of an exaggerated meal-stimulated gastrin response in pathogenesis of *Helicobacter pylori*-negative duodenal ulcer. Dig Dis Sci 2003;48(4):644–51.
39. Gillen D, Wirz AA, Ardill JE, et al. Rebound hypersecretion after omeprazole and its relation to on-treatment acid suppression and *Helicobacter pylori* status. Gastroenterology 1999;116:239–47.
40. Gillen D, Wirz AA, McColl KE. *Helicobacter pylori* eradication releases prolonged increased acid secretion following omeprazole treatment. Gastroenterology 2004;126(4):980–8.

41. Waldum HL, Arnestad JS, Brenna E, et al. Marked increase in gastric acid secretory capacity after omeprazole treatment. Gut 1996;29:649–53.
42. Labenz J, Tillenburg B, Peitz U, et al. *Helicobacter pylori* augments the pH-increasing effect of omeprazole in patients with duodenal ulcer. Gastroenterology 1996;110:725–32.
43. Verdu EF, Armstrong D, Fraser R, et al. Effect of *Helicobacter pylori* status on intragastric pH during treatment with omeprazole. Gut 1995;36:539–43.
44. Hung LC, Ching JY, Sung JJ, et al. Long-term outcome of *Helicobacter pylori*-negative idiopathic bleeding ulcers: a prospective cohort study. Gastroenterology 2005;128:1845–50.

Differences in Peptic Ulcer Between the East and the West

Rupert W. Leong, MBBS, MD, FRACP[a,b,*]

KEYWORDS

- Ulcer • Epidemiology • Asia • Caucasian • Ethnicity
- Management • Polymorphism • Race

Although the "East" and the "West" are loose terms based originally in differentiating ancient civilizations, their cultures, religions, and subsequent colonization to other parts of the world, this review differentiates the East and the West based on racial and ethnic differences, genetic ancestry, customs and lifestyles, and geography. These factors may have particular relevance in the development of peptic ulcer disease (PUD). In particular, emphasis is laid on reviewing the similarities and differences between the two based on the epidemiology, clinical manifestations, treatments, and complications of PUD.

A systematic review of the literature was performed. Publications were selected based on those that clearly distinguished populations descended from the Western civilization from their Eastern counterparts. The "West" was defined as Caucasian populations of Western and Central European ancestry. The "East" referred to populations in South, South-East, and Far-East Asia. Studies on populations from the Middle East, South and Central America, and Africa were excluded. A search of published literature was performed using PubMed from 1966 through December 2008 using the search terms "peptic ulcer," "Asia(n)," and "Western/Caucasian." In addition, in the evaluation of causative factors for PUD, the search terms "prevalence/epidemiology," "*Helicobacter pylori*," and "nonsteroidal anti-inflammatory drugs" were used. *H pylori* prevalence studies in specific disease states were excluded, because they represented highly selected populations. Only recent publications from the end of 2006 to 2008 were included to reflect the declining *H pylori* prevalence rates worldwide. The literature was reviewed for studies on PUD epidemiology,

[a] Concord Hospital, Ambulatory Care Endoscopy Unit, Level 1 West, Hospital Road, Concord, Sydney NSW 2139, Australia
[b] Department of Gastroenterology, Bankstown-Lidcombe Hospital, Level 3, Elridge Road, Bankstown, Sydney NSW 2200, Australia
* Concord Hospital, Ambulatory Care Endoscopy Unit, Level 1 West, Hospital Road, Concord, Sydney NSW 2139, Australia.
E-mail address: rupertleong@hotmail.com

Gastroenterol Clin N Am 38 (2009) 363–379
doi:10.1016/j.gtc.2009.03.010
0889-8553/09/$ – see front matter. Crown Copyright © 2009 Elsevier Inc. All rights reserved.

causes, clinical features, and management directly comparing Eastern and Western populations. Studies on neoplastic, ischemic, or infective causes of gastroduodenal ulceration, gastroesophageal reflux disease, and inflammatory bowel diseases were excluded. Relevant clinical and basic science publications were identified, and the related references were also obtained. Authors were contacted to provide further material if required. From all eligible articles, one reviewer (R.W.L.) scrutinized the abstracts to finally select the relevant publications.

PEPTIC ULCERS
Epidemiology

Few publications directly compare PUD in the East with that in the West. The definition of PUD is mostly consistent in both the East and the West, although it is not explicitly expressed in most publications. The histopathologic description of PUD encompasses an epithelial defect, usually referring to the stomach or duodenum that extends down through the muscularis mucosae into the submucosa. The endoscopic definition usually requires the ulcerated surface breach to be obvious and with perceivable depth.[1]

Accurate descriptive epidemiology of PUD is difficult to ascertain, making direct comparisons difficult between the East and the West. Most peptic ulcers are asymptomatic, and diagnosis relies on radiology or gastroscopy. The availability of these tests varies according to local health care systems and accessibility to these tests by patients. Reported incidence rates may be biased toward symptomatic presentations, development of overt clinical complications such as hemorrhage or perforation, and mortality. As such, there is an underestimate of the true disease prevalence. The true point prevalence of PUD can be obtained only through invasive diagnostic procedures, such as with gastroscopy, on the general population. There are, however, few such studies given the risks and discomfort associated with this investigation. A Swedish adult study that performed gastroscopies on random population samples found the prevalence of PUD to be 4.1% with equal proportions of GUs and DUs. The presence of PUD also correlated poorly with symptoms.[2] A population-based endoscopy survey conducted in rural China found the PUD rate to be 9.3%. A total of 2423 individuals underwent gastroscopy. Of these, 137 had DUs (5.7%), 82 had non-malignant GUs (3.4%), and five had both DUs and GUs (0.2%).[3] These population-based studies may be representative of the Western and Eastern populations respectively, but there is probably greater heterogeneity in different populations within these regions. Differences in the background risk factors, especially with the *H pylori* infection rate and use of ulcerogenic drugs, are the likely causes of heterogeneity of these results.

In the past, many Asian countries tended to have a higher DU-to-GU ratio.[4] However, in many Asian countries there has been a gradual decline in this relationship. This most likely represents the declining prevalence of *H pylori* infection, which decreases DU risk and increasing use of aspirin and NSAIDs, which correspondingly increase the rate of GUs. A South Korean study of 895 patients with newly diagnosed PUD from Sep 2004 to Feb 2005 showed that the proportion of GU significantly increased from 44% to 48% with a corresponding decrease of DU from 45% to 39%.[5] In a retrospective review of 15,341 endoscopies performed in the Philippines, the overall prevalence of PUD and *H pylori* infection have decreased over the past 7 years from 36% to 19%. The study also noted a significant increase in GUs presenting over time.[6] In the pediatric population, upper gastrointestinal tract bleeding (UGIB) in Asia is more frequently caused by DUs. In the study by Guo and Zhan in China, DUs accounted for 54% of children with UGIB.[7] Recent studies from Hong Kong found that DUs accounted for 75% of UGIB, with the majority being caused by *H pylori*.[8] There is a male predisposition in presentation with UGIB in Asia, with a rate ranging from 1.9:1[7] to 2.6:1.[8] Similarly, the endoscopic finding of PUD has decreased in Australia. A retrospective review from 1990 to 1998 showed the prevalence of PUD decreasing significantly from 22% to 13%.[9] Despite the retrospective nature of these studies, there is agreement that PUD is decreasing in recent years in both the East and the West.

Historical Perspectives

PUD natural history has changed over the last 2 centuries. Data from the West show PUD to be rare before the 1800s. From the mid 1800s, GUs predominated over DUs. In the 1900s the prevalence of DUs increased to several times that of GUs.[10] In the United States and Canada, hospitalization for PUD declined in the 1950s to 1970s, especially in males with PUD hemorrhage. Then there were increasing proportions of females and the elderly who presented with complicated PUD.[11,12] In the United Kingdom, in a population study of 7590 incident PUD cases (DUs, 5564; GUs, 2026) from 1977 to 2001, presentation peaked in 1982 to 1986 and declined thereafter. There is a falling male preponderance, and GU patients tended to be older than DU patients. The mean age of both GU and DU patients increased over time.[13] In the 1990s, there was a rise in PUD hemorrhage in the elderly, particularly from DU. GU perforations declined, but DU perforations increased among elderly men.[14]

In an analysis of PUD mortality data from 1921 to 2004 from 6 European countries, there was a high correlation of data on PUD. The mortality rate of PUD increased among consecutive generations during the second half of the nineteenth century until shortly before the turn of the century and then decreased in all successive generations. The time trends of GU preceded those of DU by 10 to 30 years.[15] There are fewer epidemiology studies from Asia. In Japan, the risk of PUD also increased in birth cohorts born before the twentieth century and declined in subsequent generations, similar to Western data.[16] Declining PUD mortality occurred in both the East and the West but occurred later in the East.[17] A decline in DU with corresponding increase in GU, similar to the changes in the West, has been noted in Korea.[5]

Temporal Trend Changes in Peptic Ulcer Disease

The initial increase in PUD between 1850 and 1950 was thought to be due to a shift in the age of acquisition of *H pylori*. With the improvement in community hygiene, acquisition of infection tended to be later in life during adolescence. As opposed to acquisition of *H pylori* in early childhood, which leads to pangastritis, gastric atrophy, and reduced acidity, acquisition of *H pylori* later in life in a mature acid-secreting mucosa tends to confine the bacteria to the gastric antrum, where the bacteria inhibits D-cell function, further increasing gastric acid secretion.[18] This increase in gastric acidity would increase PUD prevalence and in particular DUs. The decrease in PUD death rates among generations born during the twentieth century is usually attributed to the improving standards of hygiene in developed countries and receding infection by *H pylori*. The increase in aspirin and/or NSAID consumption and the introduction of potent antisecretory medications probably have not affected the long-term downward trends of ulcer mortality. The use of ulcerogenic drugs, however, has contributed to the increased proportion of the GU component of PUD in recent years. Overall, data from the East and West support a birth-cohort effect of PUD.

RISK FACTORS
Gastric Physiology

Previous studies had found lower parietal cell mass in the Chinese[19] compared with Caucasians.[20] Parietal cell mass and maximal acid output after pentagastrin stimulation are higher in Caucasians than those in the Chinese. This difference was still present when the acid output was corrected for body weight with an acid output of 0.25 ± 0.11 mmol/h/kg for the Chinese and 0.30 ± 0.10 for Scots ($P<.01$) as well as after controlling for sex and age.[21] A higher *H pylori* prevalence in the Chinese, causing atrophic gastritis, may also contribute toward racial differences in gastric physiology.

Helicobacter pylori

H pylori infection plays an important part in the development of PUD. Because infection with the organism is typically subclinical, information on its prevalence is based mainly on serologic studies. Infection with *H pylori* in developing countries occurs at an earlier age than that in developed countries.[22,23]

Given the geographic variability and recent changes in *H pylori* prevalence, a review was conducted on recent publications on *H pylori* prevalence in the East and West. From a total of 725 articles from a Pubmed search using the terms "*Helicobacter pylori*" and "prevalence" published in late 2006 to 2008, 12 relevant prevalence studies from Asia and 13 from the West were found. An additional 17 articles on *H pylori* prevalence in other parts of the world or studies performed in highly selected populations were excluded. The prevalence of *H pylori* from these studies is summarized in **Table 1**.

The prevalence of *H pylori* infection varies widely both between and within populations based on geography, age, race, ethnicity, and socioeconomic status (SES). Overall, inadequate sanitation practices, low social class, crowded or high-density living conditions, and inadequate nutritional status are associated with a higher prevalence of infection.[24] Based on this, the rate of acquisition is generally higher in developing countries than that in industrialized countries.

Helicobacter pylori *in the East*

Traditionally, Asian countries demonstrated overall higher prevalence rates of *H pylori* compared with those in Western countries. In a study of 500 hospital patients from South India, the overall prevalence of *H pylori* was 80%. The prevalence rate varied according to the source of drinking water (prevalence of 92% when water came from wells compared with 74.8% from taps), socioeconomic status (SES; 86.1% with lower SES compared with 70% from higher SES), and crowded living conditions (high density, 83.7%; medium density, 76.6%; low density, 71.3%; all statistically significant). The greatest contribution toward *H pylori* prevalence was the clean water index (CWI), with a prevalence rate of 88.2% in those with access to low CWI and as low as 33.3% from those with high CWI.[25] The CWI reflected whether water is stored and reused, frequency of bathing, and whether water is boiled before drinking. These practices are highly variable within Asia and even within communities. Cultural practices and ethnicity may play additional roles in the higher rates of *H pylori* infection in Asia and other developing countries. In rural areas of China, the rate of mother-to-child transmission of *H pylori* may increase due to the traditional practice of close maternal contact with their children, including sharing the same bed, eating from the same bowls, using the same chopsticks, and even feeding infants by prechewing their food.[24] Cultural practices and local environmental conditions are likely to perpetuate the high rates of infection in Asia.

There are ethnic differences in the pattern of H pylori gastritis. Koreans and Japanese are more likely to have antral involvement compared with Americans and more likely to develop interstitial neutrophilic infiltration, intestinal metaplasia, and atrophy.[26] In patients with DUs, H pylori infection in the stomach usually results in antral-predominant gastritis, with a lower likelihood of corpus gastritis and intestinal metaplasia. Geographically, however, there is a difference in the risk of intestinal metaplasia in patients with DUs, with a significantly higher rate of intestinal metaplasia in Korea (38%) compared with that in Caucasian populations (10%, P = .018), indicating variability in the effects of H pylori.[27]

Within countries, there are also differences in H pylori prevalence rates between races. In Malaysia, differential prevalence rates of H pylori are noted among the Malay, Chinese, and Indian populations, with prevalence rates lowest in Malays (11.9%–29.2%), intermediate in the Chinese (26.7%–57.5%) and highest in Indians (49.4%–52.3%).[28] In contrast to other parts of Asia, Indonesia has a disproportionately low prevalence rate of H pylori infection. Over a 14-year period from 1998 to 2005, the prevalence of H pylori decreased from 12.8% to 2.9%.[29] Similarly low H pylori prevalence rates of 4% to –8% have also been described in the Malay population in Malaysia.[30] These prevalence rates are unexpected from a developing Asian country, and it is hypothesized that such populations with unexpectedly low prevalence or absence of H pylori may have descended from uninfected founding populations.[31] Alternatively, there may be as yet unknown host mechanisms that resist transmission and acquisition of the organism.

With the economic development of many parts of Asia, increasing prosperity and industrialization, and improving hygienic practices, several longitudinal studies from Asia have demonstrated declining H pylori seroprevalence. Serum from the National Institute of Infectious Diseases in Tokyo revealed a declining H pylori seroprevalence from 73% in 1974 to 55% in 1984 and to 39% in 1994.[32] In South Korea, the infection rate was 50.0% in 1997 but declined down to 40.6% in 2005 (P<.001).[33] In Guangzhou, southern China, the age-standardized seroprevalence of H pylori decreased from 62.5% in 1993 to 49.3% in 2003.[34] A decrease in H pylori prevalence in children represents a true decline in H pylori, especially in the coming years given the age-cohort effect in the acquisition of infection. In the pediatric population, many parts of China now report decrease in H pylori prevalence. In Linqu County of northeast China, the prevalence rate increased from 50% at ages 3 to 4 years to 85% at ages 9 to 10 years before falling to 67% at ages 11 to 12 years.[35] Previously, the high prevalence of H pylori at an early age was linked to the high rate of chronic atrophic gastritis and progression to gastric cancer in adults, especially in this region.[36] In Guangzhou, the prevalence of children with H pylori decreased from 30.8% to 19.4% during 10 years.[34] Hong Kong, in southern China, is characterized by rapid Westernization and industrialization. The H pylori prevalence has remained stable at 25% over time.[37] In this region, there is a high standard of hygiene, but overcrowding and familial clustering are thought to play important roles perpetuating H pylori transmission. H pylori either alone or in combination with ulcerogenic drugs is still a major cause of UGIB and accounted for 73.5% to 90.2% of bleeding in the pediatric population.[8,38]

Helicobacter pylori *in the West*
In contrast, Western countries generally have a lower rate of H pylori infection in comparison with Asia. Based on 13C urea breath test, the rate of H pylori infection in the Switzerland-born population was 11.9%, which was significantly lower than 26.6% (P = .003) for those residing in Switzerland but born outside of the country.[39]

Table 1
Recent prevalence data on *Helicobacter pylori* from the East and the West

Authors and Reference	Population	Region and Sample Size	Age Range (y)	Diagnostic Test	Prevalence (%)
Asia					
Ahmed et al.[25]	Hospital based	South India (500)	30–79	Gastric biopsy, 16S rRNA	80.0
Saragih et al.[29]	Endoscopy based	Indonesia	—	Histology	2.9
Lee at al.[33]	Endoscopy based	South Korea (8646)	>/=16	RUT	40.6
Chen et al.[34]	Population based	South China (1471)	Total	Serology	47.0
		(180)	1–4	—	19.4
		(105)	5–9	—	22.9
		(185)	10–19	—	36.8
		(253)	20–29	—	53.4
		(196)	30–39	—	54.6
		(204)	40–49	—	63.2
		(163)	50–59	—	57.7
		(185)	60–69	—	54.1
Fujimoto et al.[41]	Population based	3 areas, Japan (3819)	20–70+	Serology	55.4
Lin et al.[42]	Community based	Central Taiwan healthy school children (1625)	9–12	Serology	11.0
		Healthy school children (325)	13–15	—	12.3
		Teacher (253)	>/=25	—	45.1
Okuda et al.[43]	Birth cohort	Japan (108)	2	Stool antigen	3.7
Yim et al.[44]	Population based	South Korea (15,916)	16	Serology	56.0
Shi et al.[45]	Population based	Jiangsu province, China (1371)	5–100	UBT, serology	62.1
Tam et al.[46]	Population based	Hong Kong (2480)	6–19	UBT	13.1
Yanaoka et al.[47]	Population based, males	Western Japan (5,209)	40–60	Serology	70.1
Bhuiyan et al.[48]	Birth cohort study	Bangladesh (238)	0–2	Fecal antigen	50
				Serology	60

Caucasian					
Moujaber et al.[40]	Laboratory blood samples	Australians (2413)	1-59	Serology	15.4
Gruber et al.[39]	Hospital based	Swiss-born (101)	18-85	UBT	11.9
		Non-Swiss-born (252)	—		26.6
Mourad-Baars et al.[49]	Population based	Zuid-Holland, The Netherlands (1258)	2-4	Serology	1.2%
Dinic et al.[50]	School based	Nis, Serbia (283)	7-18	Serology	36.4
Boyanova et al.[51]	Endoscopy based	Bulgaria (658)	1-17	RUT, histology, culture	61.7
Thjodleifsson et al.[52]	Population based	Tartu, Estonia (240)	25-50	Serology	69
		Reykjavik, Iceland (447)	—		36
		Uppsala, Sweden (359)	—		11
Naja et al.[53]	Population based	Ontario, Canada (1306)	50-80	Serology	23.1
Weck et al.[54]	Population based	Saarland, Germany (9444)	50-74	Serology	48.8
Sterzl et al.[55]	Population based	Czech Republic (1621)	Mean age, 27	Serology	35.6
Segal et al.[56]	Endoscopy based	Canadians (204)	5-18	Histology, RUT, UBT, HpSA	7.1
Monno et al.[57]	Healthy volunteers	Albanians (1088)	16-64	Serology	70.7
Rejchrt et al.[58]	Hospital-based	Czech Republic (1810)	5-100	UBT	42.1
Gruber et al.[39]	Hospital-based	—	18-85	UBT	—
		Non-Swiss-born (252)	—		26.6
		Swiss-born (101)	—		11.9

Abbreviations: UBT, urea breath test; RUT, rapid urease test; HpSA, *H pylori* stool antigen test.

In Australia, the overall seroprevalence of *H pylori* infection was 15.1% in 2002 with no difference between genders. Seropositivity rates increased progressively with age from 4% in 1- to 4-year-olds to 23.3% in 50- to 59-year-olds.[40]

In general, there has been a decline in the rate of *H pylori* infection in many parts of the world. The risk of infection remains the same—overcrowding, unclean water sources, and possibly cultural behaviors that increase the rate of transmission between mother and babies maintain the higher prevalence rates in Asia. Asian countries that have become more Westernized have demonstrated reduction in the prevalence of *H pylori* infection, especially in the pediatric population. In the peak prevalence age group of 50- to 59-year-olds, however, the infection rate continues to be more than 50%. This group of patients therefore are at risk of developing PUD and other complications of *H pylori* infection. **Fig. 1** illustrates the varied and overlapping *H pylori* prevalence rates in the East and the West and their references.

DRUG-INDUCED

Aspirin and NSAIDs are important causes of PUD and are extensively used worldwide for their antiplatelet and anti-inflammatory properties, respectively. Unfortunately, these drugs are well known to cause PUD, including complications of UGIB and perforations.[59] Endoscopic studies of patients commencing NSAIDs show a similar risk of ulcer development in Eastern and Western populations. The observed prevalence of endoscopic GUs among NSAID users was 15.6% in a Japanese study,[60] which is similar to a Western study in which the point prevalence of the endoscopic finding of PUD was 15.4%.[61]

Few data are available on the development of complicated PUDs that are comparable between the East and the West. Data from a UK nested, case control study found the incidence of adverse upper GI events to be 1.36 per 1000 person years (95% confidence interval [CI], 1.34–1.39). The odds ratio

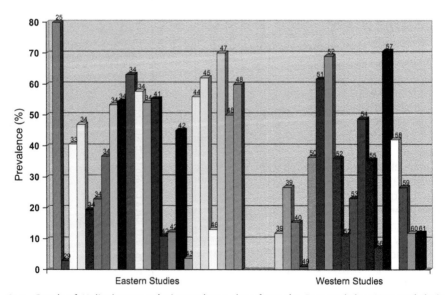

Fig. 1. Graph of *Helicobacter pylori* prevalence data from the East and the West and their references.

(OR) of GI events with naproxen is 2.12 (95% CI, 1.73–2.58).[62] A Japanese case control study found that the OR of UGIB was 5.5 (95% CI, 2.5–11.9) for aspirin and 6.1 (95% CI, 2.7–13.4) for NSAIDs. The OR of UGIB in regular users of aspirin as opposed to intermittent users was as high as 7.7 (95% CI, 3.2–18.7).[63] The risk of NSAIDs and in particular low-dose aspirin in causing major GU bleeding appeared to be relatively high in the Japanese population. However, more prospective studies from Asia are required, and aspirin or NSAID may need to be used with extra caution in Asian countries.[64] Sakamoto's study was based on an older population with a median age of 60 years, and the older population may have been more prone to drug-induced PUD. The incidence of serious UGIB in patients was further assessed in patients who were on histamine-2 receptor antagonists (H2RA) or proton pump inhibitors (PPIs). Of 17,270 patients commencing NSAIDs, bleeding PUD occurred in only 0.05%, with a pooled incidence rate of 2.65 (95% CI, 2.56–2.74) and 1.29 (95% CI, 1.27–1.31) per 1000 patient years for low-dose aspirin and NSAID users, respectively.[65] Genetic susceptibility to NSAID-related gastroduodenal bleeding through cytochrome P450 2C9 (CYP2C9) polymorphisms may underlie racial differences in the development of such adverse drug effects.[66]

Despite decreasing prevalence of H pylori in Western countries and increasing use of eradication regimens, the hospitalization rate for PUD has not shifted. In five large hospitals in the United States, an analysis of data over a 10-year span from 1996 to 2005 did not show a statistically significant trend in the number of GUs and DUs based on discharge diagnoses. This finding supports the increasing role played by other etiologies in the development of PUD such as NSAID and idiopathic ulcers in developed nations.[67] The risk factors of NSAIDs and H pylori are at least additive when combined together.[68] In the Japanese population, there was also no evidence of any interaction between NSAIDs and H pylori infection, with the two risk factors having only additive effects in the development of PUD.[63]

IDIOPATHIC PEPTIC ULCER DISEASE

The differences in H pylori prevalence of 15% in developed countries to over 80% in less developed areas, however, do not parallel the development of PUD. There are other genetic, environmental, and cultural factors influencing the geographic differences.[69] In Western countries, non-H pylori idiopathic ulcers are well-described. In Australia, idiopathic, non-H pylori, non-NSAID GUs occurred in younger patients than in NSAID ulcer patients (mean age, 48 years and 68 years, respectively, P = .02).[9] In the United States, 27% of endoscopically diagnosed DU patients had idiopathic, non-H pylori ulcers.[70] In a random gastroscopy survey of 1001 adults in the general Swedish population, the rate of idiopathic GU was 25% and idiopathic DU was 19%.[2]

Up to a quarter of peptic ulcers in some Asian countries may be non-H pylori, idiopathic ulcers. This increase has taken place in the past decade following a decrease in the background prevalence of H pylori infection. It may be difficult, however, to completely exclude past bacterial infection.[71] The phenomenon is consistently reported across Asia and appears to be a true increase in these ulcers rather than a proportional increase due to falling rates of H pylori infection. In Hong Kong, a 4.5-fold increase in the incidence of H pylori-negative, idiopathic, bleeding ulcers was noted from 4.2% in 1997 to 1998[72] to 18.8% in 2000 (P<.001).[73] In South Korea, the rate of idiopathic ulcers has increased to 22.2%.[5]

DIET AND GENETICS

Dietary lipids and carbohydrates have been implicated in causing the regional variability in DU prevalence in parts of Asia. Despite similarities in the background prevalence of *H pylori* and other environmental factors, DUs are significantly more common in the rice-eating areas of southern India than in the northern wheat-eating areas.[74] In animal peptic ulcer models, unrefined wheat, wheat bran, some millets and pulses containing certain lipid fractions are ulceroprotective. Sterol esters were protective in chronic ulcer models but not sterols, free fatty acids, and triglycerides. In contrast, sterols were protective in acute ulcer models and not long-term chronic models.[75] The southern regions of China have a 2.4-fold higher rate of DU compared with that in northern regions. This correlated with the daily rice intake (r = 0.855; P = .029) and inversely correlated with the daily wheat flour intake (r = -0.8472; P = .033).[76] In a Swedish study of 332 patients with confirmed PUD from a population dietary survey of 1135 people, lower intake of fermented milk products and vegetables and high intake of milk, meat, and bread were associated with ulcer risk.[77] However, this retrospective dietary assessment may have been biased from dietary modification in symptomatic PUD or following diagnosis or inaccurate recall. Chilli, despite its ability to cause dyspepsia, has been found to have a protective effect against the development of PUD.[78]

Genetic factors play a role in the development of PUD. A registry twin study revealed that genetic effects are of moderate importance for the development of PUD, and it is independent of genetic influences that are important for acquiring *H pylori*.[79]

PEPTIC ULCER TREATMENT
Helicobacter pylori *Eradication*

The eradication of *H pylori* may be influenced by ethnicity. In Singapore, the eradication rate using the standard 1-week lansoprazole, amoxicillin and clarithromycin regimen was 87% by intention to treat and 92% per protocol. The eradication rate was significantly higher in the Chinese on both intention to treat and per protocol compared with that in the non-Chinese.[80] There may be differences in strains of *H pylori* in different ethnicities, but the overall eradication rates are within the range of Western studies.[81]

Helicobacter pylori *Recurrence*

H pylori recurrence is said to be rare in developed countries and frequent in developing countries. Most cases of recurrence are attributed to recrudescence, that is, recolonization of the same strain within 12 months, rather than reinfection with a new strain. A meta-analysis of 17 studies showed that the annual recurrence rate of *H pylori* infection in developed countries was 2.67% in comparison with 13.0% in developing countries.[82] The variability in *H pylori* recurrence rates in developing countries may relate to background-infection prevalence levels, sanitation, and other factors that increase the risk of PUD relapse.

Helicobacter pylori *Antibiotic Resistance*

H pylori eradication treatment tends to be internationally standardized, evidence-based, and supported by consensus statements and recommendations. Eradication therapy, in general, is safe and well tolerated. The development of resistance may be associated with the background and prior use of antibiotics.[81] *H pylori* antibiotic resistance is a key factor in the failure of eradication and recrudescence of PUD. Metronidazole and clarithromycin resistance rates were 28.6% and 8.3%, respectively, from a total of 1310 isolates from Wales and south-east England, with increasing rates during the 6-year follow-up period from 2000 to 2005.[83] In France, primary resistant strains among 377 isolates in children from 1994 to 2005 demonstrated resistance to metronidazole in 36.7%, clarithromycin in 22.8%, and both metronidazole and clarithromycin in 7.9%. All strains were susceptible to amoxicillin. Resistance to clarithromycin did not change over the 11 years, but metronidazole resistance decreased from 43.3% to 32%.[84] In Italy, the resistance rate for clarithromycin doubled from 10.2% to 21.3% during a 15-year period from 1989 to 2004 ($P<.01$).[85]

H pylori antibiotic resistance rates tend to be higher in Asia but once again highly variable. A Japanese study of 3707 H pylori strains from 2002 to 2005 showed that the clarithromycin resistance as defined by minimal inhibitor concentration 80 had increased to 27.7%, whereas amoxicillin and metronidazole resistance remained stable over this time period.[86] Resistance rates to metronidazole, clarithromycin, and amoxicillin were 51.9%, 13.5%, and 36.1%, respectively, in eastern Taiwan on testing of 133 isolates with a triple-drug resistance rate of 3%.[87]

Resistance to both clarithromycin and metronidazole severely reduces the rate of successful eradication using standard first-line treatments. Therefore, alternative regimens may have to be tried.[81] The efficacy of rifabutin-based salvage treatments is associated with the number of previous failed eradication attempts but is independent of ethnicity. The eradication rate was as high as 95% when used as second-line therapy but fell to 68% when multiple agents had already failed.[88]

Proton Pump Inhibitors

PPIs vary according to pharmacogenetics, which refers to the relationship between genetics and drug response. This in turn may result in differences in PUD treatment efficacy between the West and East. Polymorphisms in the CPY2C19 genes of the cytochrome P450 superfamily affect the hepatic metabolism of PPIs. The frequency of the poor-metabolizer genotype of CPY2C19 is higher in Asian populations (13%–23%) than that in Western populations (3%–5%), resulting in higher plasma levels of PPI in Asians.[89] Omeprazole area under curve is 2.5-fold higher, and clearance, 50% lower in Chinese extensive metabolizers (EMs) than that in Swedish Caucasian EMs.[90,91] These genetic differences in PPI metabolism affect the H pylori eradication rate using omeprazole dual therapy with amoxicillin. PUD healing rates paralleled the eradication rates of H pylori and varied according to the CYP2C19 polymorphisms. Ulcer healing rates were significantly higher in poor metabolizers (100.0%) compared with intermediate- (75.3.0%) and rapid (27.7%) metabolizers.[89] Therefore, the variability in the metabolism of drugs in the East and the West may influence the efficacy of PUD treatment.

Studies on treatment of bleeding and prevention of rebleeding in PUD show geographic variability in the efficacy of PPIs. A European study did not find omeprazole 80 mg followed by 40 mg three times a day injections to be effective in the prevention of peptic ulcer rebleeding,[92] but a high dose was required with intravenous (IV) omeprazole 80 mg bolus followed by 8 mg/h infusion for 72 hours to achieve therapeutic efficacy.[93] In contrast, while IV omeprazole infusion is highly efficacious in Asians,[94] oral omeprazole 80 mg/d alone successfully reduced ulcer rebleeding rates in India.[95,96] In Korea, pantoprazole 40 mg twice a day was sufficient to maintain pH greater than 6.0, except in EMs of CYP2C19.[97] CYP2C19 polymorphisms, high H pylori prevalence, and a lower gastric parietal cell mass may all account for greater efficacy of PPIs in Asians compared with Caucasians.

Histamine-2 Receptor Antagonists

In parts of Asia, H2RAs are considered effective in the prevention of aspirin-induced ulcers due to the lower parietal cell mass.[98] Other small-scale studies conducted in Asia consider H2RA cost effective compared with PPIs. There are, however, no large-scale equivalence studies to conclusively confirm this, and PPIs are considered the gold standard in the prophylaxis of gastroduodenal events in patients taking ulcerogenic drugs.

SUMMARY

PUD affects both the East and the West. The magnitude of the problem, however, varies within these regions. The study of peptic ulcer epidemiology is impeded by the paucity of general population-based data, invasiveness of diagnostic tests, and variable access to testing facilities. As such, direct comparisons of PUD epidemiology between the East and the West are difficult. The prevalence rates of *H pylori* are highly variable and depend greatly on the local sanitation conditions. The use of NSAIDs and aspirin is ubiquitous and increasing especially for the antiplatelet activity of aspirin in the prophylaxis of cardiovascular events. There is evidence that pharmacogenetics play a role in susceptibility to the ulcerogenic properties of NSAIDs. The prevalence of PUD parallels the risk factors, but emerging in both the East and the West is idiopathic PUD, now a substantial proportion of ulcers in areas of declining *H pylori* infection. Genetic polymorphisms affect the efficacy of treatment using PPIs. Local *H pylori* resistance rates also influence the eradication success rates.

REFERENCES

1. Leong RWL, Chan FKL. Duodenal ulcer. In: Johnson LR, editor. Encyclopedia of gastroenterology. 1st edition. Memphis (USA): Academic Press; 2004. p. 645–52.
2. Aro P, Storskrubb T, Ronkainen J, et al. Peptic ulcer disease in a general adult population: the Kalixanda study: a random population-based study. Am J Epidemiol 2006;163(11):1025–34.
3. Wong BC, Lam SK, Wong WM, et al. *Helicobacter pylori* eradication to prevent gastric cancer in a high-risk region of China: a randomized controlled trial. JAMA 2004;291(2):187–94.
4. Lam SK. Differences in peptic ulcer between East and West. Baillieres Best Pract Res Clin Gastroenterol 2000;14(1):41–52.
5. Jang HJ, Choi MH, Shin WG, et al. Has peptic ulcer disease changed during the past ten years in Korea? A prospective multi-center study. Dig Dis Sci 2008;53(6): 1527–31.
6. Wong SN, Sollano JD, Chan MM, et al. Changing trends in peptic ulcer prevalence in a tertiary care setting in the Philippines: a seven-year study. J Gastroenterol Hepatol 2005;20(4):628–32.
7. Guo Q, Zhan L [Analysis of 136 children with gastrointestinal hemorrhage]. Hunan Yi Ke Da Xue Xue Bao 2001;26:566–8 [Chinese].
8. Houben CH, Chiu PW, Lau JY, et al. Duodenal ulcers dominate acute upper gastrointestinal tract bleeding in childhood: a 10-year experience from Hong Kong. J Dig Dis 2008;9(4):199–203.
9. Xia HH, Phung N, Kalantar JS, et al. Demographic and endoscopic characteristics of patients with *Helicobacter pylori* positive and negative peptic ulcer disease. Med J Aust 2000;173(10):515–9.

10. Langman MJS. Aetiology of peptic ulcer. In: Murphy M, Rawlins MD, Venebles CW, editors. Diseases of the gut and pancreas. Oxford (UK): Blackwell; 1987. p. 268–81.

11. Elashoff JD, Grossman MI. Trends in hospital admissions and death rates for peptic ulcer in the United States from 1970 to 1978. Gastroenterology 1980; 78(2):280–5.

12. Preshaw RM. Sex differences in morbidity and mortality from peptic ulcer in Canada, 1950-1981. Clin Invest Med 1985;8(1):62–7.

13. Bardhan KD, Royston C. Time, change and peptic ulcer disease in Rotherham, UK. Dig Liver Dis 2008;40(7):540–6. Epub 2008 Apr 14.

14. Higham J, Kang JY, Majeed A. Recent trends in admissions and mortality due to peptic ulcer in England: increasing frequency of haemorrhage among older subjects. Gut 2002;50(4):460–4.

15. Sonnenberg A. Time trends of ulcer mortality in Europe. Gastroenterology 2007; 132(7):2320–7. Epub 2007 Apr 14.

16. Sonnenberg A. Time trends of ulcer mortality in non-European countries. Am J Gastroenterol 2007;102(5):1101–7.

17. Tango T, Kurashina S. Age, period and cohort analysis of trends in mortality from major diseases in Japan, 1955 to 1979: peculiarity of the cohort born in the early Showa Era. Stat Med 1987;6(6):709–26.

18. Graham DY. *Helicobacter pylori*: its epidemiology and its role in duodenal ulcer disease. J Gastroenterol Hepatol 1991;6:105–13.

19. Cheng FCY, Lam SK, Ong GB. Maximum acid output to graded doses of pentagastrin and its relation to parietal cell mass in Chinese patients with duodenal ulcer. Gut 1977;18:827–32.

20. Card WI, Marks IN. The relationship between the acid output of the stomach following 'maximal' histamine stimulation and the parietal cell mass. Clin Sci 1960;19:147–63.

21. Lam SK, Hasan M, Sircus W, et al. Comparison of maximal acid output and gastrin response to meals in Chinese and Scottish normal and duodenal ulcer subjects. Gut 1980;21(4):324–8.

22. Mitchell HM, Li YY, Hu PJ, et al. Epidemiology of *Helicobacter pylori* in southern China: identification of early childhood as the critical period for acquisition. J Infect Dis 1992;166:149–53.

23. Pounder RE, Ng D. The prevalence of *Helicobacter pylori* infection in different countries. Aliment Pharmacol Ther 1995;9(Suppl 2):33–9.

24. Brown LM. *Helicobacter pylori*: epidemiology and routes of transmission. Epidemiol Rev 2000;22:283–97.

25. Ahmed KS, Khan AA, Ahmed I, et al. Impact of household hygiene and water source on the prevalence and transmission of *Helicobacter pylori*: a South Indian perspective. Singapore Med J 2007;48(6):543–9.

26. Lee I, Lee H, Kim M, et al. Ethnic difference of *Helicobacter pylori* gastritis: Korean and Japanese gastritis is characterized by male- and antrum-predominant acute foveolitis in comparison with American gastritis. World J Gastroenterol 2005;11(1):94–8.

27. El-Zimaity HMT, Gutierrez O, Kim JG, et al. Geographic differences in the distribution of intestinal metaplasia in duodenal ulcer patients. Am J Gastroenterol 2001;96(3):666–72.

28. Goh KL, Parasakthi N. The racial cohort phenomenon: seroepidemiology of *Helicobacter pylori* infection in a multiracial South-East Asian country. Eur J Gastroenterol Hepatol 2001;13(2):177–83.

29. Saragih JB, Akbar N, Syam AF, et al. Incidence of *Helicobacter pylori* infection and gastric cancer: an 8-year hospital based study. Acta Med Indones 2007; 39(2):79–81.

30. Uyub AM, Raj SM, Visvanathan R, et al. *Helicobacter pylori* infection in northeastern Peninsular Malaysia – evidence for an unusually low prevalence, Scand. J Gastroenterol 1994;29:209–13.

31. Graham DY, Yamaoka Y, Malaty HM. Thoughts about populations with unexpected low prevalences of *Helicobacter pylori* infection. Trans R Soc Trop Med Hyg 2007;101(9):849–51.

32. Fujisawa T, Kumagai T, Akamatsu T, et al. Changes in seroepidemiological pattern of *Helicobacter pylori* and hepatitis a virus over the last 20 years in Japan. Am J Gastroenterol 1999;94:2094–9.

33. Lee SY, Park HS, Yu SK, et al. Decreasing prevalence of *Helicobacter pylori* infection: a 9-year observational study. Hepatogastroenterology 2007;54(74): 630–3.

34. Chen J, Bu XL, Wang QY, et al. Decreasing seroprevalence of *Helicobacter pylori* infection during 1993–2003 in Guangzhou, southern China. Helicobacter 2007; 12(2):164–9.

35. Ma JL, You WC, Gail MH, et al. *Helicobacter pylori* infection and mode of transmission in a population at high risk of stomach cancer. Int J Epidemiol 1998;27(4): 570–3.

36. Zhang L, Blot WJ, You WC, et al. *Helicobacter pylori* antibodies in relation to precancerous gastric lesions in a high-risk Chinese population. Cancer Epidemiol Biomarkers Prev 1996;5:627–30.

37. Wong KKY, Chung PHY, Lan LCL, et al. Trends in the prevalence of *Helicobacter pylori* in symptomatic children in the era of eradication. J Pediatr Surg 2005;40: 1844–7.

38. Wong BPY, Chao NSY, Leung MWY, et al. Complications of peptic ulcer disease in children and adolescents: minimally invasive treatments offer feasible surgical options. J Pediatr Surg 2006;41:2073–5.

39. Gruber D, Pohl D, Vavricka S, et al. Swiss tertiary care center experience challenges the age-cohort effect in *Helicobacter pylori* infection. J Gastrointestin Liver Dis 2008;17(4):373–7.

40. Moujaber T, MacIntyre CR, Backhouse J, et al. The seroepidemiology of *Helicobacter pylori* infection in Australia. Int J Infect Dis 2008;12(5):500–4. Epub 2008 Apr 8.

41. Fujimoto Y, Furusyo N, Toyoda K, et al. Intrafamilial transmission of *Helicobacter pylori* among the population of endemic areas in Japan. Helicobacter 2007;12(2): 170–6.

42. Lin DB, Lin JB, Chen CY, et al. Seroprevalence of *Helicobacter pylori* infection among schoolchildren and teachers in Taiwan. Helicobacter 2007;12(3): 258–64.

43. Okuda M, Miyashiro E, Booka M, et al. *Helicobacter pylori* colonization in the first 3 years of life in Japanese children. Helicobacter 2007;12(4):324–7.

44. Yim JY, Kim N, Choi SH, et al. Seroprevalence of *Helicobacter pylori* in South Korea. Helicobacter 2007;12(4):333–40.

45. Shi R, Xu S, Zhang H, et al. Prevalence and risk factors for *Helicobacter pylori* infection in Chinese populations. Helicobacter 2008;13(2):157–65.

46. Tam YH, Yeung CK, Lee KH, et al. A population-based study of *Helicobacter pylori* infection in Chinese children resident in Hong Kong: prevalence and potential risk factors. Helicobacter 2008;13(3):219–24.

47. Yanaoka K, Oka M, Yoshimura N, et al. Risk of gastric cancer in asymptomatic, middle-aged Japanese subjects based on serum pepsinogen and *Helicobacter pylori* antibody levels. Int J Cancer 2008;123(4):917–26.

48. Bhuiyan TR, Qadri F, Saha A, et al. Infection by *Helicobacter pylori* in Bangladeshi children from birth to two years: relation to blood group, nutritional status, and seasonality. Pediatr Infect Dis J 2009;28:79–85.

49. Mourad-Baars PE, Verspaget HW, Mertens BJ, et al. Low prevalence of *Helicobacter pylori* infection in young children in the Netherlands. Eur J Gastroenterol Hepatol 2007;19(3):213–6.

50. Dinić M, Tasić G, Stanković-Dordević D, et al. Serum anti-*Helicobacter pylori* IgA and IgG antibodies in asymptomatic children in Serbia. Scand J Infect Dis 2007; 39(4):303–7.

51. Boyanova L, Lazarova E, Jelev C, et al. *Helicobacter pylori* and *Helicobacter heilmannii* in untreated Bulgarian children over a period of 10 years. J Med Microbiol 2007;56(Pt 8):1081–5.

52. Thjodleifsson B, Asbjörnsdottir H, Sigurjonsdottir RB, et al. Seroprevalence of *Helicobacter pylori* and cagA antibodies in Iceland, Estonia and Sweden. Scand J Infect Dis 2007;39(8):683–9.

53. Naja F, Kreiger N, Sullivan T. *Helicobacter pylori* infection in Ontario: prevalence and risk factors. Can J Gastroenterol 2007;21(8):501–6.

54. Weck MN, Stegmaier C, Rothenbacher D, et al. Epidemiology of chronic atrophic gastritis: population-based study among 9444 older adults from Germany. Aliment Pharmacol Ther 2007;26(6):879–87.

55. Sterzl I, Hrdá P, Matucha P, et al. Anti-*Helicobacter pylori*, anti-thyroid peroxidase, anti-thyroglobulin and anti-gastric parietal cells antibodies in Czech population. Physiol Res 2008;57(Suppl 1):S135–41.

56. Segal I, Otley A, Issenman R, et al. Low prevalence of *Helicobacter pylori* infection in Canadian children: a cross-sectional analysis. Can J Gastroenterol 2008; 22(5):485–9.

57. Monno R, Volpe A, Basho M, et al. *Helicobacter pylori* seroprevalence in selected groups of Albanian volunteers. Infection 2008;36(4):345–50. Epub 2008 Jun 20.

58. Rejchrt S, Koupil I, Kopácová M, et al European society for primary care gastroenterology. Prevalence and sociodemographic determinants of uninvestigated dyspepsia in the Czech Republic. Eur J Gastroenterol Hepatol 2008;20(9): 898–905.

59. Leong RWL, Chan FKL. Drug-induced side effects affecting the gastrointestinal tract. Expert Opin Drug Saf 2006;5:585–92.

60. Shiokawa Y, Nobunaga M, Saito T, et al [Epidemiology study on upper gastrointestinal lesions induced by non-steroidal anti-inflammatory drugs]. Ryumachi 1991;31(1):96–111 [Japanese].

61. Larkai EN, Smith JL, Lidsky MD, et al. Gastroduodenal mucosa and dyspeptic symptoms in arthritic patients during chronic nonsteroidal anti-inflammatory drug use. Am J Gastroenterol 1987;82(11):1153–8.

62. Hippisley-Cox J, Coupland C, Logan R. Risk of adverse gastrointestinal outcomes in patients taking cyclo-oxygenase-2 inhibitors or conventional nonsteroidal anti-inflammatory drugs: population based nested case-control analysis. BMJ 2005;331(7528):1310–6.

63. Sakamoto C, Sugano K, Ota S, et al. Case-control study on the association of upper gastrointestinal bleeding and nonsteroidal anti-inflammatory drugs in Japan. Eur J Clin Pharmacol 2006;62(9):765–72.

64. Shiotani A, Kamada T, Haruma K. Low-dose aspirin-induced gastrointestinal diseases: past, present, and future. J Gastroenterol 2008;43(8):581–8.
65. Ishikawa S, Inaba T, Mizuno M, et al. Incidence of serious upper gastrointestinal bleeding in patients taking non-steroidal anti-inflammatory drugs in Japan. Acta Med Okayama 2008;62(1):29–36.
66. Pilotto A, Seripa D, Franceschi M, et al. Genetic susceptibility to nonsteroidal anti-inflammatory drug-related gastroduodenal bleeding: role of cytochrome P450 2C9 polymorphisms. Gastroenterology 2007;133(2):465–71.
67. Manuel D, Cutler A, Goldstein J, et al. Decreasing prevalence combined with increasing eradication of *Helicobacter pylori* infection in the United States has not resulted in fewer hospital admissions for peptic ulcer disease-related complications. Aliment Pharmacol Ther 2007;25(12):1423–7.
68. Huang JQ, Sridhar S, Hunt RH. Role of *Helicobacter pylori* infection and non-steroidal anti-inflammatory drugs in peptic-ulcer disease: a meta-analysis. Lancet 2002;359:14–22.
69. Genta RM, Gürer IE, Graham DY. Geographical pathology of *Helicobacter pylori* infection: is there more than one gastritis? Ann Med 1995;27(5): 595–9.
70. Ciociola AA, McSorley DJ, Turner K, et al. *Helicobacter pylori* infection rates in duodenal ulcer patients in the United States may be lower than previously estimated. Am J Gastroenterol 1999;94:1834–40.
71. Tokudome S, Ando R, Ghadimi R, et al. Are there any real *Helicobacter pylori* infection-negative gastric cancers in Asia? Asian Pac J Cancer Prev 2007;8(3): 462–3.
72. Chan HLY, Wu JCW, Chan FKL, et al. Is non-*Helicobacter pylori*, non-NSAID peptic ulcer a common cause of upper GI Bleeding? A prospective study of 977 patients. Gastrointest Endosc 2001;53:438–42.
73. Hung LC, Ching JY, Sung JJ, et al. Long-term outcome of *Helicobacter pylori*-negative idiopathic bleeding ulcers. A prospective cohort study. Gastroenterology 2005;129:1845–50.
74. Tovey FI, Hobsley M, Kaushik SP, et al. Duodenal gastric metaplasia and *Helicobacter pylori* infection in high and low duodenal ulcer-prevalent areas in India. J Gastroenterol Hepatol 2004;19(5):497–505.
75. Paul Jayaraj A, Tovey FI, Hobsley M. Duodenal ulcer prevalence: research into the nature of possible protective dietary lipids. Phytother Res 2003;17(4): 391–8.
76. Wong BC, Ching CK, Lam SK, et al. Differential north to south gastric cancer-duodenal ulcer gradient in China. China Ulcer Study Group. J Gastroenterol Hepatol 1998;13(10):1050–7.
77. Elmståhl S, Svensson U, Berglund G. Fermented milk products are associated to ulcer disease. Results from a cross-sectional population study. Eur J Clin Nutr 1998;52(9):668–74.
78. Kang JY, Yeoh KG, Chia HP, et al. Chili–protective factor against peptic ulcer? Dig Dis Sci 1995;40(3):576–9.
79. Malaty HM, Graham DY, Isaksson I, et al. Are genetic influences on peptic ulcer dependent or independent of genetic influences for *Helicobacter pylori* infection? Arch Intern Med 2000;160(1):105–9.
80. Kaushik SP, Vu C. *Helicobacter pylori* eradication with lansoprazole, amoxycillin and clarithromycin: testing an ideal regimen in a multicultural south east Asian population and examining factors potentially influencing eradication. Aust N Z J Med 2000;30(2):231–5.

81. Kwok A, Lam T, Katelaris P, et al. *Helicobacter pylori* eradication therapy: indications, efficacy and safety. Expert Opin Drug Saf 2008;7(3):271–81.

82. Niv Y, Hazazi R. *Helicobacter pylori* recurrence in developed and developing countries: meta-analysis of 13C-urea breath test follow-up after eradication. Helicobacter 2008;13(1):56–61.

83. Chisholm SA, Teare EL, Davies K, et al. Surveillance of primary antibiotic resistance of *Helicobacter pylori* at centres in England and Wales over a six-year period (2000–2005). Euro Surveill 2007;12(7):E3–4.

84. Kalach N, Serhal L, Asmar E, et al. *Helicobacter pylori* primary resistant strains over 11 years in French children. Diagn Microbiol Infect Dis 2007;59(2):217–22.

85. De Francesco V, Margiotta M, Zullo A, et al. Prevalence of primary clarithromycin resistance in *Helicobacter pylori* strains over a 15 year period in Italy. J Antimicrob Chemother 2007;59(4):783–5. Epub 2007 Feb 28.

86. Kobayashi I, Murakami K, Kato M, et al. Changing antimicrobial susceptibility epidemiology of *Helicobacter pylori* strains in Japan between 2002 and 2005. J Clin Microbiol 2007;45(12):4006–10. Epub 2007 Oct 17.

87. Hu CT, Wu CC, Lin CY, et al. Resistance rate to antibiotics of *Helicobacter pylori* isolates in eastern Taiwan. J Gastroenterol Hepatol 2007;22(5):720–3.

88. Van der Poorten D, Katelaris PH. The effectiveness of rifabutin triple therapy for patients with difficult-to-eradicate *Helicobacter pylori* in clinical practice. Aliment Pharmacol Ther 2007;26(11–12):1537–42.

89. Furuta T, Ohashi K, Kamata T, et al. Effect of genetic differences in omeprazole metabolism on cure rates for *Helicobacter pylori* infection and peptic ulcer. Ann Intern Med 1998;129(12):1027–30.

90. Andersson T, Regårdh CG, Lou YC, et al. Polymorphic hydroxylation of S-mephenytoin and omeprazole metabolism in Caucasian and Chinese subjects. Pharmacogenetics 1992;2(1):25–31.

91. Ishizaki T, Sohn D, Kobayashi K, et al. Interethnic differences in omeprazole metabolism in the two S-mephenytoin hydroxylation phenotypes studied in Caucasians and Orientals. Ther Drug Monit 1994;16(2):214–5.

92. Daneshmend TK, Hawkey CJ, Langman MJ, et al. Omeprazole versus placebo for acute upper gastrointestinal bleeding: randomised double blind controlled trial. BMJ 1992;304:143–7.

93. Schaffalitzky de Muckadell OB, Havelund T, Harling H, et al. Effect of omeprazole on the outcome of endoscopically treated bleeding peptic ulcers. Randomized double-blind placebo-controlled multicentre study. Scand J Gastroenterol 1997;32:320–7.

94. Lau JY, Sung JJ, Lee KK, et al. Effect of intravenous omeprazole on recurrent bleeding after endoscopic treatment of bleeding peptic ulcers. N Engl J Med 2000;343:310–6.

95. Khuroo MS, Yattoo GN, Javid G, et al. A comparison of omeprazole and placebo for bleeding peptic ulcer. N Engl J Med 1997;336:1054–8.

96. Javid G, Masoodi I, Zargar SA, et al. Omeprazole as adjuvant therapy to endoscopic combination injection sclerotherapy for treating bleeding peptic ulcer. Am J Med 2001;111:280–4.

97. Oh JH, Choi MG, Dong MS, et al. Low-dose intravenous pantoprazole for optimal inhibition of gastric acid in Korean patients. J Gastroenterol Hepatol 2007;22(9):1429–34. Epub 2007 Jul 20.

98. Nakashima S, Arai S, Mizuno Y, et al. A clinical study of Japanese patients with ulcer induced by low-dose aspirin and other non-steroidal anti-inflammatory drugs. Aliment Pharmacol Ther 2005;21(Suppl 2):60–6.

Index

Note: Page numbers of article titles are in **boldface** type.

Gastroenterol Clin N Am 38 (2009) 381–391
doi:10.1016/S0889-8553(09)00049-1
0889-8553/09/$ – see front matter © 2009 Elsevier Inc. All rights reserved.

gastro.theclinics.com

Moving?

Make sure your subscription moves with you!

To notify us of your new address, find your **Clinics Account Number** (located on your mailing label above your name), and contact customer service at:

E-mail: elspcs@elsevier.com

800-654-2452 (subscribers in the U.S. & Canada)
314-453-7041 (subscribers outside of the U.S. & Canada)

Fax number: 314-523-5170

Elsevier Periodicals Customer Service
11830 Westline Industrial Drive
St. Louis, MO 63146

*To ensure uninterrupted delivery of your subscription, please notify us at least 4 weeks in advance of move.

Printed and bound by CPI Group (UK) Ltd, Croydon, CR0 4YY

03/10/2024

01040463-0017